EAT THIS NOT THAT! 2011

The No-Diet Weight Loss Solution
Completely Updated and Expanded

BY DAVID ZINCZENKO
WITH MATT GOULDING

RODALE

Eat This, Not That! is a registered trademark of Rodale Inc.

© 2010, 2009, 2008 by Rodale Inc.

All rights reserved. No part of this publication may be reproduced or transmitted in any form
or by any means, electronic or mechanical, including photocopying, recording, or any other information
storage and retrieval system, without the written permission of the publisher.

Rodale books may be purchased for business or promotional use or for special sales. For information,
please write to: Special Markets Department, Rodale Inc., 733 Third Avenue, New York, NY 10017

Printed in the United States of America

Rodale Inc. makes every effort to use acid-free ♾, recycled paper ♻

Book design by George Karabotsos

Cover photos by Jeff Harris / Cover food styling by Ed Gabriels for Halley Resources

Interior photo direction by Tara Long

All interior photos by Mitch Mandel and Thomas MacDonald/Rodale Images
with the exception of the following: pages 49-50, 289-295 © Jeff Harris;
pages 104-105, 108-109, 134-135, 136-137 © Orly Catz; pages 130-131 © Lisa Adams;
pages 184-185 © Shawn Taylor; pages ix-xv courtesy of all the subjects

Rodale Images food styling by Melissa Reiss
with the exception of pages 315, 317, 319, 321, 323, 325, 327, 329, 331, 332 by Diane Simone Vezza

Library of Congress Cataloging-in-Publication Data is on file with the publisher
ISBN-13: 978-1-60529-313-4 paperback

Distributed to the trade by Macmillan

2   4   6   8   10   9   7   5   3   1   paperback

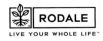

RODALE
LIVE YOUR WHOLE LIFE™

We inspire and enable people to improve their lives and the world around them.

EAT THIS NOT THAT! 2011

DEDICATION

To the six million men and women who have made **EAT THIS, NOT THAT!**
a publishing phenomenon and who have spread the word to friends
and relatives about the importance of knowing what's really in our food.
Because of your passionate efforts, food manufacturers and restaurant
chains have woken up to the fact that more and more of us demand good,
solid information about our food, and healthy choices that will let us
drop pounds and stay lean for life.

And to the men and women working in America's fields, farms, and
supermarkets, waiting tables, and toiling in kitchens everywhere:
It is because of your hard work that Americans have so many options.
This book is designed to help us choose the best of what you've created.

—Dave and Matt

ACKNOWLEDGMENTS

This book is the product of thousands of meals, hundreds of conversations with nutritionists and industry experts, and the collective smarts, dedication, and raw talent of dozens of individuals. Our undying thanks to all of you who have inspired this project in any way. In particular:

To Maria Rodale and the Rodale family, whose dedication to improving the lives of their readers is apparent in every book and magazine they put their name on.

To George Karabotsos and his crew of immensely talented designers, including Courtney Eltringham, Laura White, Mark Michaelson, Elizabeth Neal, and Rob Campos. You're the reason why each book looks better than the last.

To Clint Carter, the Rainman of the calorie-counting world: Thanks for another huge effort. And to Carolyn Kylstra and Andrew Del-Colle: Your willingness to take on any task is vital to these books.

To Tara Long, who spends more time in the drive-thru and the supermarket aisles than anyone on the planet, all in the name of making us look good.

To Debbie McHugh, whose ability to keep us sane and focused under the most impossible circumstances cannot be overstated.

To John DeLucie, chef extraordinaire—you've enlightened our palate in ways I could have never imagined.

And to Dan Abrams, Mark, Sean, and the rest of the team at The Lion: We look forward to eating up more great times with you all.

To the Rodale book team: Steve Perrine, Karen Rinaldi, Chris Krogermeier, Erin Williams, Nancy Bailey, Sara Cox, Mitch Mandel, Tom MacDonald, Troy Schnyder, Melissa Reiss, Nikki Weber, Jennifer Giandomenico, Wendy Gable, Keith Biery, Liz Krenos, Brooke Myers, Sean Sabo, and Caroline McCall. You continue to do whatever it takes to get these books done. As always, we appreciate your heroic efforts.   —Dave and Matt

Check out the other informative books in the **EAT THIS, NOT THAT!** and **COOK THIS, NOT THAT!** series:

Eat This, Not That! for Kids! (2008)

Eat This, Not That! Supermarket Survival Guide (2009)

Eat This, Not That! Restaurant Survival Guide (2009)

Cook This, Not That! Kitchen Survival Guide (2010)

Drink This, Not That! (2010)

CONTENTS

Introduction vi

Chapter 1
The Truth about Your Food 1
The dirty little secrets of the food industry, revealed!
PLUS: *The Year in Food 2010*

Chapter 2
Foods That Cure 35
The best and worst foods to boost brain power, fight disease, and more!
PLUS: *10 Foods for a Longer, Healthier Life!*

Chapter 3
At Your Favorite Restaurants 55
The newest picks and pans from more than 50 fast food and sit-down restaurants
PLUS: *The 20 Worst Foods in America*

Chapter 4
At the Supermarket 191
Learn to stock your pantry, fridge, and freezer with America's best packaged foods

Chapter 5
Holidays & Special Occasions 261
Lose weight while indulging, from the Thanksgiving table to the vending machine

Chapter 6
For Kids 279
Everything you need to know to raise the leanest, fittest family on the block
PLUS: *The easiest way to get kids to eat more fruits and vegetables*

Chapter 7
On a Budget 307
Cut calories and save cash with these savvy strategies and delicious recipes

Index 334

Your new body is here.

It's here in these pages: that brand-new physique you've been waiting for, the leaner, fitter, healthier body you thought you'd never have. It's coming to you express delivery, without the need for dieting, for going hungry, for giving up anything. *EAT THIS, NOT THAT!* is ready to start stripping extra pounds from your body today. And once you lose that weight, you're going to keep it off. Forever.

I know what you're thinking: All that, just from a book? Won't I need something else to go with the book, like maybe a fancy home gym, a pricey personal trainer, a rice-cake-and-cottage-cheese diet, 5 hours a day of marathon training, a thousand bucks' worth of nutritional supplements, and an instruction manual that tells me how to turn my vacuum cleaner into a makeshift liposuction machine?

Nope. Just this book.

See, **EAT THIS, NOT THAT!** isn't a typical book. Sure, it's made of paper, with lots of photos and plenty of words. But the fact is, **EAT THIS, NOT THAT!** is so revolutionary, so amazingly effective, you can lose weight without even reading it!

Really? I don't have to read it? What do I do, rub it on my belly?

Well, no: Of course I want you to read it—I worked hard on every word! And if you read it cover to cover, you'll discover it's packed with tons of information about the foods you eat that will shock and amaze you—and maybe even creep you out. But **EAT THIS, NOT THAT!** wasn't created to be a sit-down-and-read-it type of book.

Eat This, Not That! is a tool.

A peek-at-it-in-the-restaurant tool. A consult-it-in-the-grocery-store tool. A whip-it-out-at-the-drive-thru tool. A veritable Swiss Army knife of fat fighting, a weight-loss coach in your pocket. It's designed to make smart food choices easier, no matter where you're making them. And it just might be the best health-boosting, fat-fighting investment you'll ever make. Consider just a handful of real stories from real people who've shed 25, 50, 75 pounds—

or more!—of unwanted, unhealthy flab, and you'll understand why I call it "The no-diet weight-loss solution":

▶ **MICHAEL COLOMBO of Staten Island, New York,** _shed 91 pounds_ in just over 8 months and conquered life-threatening sleep apnea, after picking up a copy of **EAT THIS, NOT THAT!** "My confidence has sky-rocketed!" he says. (Read his full story on the opposite page). And Colombo never had to go on a diet or skip a meal!

▶ **ERIKA BOWEN of Minneapolis, Minnesota,** _dropped 84 pounds_--without dieting. "I feel like I've always wanted to feel," Bowen reports. Once she discovered the truth about her food, she learned she could lose weight and never feel hungry. (You'll find her true-life tale on page xi.)

▶ **DANA BICKELMAN of Waltham, Massachusetts,** _lost 70 pounds_ after discovering the shocking truth about the foods she was eating. Her secret: She learned to indulge—even at her favorite restaurants—but to do it more smartly. "Boys want to say hi to me now, and that's awesome," she says. "I've never had this kind of attention before!" (Read her whole tale on page xiii.)

Never dieting, never skipping meals, never going hungry? Always eating what you want, when you want, where you want? And still losing all the weight you want?

Sounds impossible, right? Like I'm trying to sell you a bridge to Brooklyn or some swampland in Florida?

Well, it's not impossible. In fact, it's scientifically proven. And here's why:

Many of the foods we eat today—from common supermarket products to drive-thru snacks to sit-down dinners at chain restaurants, and even some popular "health" foods—are far, far worse for our waistlines than we could ever imagine. See, food marketers have spent the past few generations devising

"I'm finally happy when I look in the mirror."

Michael Colombo, a long-time *Men's Health* magazine reader, had always been bigger than his buddies. "I was always the type of person whom you'd describe as 'chunky,'" he says. "I liked to say I was big boned." But it was when he moved out of his parents' house and began to live on his own that he grew much larger, and "big boned" transitioned from a wink-wink euphemism into a big form of denial.

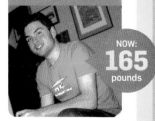

BEFORE: 256 pounds

THE "A-HA!" MOMENT

Even after Michael tipped the scales past 250 pounds, he never considered himself obese. "I turned to food for pleasure and comfort, and my weight spiraled downhill to the point where I didn't even realize I'd gotten as heavy as I did," he says. His moment of inspiration to lose weight came after a trip to Chicago with friends. "I saw pictures from the vacation after we got back, and I couldn't believe that was me, that I was that big." Those pictures were all it took—the same week he returned from Chicago, he joined a gym and bought his first *Eat This, Not That!* book, which he'd read about in *Men's Health*. "I decided this was going to be it, and I would turn my weight around, no matter how hard it was."

THE TURNING POINT

For the first 2 weeks of Michael's new routine, he refused to step on a scale. "I was afraid I wouldn't have lost much weight and I'd be discouraged and give up," he says. "But when I got on the scale, I had lost 5 pounds—and that made such a difference in my motivation."

HIS NEW LIFE

Michael says he feels like a different person after having lost more than 90 pounds. For starters, he's sleeping much better. "I used to have sleep apnea, and would wake up in the middle of the night. But now I sleep all the way through." He says he doesn't even snore anymore.

Even more impressive to Michael is the effect it's had on his self-esteem. "I'm finally happy when I look in the mirror," he says. "I have a lot more confidence to meet new people, because I'm not concerned with how I look, or how they'll perceive me when we're first introduced. My confidence has skyrocketed."

HOW *EAT THIS, NOT THAT!* HELPED

Before Michael began his new lifestyle, he says he was concerned that he'd have to starve himself in order to lose weight. "*Eat This, Not That!* showed me that you don't have to go completely crazy with your diet—it taught me that there are good options out there other than tiny salads or crazy 'health food' fads."

He says that the Worst Drinks in America was a life-saver. "I have a sweet tooth, and I've always loved soda and smoothies. But the list showed me that while restaurants might market smoothies as the healthier alternatives, they're really not."

VITALS:
Michael Colombo, 24, Staten Island, New York
HEIGHT: 5'11"
TOTAL WEIGHT LOST: 91 lbs
TIME IT TOOK TO LOSE THE WEIGHT: 8½ months

NOW: 165 pounds

"Eat This, Not That! *taught me that there are options out there other than tiny salads and crazy 'health food' fads.*"

ever more creative ways to pack our food with fat, salt, and sugar in an effort to hit the ultimate sweet spot on our palates, the bull's-eye on our tongues. That's why so many of our foods now have ingredients that, when read aloud, sound like characters from a science-fiction novel—characters like Trans-Fatty Acid (sounds like a cross-dressing hippie, but in fact it's a cholesterol-promoting fat) and Soy Isolate (could be the name of a Yiddish time traveler who's chronically behind schedule but is in fact a refined protein that may actually undermine testosterone). It's all part of an effort on the part of food manufacturers to make us rush out to buy more. But the unnatural foods they've created trigger unnatural hunger and unnatural cravings. And those unnatural cravings for unnatural foods lead to something else: unnatural weight gain. Today's food is far higher in fat, salt, sugar, and calories than the foods our grandparents ate. In fact, we now consume an average of 300 calories a day more than we did in 1985. No wonder we're in the throes of an obesity epidemic beyond the scope of anything humankind has ever seen. And look at what it's doing to our world:

Fat in the sky! After a plane crash in 2003, Federal Aviation Administration investigators figured out the cause: excessive passenger weight. In fact, the FAA has come to the realization that Americans simply weigh more than they did back when the Wright brothers took off from Kitty Hawk. As a result, to ensure better safety, the FAA has added 10 pounds to the estimated weight of every adult passenger.

Fat on the road! The Chicago Transit Authority ordered a fleet of new buses in 2005 and had to add a half-inch to the width of the seats—they're now 18 inches across, to compensate for riders' bigger butts.

Fat at Disneyland! The theme park's "It's a Small World After All" had to be closed for 10 months in 2007 to replace the boats and the flume they travel down. The boats had been increasingly getting stuck in the middle of the ride, and some observers speculated the problem was that the ride was built back in 1963—before 200-pound riders became a common occurrence.

"I needed a way to make this weight loss last."

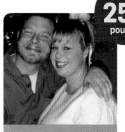

BEFORE: 250 pounds

Growing up, **Erika Bowen** had been athletic—she played volleyball and ran track-and-field in high school, and barely ever thought about her weight. She began to gain more in college, but even then didn't consider herself fat. "Even when I hit 200 pounds, I didn't think it was such a big deal," she says.

THE "A-HA!" MOMENT

In reality, though, Erika's weight was affecting several aspects of her life. She began to have to shop online, because stores no longer carried clothing in her size. And when she turned 27, she and her husband started trying to have a baby—and were unsuccessful. "There wasn't any real medical reason for why we couldn't get pregnant, but one theory was that I needed to get my weight under control. My BMI was 40 percent, and the doctors said that might affect successful conception."

Just two weeks before she turned 29, she went to the doctor for a checkup and learned that she weighed 250 pounds. "That was a huge eye-opener for me. I thought: Oh my gosh, I've wasted my 20s. So that's when I decided I had to do something."

THE TURNING POINT

After losing 6 pounds with the help of a trainer, Erika bought the first edition of **Eat This, Not That!** Once she began incorporating healthy eating with exercise, she saw the weight start to melt off. "My original goal was to lose 50 pounds," she says. Eighty-four pounds later, she's 10 pounds away from her goal weight: 155 pounds.

The most notable point for her, she says, is the first time she ran outside. "When I first ran outside, I realized, I'm one of those people. But now I look forward to my run with my dog every day. "

HER NEW LIFE

"There was a time when I refused to wear tank tops," she says. "But now I'm very comfortable in my own skin, and I'm wearing things I'd never have worn before." Her husband has told her she acts like a happier person now, and her friends leave ego-boosting comments on her Facebook wall. "They tell me my outward appearance now reflects my inner beauty," she says. "I feel like I've always wanted to feel. Other people are finally seeing me the way I've always seen myself."

HOW EAT THIS, NOT THAT! HELPED

"I knew I couldn't do Atkins or South Beach or Weight Watchers, because I like to be in control of things—I want to eat what I want to eat," Erika says. The concept of **Eat This, Not That!** appealed to her because of the freedom it allowed. "I love chips. And the books taught me that I don't have to give them up—I discovered Popchips, and I love them!

"I need a way to make this weight loss last. It might have come off quicker, but I wouldn't have maintained it as much as I have. **Eat This, Not That!** is more about lifestyle."

VITALS:
Erika Bowen, 30,
Minneapolis, Minnesota

HEIGHT: 5'7"

TOTAL WEIGHT LOST: 84 lbs

TIME IT TOOK TO LOSE THE WEIGHT: 17 months

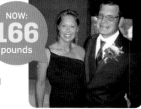

NOW: 166 pounds

"Other people are finally seeing me the way I've always seen myself."

Fat in the hospital! A survey of 900 nurses and X-ray technicians found that the majority of them had sustained injury or chronic pain from having to lift obese patients. At Barnes-Jewish Hospital in St. Louis, Missouri, doctors discovered that their 4½-inch syringes could no longer penetrate the majority of patients' oversize backsides. (The same hospital had to upgrade many of their beds to accommodate patients up to 500 pounds—standard 350-pound beds were no longer strong enough!)

Fat at the table! In the 1950s, the average dinner plate measured 9 inches in diameter. In the 1980s, that plate had grown to 11 inches. And today, we eat off dinner plates that measure 13 inches in diameter. No wonder many serving sizes from that old standby, *The Joy of Cooking,* are now 62 percent larger than when the book was originally published in 1931.

Fat in the back seat! Obesity rates among infants—infants!—have increased 73 percent over the past quarter century. Traditional car seats, for example, were built to accommodate little kids up to 40 pounds. Today, that just won't cut it; there are more than a dozen car seats on the market built for scale-tipping toddlers.

Fat from the cradle to the grave! Goliath Caskets is doing a booming business in plus-size caskets, the biggest of which is designed to hold a corpse weighing up to 1,000 pounds. (How do they get you to the morgue? In the new extreme-weight ambulance stretcher made by Stryker Corp., which holds up to 1,600 pounds of fleshy deadweight.)

In fact, we're now eating so much, and getting so fat, that we don't even recognize our fat selves as fat. One study found that between 1988 and 1994, about 14.5 percent of overweight women identified themselves as "about right," as did 40.9 percent of overweight men. (Yep, it is great to be a guy. A study at the University of Kansas found that men almost always believe they're thinner than their doctors think they are.) By 2004, those misperception numbers had jumped to 20.7 percent of overweight women and 46.1 percent

"I've never gotten this kind of attention before."

Dana Bickelman says that she'd been overweight her entire life. "I always used food in reaction to every emotion, whether it was a good moment or a bad." She thought she'd tried every method of losing weight—Weight Watchers, fat camps, gym memberships—but nothing stuck. "Food used to control my life," she says. "I'd eat and eat and then feel terrible about it afterward." It was a spiral that she thought she'd never come out of.

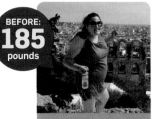

BEFORE: 185 pounds

THE "A-HA!" MOMENT

Dana saw the first edition of *Eat This, Not That!* on a shelf in Walmart and bought it impulsively. But the concept appealed to her, she says, because it wasn't as strict as a regular diet plan. "I don't like someone telling me how I should diet, exactly how much I should eat. *Eat This, Not That!* offered useful tips, rather than a strict plan."

She was shocked to learn how many calories were in foods she ate regularly. "Once I started being more aware of what I was eating, the weight started coming off."

THE TURNING POINT

Eat This, Not That! Supermarket Survival Guide taught Dana how to read food labels. "I learned all about portion control, and that so many packaged foods have a ton of added sugar and additives." Once she

finally understood what she was putting into her body, she says she started losing weight more quickly.

Portion control was also key. "I was eating this small serving size of ice cream, and I realized I was content with eating half of it. The idea that I didn't have to eat the whole thing was shocking, and made me feel so much more in control."

HER NEW LIFE

Everything in Dana's life has been affected by her weight loss. She's become better at her job: As a case manager for people with disabilities, she's brought the knowledge gained from *Eat This, Not That!* to her work, and teaches her clients how to read product labels and shop smarter. "Nutrition is something I'm really passionate about now, and I really want to help people learn about it."

And her self-esteem is the highest it's ever been.

"Boys want to say hi to me now, and that's awesome. I've never gotten this kind of attention before, and it's wonderful."

HOW *EAT THIS, NOT THAT!* HELPED

Dana brings the books to her favorite restaurants, like the Olive Garden. "It's so great that I can still eat there and enjoy the food, but know that I'm not overdoing it."

She says she incorporates the tips into her lifestyle, and feels confident that she's making smart food decisions along the way. "*Eat This, Not That!* has changed my life. I bring the books with my coworkers into Whole Foods, and we'll go around and read labels, and they're shocked. It's not just one type of person who's going to benefit from this type of stuff; it's everyone."

VITALS:
Dana Bickelman, 26, Waltham, Massachusetts

HEIGHT: 5'5"

TOTAL WEIGHT LOST: 70 lbs

TIME IT TOOK TO LOSE THE WEIGHT: 1 year

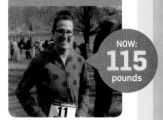

NOW: 115 pounds

"It's not just one type of person who's going to benefit from this type of stuff; it's everyone."

of overweight men. We're so used to being surrounded by fat—our own and others'—that we no longer recognize it as fat.

Now consider what this is costing us: In April 2010, a study found that 27 percent of 17- to 24-year-olds are too fat to serve in the military. Obesity and its related disease now cost the United States almost $117 billion in increased health care spending every year, and another $56 billion in disability, lost work, and premature death benefits.

Those are some overwhelming, and terrifying, numbers. But why is this happening? Is it all because we've suddenly become gluttons with nothing on our minds but eating and eating and eating some more?

No. It's because food marketers have come up with ever more sneaky ways to get us to buy more and more of their products. And there's little protection for consumers, and not nearly enough information out there to help us make smart choices.

Take the supermarket: Despite regulations that force packaged-foods manufacturers to print nutritional information on most of their goods, hijinks persist. Here's a great example: Next time you're in the frozen food section, take a look at Stouffer's White Meat Chicken Pot Pie. The company says the meal packs 580 calories a serving—that doesn't sound too horrible. Until you read the fine print and realize they consider a "serving" to be half a pie. (The real caloric toll? A whopping 1,160 calories!) Or look at foods designed to be "healthy," like Lean Cuisine's Sweet & Sour Chicken, which sneaks in nearly as much sugar as a package of Reese's Peanut Butter Cups. **EAT THIS, NOT THAT!** will tip you off to these food tricks and help make the right choice easy.

It gets even dicier in restaurants, many of which still refuse to make nutritional information available to their customers. So **EAT THIS, NOT THAT!** has gone behind the scenes, using food labs and state and local regulations to uncover hidden calorie counts, and make smart eating easier than ever.

"I look at pictures and can't believe I'm the same person."

As a computer programmer, **Jeff Small's** life was dominated by long, sedentary hours sitting in front of a computer screen. "I stayed up late, I ate fast food all the time, and I ate at all hours of the night," he says. And not because he didn't know better, but rather out of sheer lack of motivation to live more healthfully. "I knew the lifestyle I was leading wasn't a recipe for health, but I didn't know how soon it would come back to haunt me."

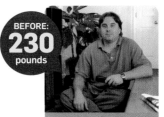

BEFORE:
230 pounds

THE "A-HA!" MOMENT
A routine doctor visit around Thanksgiving 2008 revealed a few scary facts: He weighed 230 pounds. His blood pressure and bad cholesterol were through the roof. The doctor told him that if he didn't get his weight in check, he was at high risk for heart disease and stroke.

He began by setting up a stationary bike in his garage, and he rode incrementally farther and harder each day. Soon Jeff realized: "I need to start putting better food into my body, too."

THE TURNING POINT
"The *Supermarket Survival Guide* let me take control of my life," he says. "It arms you with the ability to walk into a grocery store, spend your money, and know that you made smart eating decisions for the entire week." By May,

he had lost 70 pounds, and friends weren't recognizing him on the street.

HIS NEW LIFE
"I'm a completely different person in my job. It changed how people interacted with me at work, it changed how people wanted to invite me to meetings, and it even changed the way I participated in those meetings."

The weight loss also impacted his marriage. "I had low self-esteem and low energy, and I never wanted to go out and do things. I didn't feel that my wife found me attractive." But after the transformation, he says, all those problems disappeared. "I look at pictures of myself from before and I can't believe I'm the same person."

HOW *EAT THIS, NOT THAT!* HELPED
He learned to eat small snacks throughout the day to keep

from getting hungry and over indulging during meals. "People ask me how I stay so fit when I eat so much, and I tell them it's because I'm always eating that I can keep the weight off. I eat smart things every 2 to 3 hours, and I'm never hungry."

Jeff also loves the recent addition to the franchise: *Cook This, Not That!* "I love to cook, and the recipes are delicious. The salmon recipe is incredible. I cook all the time now—my wife loves it!"

FINAL THOUGHTS:
"I'm 43 years old and nothing has ever changed my life as much as *Eat This, Not That! Supermarket Survival Guide*. Nothing has had such an impact on my life as that book because it allowed me to shop the way I shop and eat the way I eat."

VITALS:
Jeff Small, 43,
Myrtle Beach,
South Carolina
HEIGHT: 5'10"

TOTAL WEIGHT LOST: 70 lbs

TIME IT TOOK TO LOSE THE WEIGHT: 5 months

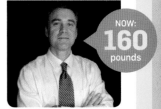

NOW:
160 pounds

"Nothing has ever had as big of an impact on my life as that book."

⭐ *Let's say you're shopping at the mall.* You pass by the food court and are taken by the wafting scent of cinnamon-dusted baked goods. On one side, Auntie Anne's is selling those delicious Cinnamon Sugar Pretzels. On the other, Cinnabon's Caramel Pecanbon beckons. Where do you go? Believe it or not, if you choose the Cinnabon, you'll ingest an additional 590 calories— almost a third of your daily allotment! (Make that wrong choice just twice a month and you'll pack an additional 4 pounds of fat onto your body in a year!)

⭐ *Or maybe you're at the ball park, and you want some ice cream.* What's the difference between an ice cream sandwich and a helping of soft-serve chocolate in one of those keepsake helmets? You get to keep the helmet—and 239 extra calories.

⭐ *Or maybe you stop at the gas station to fill up your car's tank as well as your own.* You could grab a 100 Grand bar to fix your nutty chocolate jones, or pick the old standby Snickers. But opt for the wrong one and you'll be choking down almost an extra 100 calories and nearly twice the fat. (Hint: You'd rather look like a hundred grand than have people snicker at you.)

⭐ *Or, oh my goodness, you're trying to eat right, and you grab one of Jamba Juice's Ideal Meal Chunky Strawberry breakfasts.* It's an "ideal meal," for heaven's sake! But if you had picked their Fresh Banana Oatmeal, you'd have saved 240 calories and 13 grams of fat!

For thousands of food comparisons and enough savvy nutritional advice to help you lose 10, 20, or 30 pounds in a matter of months, join the EAT THIS, NOT THAT! premium online service. Head to **EATTHIS.COM** *to find out more.*

By making smart food swaps, you can cut hundreds, even thousands, of calories out of your food intake every day, and still enjoy the treat at the mall, the nosh at the gas station, or lunch, dinner, or breakfast at your favorite restaurant. And as we've seen above, it's not just a matter of how you look; it's a matter of health, of well-being—heck, it's a matter of national security!

Smart swaps equal fewer calories. Fewer calories equal fewer pounds and a longer, healthier, happier life. It's as simple as that.

How to lose weight with this book

If you want to shed belly fat, there's only one formula you need to know, and luckily for you, it's easier than anything you encountered in ninth-grade algebra.

The magic formula is this: Calories in – calories out = total weight loss or gain. This is the equation that determines whether your body will shape up to look more like a slender 1 or a paunchy 0, a flat-bellied yardstick or a pot-bellied protractor. That's why it's absolutely critical that you have some understanding of what sort of numbers you're plugging into this formula.

On the "calories out" side, we have your daily activities: cleaning house, standing in line at the post office, hauling in groceries, and so on. Often when people discover extra flab hanging around their midsections, they assume there's something wrong with this side of the equation. Maybe so, but more likely it's the front-end of the equation—the "calories in" side—that's tipping the scale. That side keeps track of all the cookies, fried chicken, and piles of pasta that you eat every day.

In order to maintain a healthy body weight, a moderately active female between the ages of 20 and 50 needs only 2,000 to 2,200 calories per day. A male fitting the same profile needs 2,400 to 2,600. Those numbers can fluctuate depending on whether you're taller or shorter than average or whether you spend more or less time exercising, but they represent reasonable estimations for most people. (For a more accurate assessment, use the calorie calculator at mayoclinic.com.)

Let's take a closer look at the numbers: It takes 3,500 calories to create a pound of body fat. So if you eat an extra 500 per day—the amount in one Dunkin' Donuts' multigrain bagel with reduced fat cream cheese—then you'll earn 1 new pound of body fat each week. Make that a habit—like so many of us do unwittingly—and you'll gain 52 pounds of flab per year!

That's where this book comes in. Within these pages are literally hundreds of simple food swaps that will save you from 10 to 1,000 calories or more apiece. The more often you choose "Eat This" foods over "Not That!" options, the quicker you'll notice layers of fat melting away from your body. Check this out:

• A single cup of **CINNAMON TOAST CRUNCH** cereal has 173 calories. Switch to **CINNA-GRAHAM HONEY-COMBS** five times per week and you'll drop 6 pounds this year.

• A **GRANDE JAVA CHIP FRAPPUCCINO** from Starbucks has 340 calories. Switch to an **ICED COFFEE WITH MOCHA SYRUP** three times per week and you'll shed 5 pounds in 6 months.

• **BANQUET'S FRIED CHICKEN FROZEN DINNER** has 380 calories. Make the switch to **SWANSON'S** version of the same meal three times per week and you'll drop an extra 1½ pounds every 3 months.

• An **ORIENTAL CHICKEN SALAD** from Applebee's packs in an astounding 1,310 calories. Instead, order the **ASIAN CRUNCH SALAD** three times per week—or make a comparative swap at some other restaurant—and you'll blast away more than 6 pounds of body fat in just 2 months.

And here's the best news of all: These swaps aren't isolated calorie savers. If you commit yourself to just the four on this list, the cumulative calorie-saving effect will stamp out one pound of body fat every week this year. Take that, multigrain bagel! Check out 12 more of our favorite calorie-squashing, fat-melting Top Swaps on the following pages.

What Hath Eat This, Not That! Wrought?

We never set out to start a revolution.

Like those pissed-off patriots at Boston Harbor, we just wanted to call a little attention to some nagging injustices: Instead of the tax on tea, we were protesting the tax on our waistlines, caused by secretiveness, misdirection, and a simple lack of nutritional forethought on the part of the food industry.

But revolution it became, and as **EAT THIS, NOT THAT!** has continued to grow, with more than 6 million books now in print, our first nutritional volley became the shot heard 'round the food world.

✳ Maybe we didn't chase off any Redcoats, but we did scare the bejesus out of **RED LOBSTER**. When the national chain was given a Restaurant Report Card grade of F for failing to disclose its nutritional information, the folks there did an about-face and decided to post their food's calorie counts. Smart move on their part: Red Lobster is, in fact, one of the healthiest chains in America —and now it's getting the credit it deserves. (Check out page 166 for details.) Quiznos, Outback, Olive Garden, California Pizza Kitchen, and Applebee's (to name just a few) have followed suit.

* And we didn't stick a feather in our caps and call it Macaroni, but when we called on **ROMANO'S MACARONI GRILL** to get control of its ridiculous calorie counts, it stepped up to the plate—big time. It not only disclosed its nutritional info, but it also completely remade its menu to reflect Americans' desire for healthy (but still hearty) fare. In the past 2 years, it has gone from being one of the two or three worst restaurants in America (and recipient of a D- in our first report card) to being neck-and-neck with Red Lobster for the title of very best.

* And we may not have crossed the Delaware with Washington, but Washington has crossed over to our side. Indeed, 2 years after we published *EAT THIS, NOT THAT! FOR KIDS*—a book whose goal was to publicize the crisis of childhood obesity—first lady **MICHELLE OBAMA** is on the offensive, most recently with her Chefs Move to School campaign. And some of the worst kids' meals in America have been made healthier by restaurants around the country.

Of course, every revolution has casualties. Goodbye, Chili's Awesome Blossom and your 2,710 salt-dredged calories. Bon voyage, Baskin-Robbins Heath Bar Shake (2,310 slurpilicious calories). Rest in peace, Pepperidge Farm Roasted Chicken Pot Pie (1,029 calories and 64 grams of fat!), and let's hope no one remembers the full-scale assault you waged on our waistlines.

And, as the **EAT THIS, NOT THAT!** revolution continues to grow, expect to see more nutritional scoundrels run out of town. Sometimes you have to clear out the bad guys so the next generation of Americans can enjoy life, liberty, and the pursuit of happiness—without size-42 pants.

TOP SWAPS

Burgers

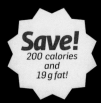

Save!
200 calories
and
19 g fat!

Eat This!
Wendy's ¼ lb Single
470 calories
21 g fat (8 g saturated,
1 g trans)
970 mg sodium

Not That!
Burger King Whopper
670 calories
40 g fat (11 g saturated,
1.5 g trans)
1,020 mg sodium

Wendy's quarter-pound creation has long been one of our favorite burgers on the block, namely because it delivers a substantial patty, along with a solid dose of produce, all for less than 500 calories and 1,000 milligrams of sodium. That's more than can be said of its burger rivals, including the Big Mac, the Quarter Pounder with Cheese, and, worst of all, the Whopper. An unthinkable 150 calories and 17 grams of fat come from BK's notoriously thick application of mayo, so if you're a helpless Whopper addict, learn to love it with ketchup and mustard only.

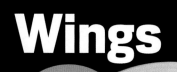

Wings

Save!
630 calories and 70 g fat!

Eat This!
Applebee's Buffalo Chicken Wings, Southern BBQ
660 calories
35 g fat
(9 g saturated)
1,070 mg sodium

Not That!
Uno Chicago Grill 3 Way Buffalo Wings
1,290 calories
105 g fat
(24 g saturated)
1,410 mg sodium

For all the chatter about them being junk food, wings can actually be a sensible start to a meal. With 61 grams of protein, these Southern-style wings from Applebee's may help you cut calories from your overall meal by frontloading your dinner with belly-filling protein. But choose the wrong chicken and you'll pay the price. Uno's version packs nearly twice the calories and triple the fat, yet for all the excess only brings 2 extra grams of protein to the table. As a rule of thumb, if you order an appetizer, make sure your portion doesn't exceed 250 calories.

Pasta

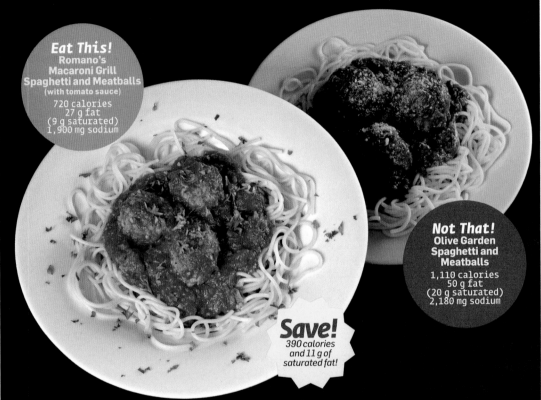

Eat This!
Romano's
Macaroni Grill
Spaghetti and Meatballs
(with tomato sauce)

720 calories
27 g fat
(9 g saturated)
1,900 mg sodium

Not That!
Olive Garden
Spaghetti and
Meatballs

1,110 calories
50 g fat
(20 g saturated)
2,180 mg sodium

Save!
390 calories
and 11 g of
saturated fat!

We firmly believe that spaghetti and meatballs is a meal best enjoyed in the comfort of your own home, preferably with a crisp salad and a recipe that stretches back through the generations. But when venturing out in search of comfort food, be aware that this Italian-American staple can swallow up an entire day's worth of saturated fat and sodium—just as it does in Olive Garden's potent rendition (and that's before you tack on their breadsticks and bottomless salad bowl). Macaroni Grill's lighter version is far from perfect, but it delivers the goods for a fraction of the calories you'll find in any other corner of the restaurant world.

Ribs

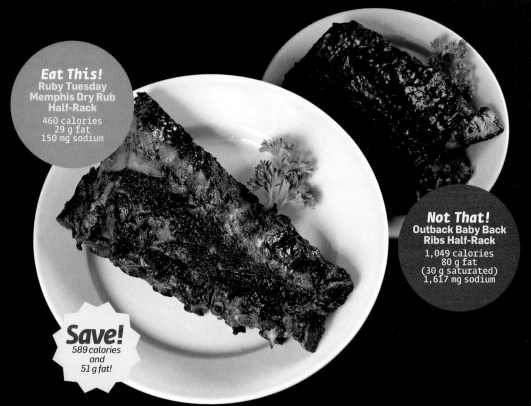

Eat This!
Ruby Tuesday
Memphis Dry Rub
Half-Rack

460 calories
29 g fat
150 mg sodium

Not That!
Outback Baby Back
Ribs Half-Rack

1,049 calories
80 g fat
(30 g saturated)
1,617 mg sodium

Save!
589 calories
and
51 g fat!

Outback has a magical way of making hunks of meat more calorie-dense than any other restaurant in the country. Hence the 1,141-calorie ribeye, the 2,144-calorie wings, and this, the worst rack in America. Inside sources tell us that it's a heavy reliance on butter and sauces, but the faux-Aussie chain might also consider finding a protein purveyor who deals in leaner cuts. Ribs will never be healthy fare, but Ruby Tuesday serves up the least-damaging version we've come across by skipping the layer of sugar-laden sauce and opting for a bold spice rub instead.

Fajitas

Fajitas are one of those foods that sound great in theory (Lean protein! Sizzling vegetables!) but rarely prove to deliver anything but a punishing blow of calories, fat, and sodium. Blame it on the accoutrements—the stacks of tortillas, the piles of cheese, the ramekins of guacamole. In the case of Chili's, tortillas and condiments account for 63 percent of the total calories. In a menu otherwise littered with potent taco platters and bulky burritos, On the Border puts out the lowest-calorie fajita platter in America, namely by skimping on the oil with the chicken and offering a restrained spread of fajita fixings. (Note: Add rice and beans and a side of cheese and you'll need to double these numbers.)

Chicken

Save!
792 calories
and 3 g of
saturated fat!

Not That!
California
Pizza Kitchen
Chicken Marsala
1,412 calories
15 g saturated fat
3,038 mg sodium

Eat This!
Romano's Macaroni
Grill Chicken Marsala
620 calories
12 g saturated fat
1,410 mg sodium

Two years ago, this would be anything but a Top Swap. Back then, Macaroni Grill was still one of the unhealthiest places to eat in America, and the chicken marsala packed 1,180 calories and 70 grams of fat. But thanks to an aggressive effort starting in 2009 to revamp and lighten its menu, Macaroni Grill has dramatically slashed the calories from many of its most popular dishes. In the case of chicken marsala, the 47 percent drop in calories means less butter, less oil, and fewer refined carbohydrates on the plate. Maybe CPK should follow suit, because so many of its salads, pastas, and chicken entrées come with quadruple-digit caloric consequences.

French Fries

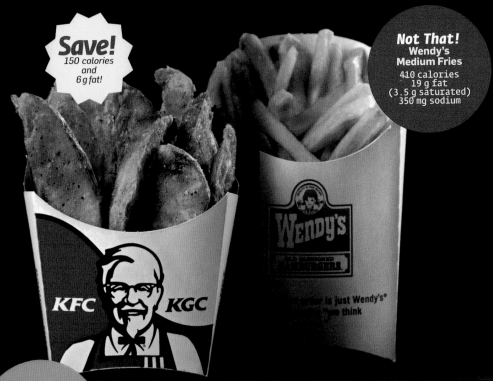

Save!
150 calories
and
6 g fat!

Not That!
Wendy's
Medium Fries
410 calories
19 g fat
(3.5 g saturated)
350 mg sodium

KFC   KGC

Eat This!
KFC
Potato Wedges
260 calories
13 g fat
(2.5 g saturated)
740 mg sodium

Yes, even hunks of fried potatoes can vary wildly in their overall nutritional profile. At some fast food joints, an order of fries is an understandable indulgence; at others, it's a knockout blow. Wendy's bulky spuds fall firmly into the latter camp, packing more calories than you'd get from a Double Stack on their Dollar Menu. (Add a medium soda and your burger just gained a 620-calorie tag team.) For all of its Kentucky-fried faults, KFC offers a range of reasonable sides. While you'd be better off with green beans or even mashed potatoes, these wedges rank at the top of the country's "healthy" fries list.

Salads

Save!
740 calories
and
50 g fat!

Not That!
Applebee's Oriental Grilled Chicken Salad
1,240 calories
77 g fat
(12 g saturated,
2.5 g trans)
2,000 mg sodium

Eat This!
Panera Bread Asian Sesame Chicken Salad
500 calories
27 g fat
(4.5 g saturated)
1,290 mg sodium

Blindfolded, you'd be hard-pressed to taste the difference between these two salads: Both contain crunchy strips, almonds, and grilled chicken, and both are dressed with a sesame vinaigrette. Yet, the Applebee's version—slightly larger, but more important, slicked with considerably more oil—packs more than twice the calories and nearly three times the fat. You could eat the Panera version and three doughnuts and still save a few hundred calories. Just goes to show, it's not always what you choose to eat, but where you choose to eat it.

Pizza

Eat This!
Domino's
Ham, Mushroom,
Green Pepper,
and Onion
(2 slices, large, thin crust)

420 calories
19 g fat
(7 g saturated)
900 mg sodium

Not That!
Pizza Hut Supreme
(2 slices, large,
Thin 'N Crispy)

660 calories
34 g fat
(14 g saturated)
1,860 mg sodium

Save!
240 calories
and
15 g fat!

In the battle between the behemoths of the pizza delivery biz, Domino's usually comes out on top. That's because its thin crust pizza produces the lowest-calorie slices in the industry. Kiss all of that goodbye if you go for one of its extreme in-house creations; instead, piece together the leanest, most satisfying pie possible by combining ham with as many veggies as you like (miraculously, the calorie counts actually go down when you add this combination of ingredients, as these healthy toppings displace some of the cheese). If Pizza Hut is your place, seek solace in its Fit 'n Delicious pies; the ham, red onion, and mushroom rendition rivals these Domino's slices.

Ice Cream

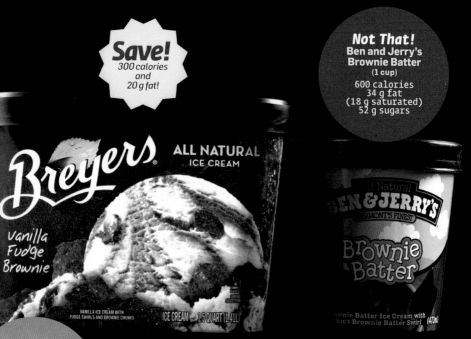

Save!
300 calories
and
20 g fat!

Not That!
Ben and Jerry's
Brownie Batter
(1 cup)
600 calories
34 g fat
(18 g saturated)
52 g sugars

Eat This!
Breyers
All Natural Vanilla
Fudge Brownie
(1 cup)
300 calories
14 g fat
(8 g saturated)
34 g sugars

More than any other sector of the food world, the ice cream industry has strived to cater to the needs and desires of the health-conscious eater who wants to have his sweets and eat them too. So there is no reason to opt for these so-called premium pints of ice cream offered by Dove, Häagen-Dazs, and Ben & Jerry's. Not only do they charge you a premium price, but they also routinely pack twice as many calories as their more affordable competitors. Breyers All Natural remains our favorite brand in the store, not just for its low calories counts and exciting flavors, but because the ingredient list is short and sweet.

Chapter

1

**THE TRUTH ABOUT
YOUR FOOD**

As with the banking industry,

the Russian political system, and the romantic liaisons on *Gossip Girl*, all is not as it seems in the world of food and drink.

Misnomers and confusing labels have been with us for generations—at least since our hungry ancestors devoured the first hamburger (with no actual ham in it) and snarfed down the first hot dog (with no actual dog in it). And how many diners and takeout places in your neighborhood claim to sell "world-famous" coffee or pizza? (Wouldn't you think being "world famous" might allow them to upgrade to neon signs that aren't missing a few letters?)

What a food seller chooses to call his product or how he chooses to advertise it has always been as much a matter of fiction and salescraft as anything else. And everybody's in on the joke. Nobody believes that Count Chocula really comes from Transylvania. Or that Aunt Jemima is out there somewhere, making pancakes. Or that there's a salty, bearded Gorton's fisherman overseeing the day's catch up in Gloucester. These silly marketing claims and characters are just part of the commercial spin of modern life, and if they make one box of frozen fish sticks look somehow more appealing than the next, so be it.

But the hype and the spin get a little more serious—and a lot more unfair—when food starts to carry words that seem to make one food "healthier" than another. Words and phrases like "lower in fat" or "all natural" or "multigrain" sure sound appealing. Who wouldn't choose the all-natural multigrain product that's lower in fat?

Problem is, none of these words and phrases really mean anything. The food that's "lower in fat" simply has less fat than the original version of the product—the "lower in fat" version is probably still bulging with unnecessary calories. (And as you'll learn in the coming chapters, the type of fat you're eating matters more than the amount.) "All natural"? So are crude oil, snake venom, and botulism, but I wouldn't want to pay to eat any of those. And "multigrain" means nothing more than "made from more than one grain"—it sounds healthy, but if all those many grains have been stripped of their fiber and nutrients, you might as well be eating a teaspoon of pure sugar.

And therein lies the rub—and the reason for this book.

While the government has made some significant strides in getting nutrition information to the public—like requiring food packaging to carry nutrition labels—there's still so much room for obfuscation and outright mendacity that knowing what's in our food is never a certainty.

Why Food Is Different Today

Two out of every three American adults are now overweight. How is this possible? You might say it's because we've all stopped exercising—except, there's a Curves or a Bally in every strip mall and downtown block in the United States and a Dick's or Sports Authority in every shopping plaza. You might say it's because we stopped watching what we eat—except that on any given week, half of the best-sellers on the *New York Times* list are diet or cookbooks. You might say it's because we all just stopped caring—except that liposuction and belly band surgery are practically an epidemic. And you know and I know that the two most common phrases in the American lexicon are "I'm trying to watch my weight" and "Does this make me look fat?"

So what's causing all this weight gain? Well, here's a clue: The Centers for Disease Control and Prevention found that American men eat 7 percent more calories than they did in 1971; American women eat a whopping 18 percent more calories (an additional 335 calories a day—enough to pack on a pound of extra flab every 11 days!). And American kids average 150 daily calories more than they did just 20 years ago. Did our stomachs get larger? Did our mouths expand?

Of course not. *We* haven't changed. The food has changed.

▶ **WE'VE ADDED EXTRA CALORIES TO TRADITIONAL FOODS.** In the early 1970s, food manufacturers, looking for a cheaper ingredient to replace sugar, came up with a substance called high-fructose corn syrup (HFCS). Today, HFCS is in an unbelievable array of foods—from breakfast cereals to bread, from ketchup to pasta sauce, from juice drinks to iced teas. According to the FDA, the average American consumes 82 grams of added sugars every day, which contribute 317 empty calories to our daily diet. HFCS might not be any worse for our bodies than normal table sugar, but its dirt-cheap cost and prevalence in processed foods has only served to intensify America's collective sweet tooth in recent years.

▶ **WE'RE SUPERSIZING OUR LIVES.** Of course we want to be smart with our money, especially in this economy. So of course when we see the word "value," especially as it pertains to a "meal," we're going to want to go for it. Supersizing it at your local fast-food restaurant gives you an average of 73 percent more calories for a mere 17 percent more in cost. Sounds like a bargain, until you realize that you don't need the 73 percent more calories!

▶ **WE'RE EATING THINGS OUR BODIES AREN'T SUPPOSED TO EAT.** A generation ago, it was hard for food manufacturers to create baked goods that would last on the store shelves. Most baked goods require oils, and oil runs and leaks at room temperature. But since the 1960s, manufacturers have been baking with—and restaurants have been frying with—something called "trans fat." Trans fat is cheap and effective: It makes potato chips crispier and Oreo cookies tastier; and it lets fry cooks make pound after pound of fries without smoking up their kitchens. But trans fat has been shown to have a horrific effect on our bodies: It raises our LDL (bad) cholesterol, lowers our HDL (good) cholesterol, and greatly increases our risk of heart disease and obesity. (If you see the words "partially hydrogenated" on the list of ingredients, you've got trans fat.)

The result of all this manipulation—manipulation of our food, to make it more appealing to our taste buds, and manipulation of our minds, to make us want to spend money on this crap—is that we absorb more calories than would have been humanly possible just a few decades ago. Our food and beverages are so calorie-dense that it's nearly impossible to eat healthy. And the way that foods are sold, in both grocery stores and restaurants, has made smart nutritional choices harder and harder to discern.

That's why ***EAT THIS, NOT THAT!*** is such an invaluable resource for those who want to eat their favorite foods and not be ambushed by hidden fat, sugar, and calories.

The ETNT! Encyclopedia

UNPACKING THE MOST MISLEADING CLAIMS OF THE FOOD INDUSTRY

LIGHTLY SWEETENED

A frequently abused claim with no formal definition, this appears most often in the cereal aisle, and many of the boxes it adorns are actually loaded with various sweeteners. Need proof? Look at Kellogg's Smart Start. It claims to be "lightly sweetened," yet it has more sugar per cup than a full serving of Oreo cookies!

GOOD SOURCE OF . . .

This packaging claim is of slightly less importance than "excellent source of." It means that the product contains between 10 and 19 percent of your daily requirement for the mentioned nutrient. In other words, you would have to eat between 5 and 10 servings to get your full day's value.

REDUCED FAT

Splashed across too many packaged goods to count, this term means that the total fat grams have been reduced by at least 25 percent. Sounds great, right? Problem is, that reduction in fat often comes with an increase in sugar and sodium and, ultimately, no net nutritional gain to speak of.

MULTIGRAIN

This simply means that more than one type of grain was used in processing (e.g., wheat, rye, barley, and rice). It doesn't, however, make any claim about the degree of processing used on those grains. Also, beware of the equally ambiguous "wheat bread," a claim that simply means the loaf was made from wheat flour, which might very well be refined and colored with molasses to appear darker. The only trustworthy claim for whole grains is "100 percent whole grain."

LIGHTLY BREADED

The phrase most restaurants use to

distract diners from the fact that the food they're about to eat has been rolled in flour, egg, and bread crumbs and let loose in a vat of bubbling fat. Doesn't matter how light the breading is; it's the oil part that will get you.

NATURAL

This term is used almost entirely at the discretion of food processors. With the exception of meat and poultry products, the USDA has set no definition and imposes no regulations on the use of this term, making it essentially meaningless.

COMPLIMENTARY

Usually attached to one of the following words: chips, bread, desserts, refills. In any case, the act of giving away low-cost, high-calorie foods is a common tactic restaurants use to add value to the "customer experience." Remember, just because

it's free doesn't mean it won't cost you—these empty calories add up fast.

REDUCED SODIUM

Used when the sodium level is reduced by 25 percent or more, regardless of the total amount. "Low sodium," on the other hand, can be used only when the product contains no more than 140 milligrams per serving.

TRANS FAT–FREE

Food processors can make this claim so long as their product contains less than 0.49 gram of trans fat per serving. Considering the American Heart Association recommends capping daily intake at 2 grams, this is no small amount. So even if the label reads "0 g trans fat," that's no guarantee that you're in the clear. Instead, read the ingredients list; if shortening or partially hydrogenated oil is listed, then you need to find another product.

The Year in Food 2010

THE BEST AND WORST CHANGES TO THE FOOD INDUSTRY—AND WHAT THEY MEAN TO YOU

Soda taxes become sin taxes

Despite the vigor and vitriol driving this national discussion, the idea of taxing our soda addiction is nothing new. Soda taxes have been a part of policy discourse for decades, and more than half of states already leverage some sort of tax on soda. But in 2010 a steeper crop of "sin taxes," intended to curb unhealthy behaviors, rose from the powerful, double-edged impetus of escalating obesity rates and states' needs for increased revenue. The leader in the fight for soda taxes is New York Governor David Paterson, who, after failing to get a tax passed in 2009, re-introduced it into New York's budget in January 2010. The message was clear: He wasn't going to let the soft drink issue fizzle.

Would this soda tax really affect you? Consider the stakes: The average American today drinks about a gallon of soda each week—more than 1,500 calories of pure liquid sugar. That amounts to approximately 22 pounds of flab added to every man, woman, and child per year, and it implicates soda as one of the biggest culprits behind rising obesity rates. We believe the soda tax has the potential to create long-term changes in public habit, but only if it's bolstered to a level higher than the current average of roughly 4 percent. A recent study from the Rand Corporation reveals that, in order for a soda tax to be effective, it has to push closer to the tax proposed by Governor Paterson. His penny-per-ounce tax works out to be about 30 percent on a 12-pack. That might be just enough to push consumers to choose fruit juice—or even better—H_2O, instead.

KFC introduces the Double Down Sandwich

The single biggest food launch this year came in the form of a farcical Frankenfood that replaces the traditional sandwich bun with two fried chicken filets wrapped around cheese, slices of bacon, and a mayo-based sauce. The sandwich was intended as a short-run publicity stunt, but because of overwhelming popularity, KFC decided to give it a permanent home on the menu. Bloggers called it names ranging from "a disgusting meal, a must avoid," to "the vilest food product created by man." Yet within two months of its launch, 10 million had been sold.

So how bad is it, really? Well, one sandwich carries 540 calories, which makes it 130 calories lighter than a Whopper from Burger King, 210 calories lighter than a Bacon Swiss Crispy Chicken Sandwich from Carl's Jr., and 880 calories lighter than a Quesadilla Burger from Applebee's. The fact that a sandwich built on deep fried chicken pieces instead of buns still manages to win nutritional battles against so many of the most popular sandwiches in American says something about the way we eat. Namely, that we can do much better.

New York declares a war on sodium

In 2009, the New York City Health Department announced it was spearheading a serious shakedown on salt, and by early 2010, the final plans were in motion. The National Salt Reduction Initiative has the ambitious goal of reducing America's sodium intake by 20 percent over the next five years, and to do so, it's asking food processors to willingly commit themselves to the target. That could have massive implications considering the Center for Science in the Public Interest's estimate that Americans consume more than 4,000 milligrams of sodium a day. Ideally we should take in just over half of that. And the vast majority of that sodium—nearly 80 percent—comes from foods prepared outside the home, putting us all at higher risk for stroke and heart disease.

In light of the bill, companies such as Heinz and Campbell's have already begun making the necessary cuts, and many others have committed themselves to doing so. Among them are

Mars, Boar's Head, Starbucks, Subway, and Uno Chicago Grill. Other companies, such as Burger King, PepsiCo, and McDonald's, have opted to pass. Perhaps because of this, the Institute of Medicine has recommended backing sodium restrictions with hard legislation, noting that doing so could prevent more than 100,000 deaths each year. Now in New York—home of calories counts on menu boards and trans fat-free restaurants—legislators are discussing a radical bill to completely eliminate the use of salt in restaurants. New York chefs, predictably, are not pleased. But whether or not this bill passes, it's likely the first of many legislative attempts to slash the amount of sodium in the American diet.

Subway unveils the nation's leanest line of fast-food breakfast sandwiches

Although some locations have been selling it for years, it wasn't until April 2010 that Subway pushed its low-cal breakfast lineup into every shop in the franchise. Now 23,000 US locations offer a roster of morning sandwiches that pair meats such as black forest ham, bacon, and steak with breads like English muffins and 6-inch heroes. But here's what's really impressive: Only one sandwich on the menu breaks 500 calories (the 6-inch Double Bacon, Egg, and Cheese), and if you order a Muffin Melt—one of the English muffin sandwiches—the worst you can do is 220 calories.

Compare that with Carl's Jr., where you can't get a breakfast sandwich with fewer than 470 calories. Or McDonald's, where a Big Breakfast with hotcakes will cost you well over 1,000. Sure, other fast-food joints offer one or two lean options, but Subway is the first to ensure that every item adheres to the same stringent nutritional criteria. That means eschewing sausage, buttery spreads, and carb-heavy breads like bagels and croissants. And to sweeten the deal, Subway gives you the option to dress any sandwich with the same roundup of produce it provides for the lunch sandwiches. Keep your fingers crossed: If the Subway approach proves profitable, other chains might follow.

Health care reform makes menu-board calorie counts mandatory

In March 2010, President Obama signed legislation that will expand health care coverage to millions of Americans and folded deep inside the massive bill was a little mandate that few discussed but that comes with major implications. It says that any restaurant chain with 20 or more outlets must print calorie information alongside items on menus, menu boards, and drive-thru signs. That means, starting next year, more than 200,000 restaurants nationwide will begin empowering customers to make healthier decisions.

Here's why we support the legislation: First, and most important, it helps consumers avoid inflicting involuntary blows to their waistlines. Research from Stanford shows that, when provided with accurate information, diners consume fewer calories than when they have no information at all. (Suddenly, that Italian sub is less tempting when it's sitting next to a number like 1,250). Also, it forces restaurants to think twice about serving up the same caloric calamities they've been serving for years with impunity. Some restaurants in New York that have been subject to this law since 2008 have already shown signs of improving their offerings, a trend we hope soon sweeps the nation.

Applebee's and Outback Steakhouse reveal nutrition information

A restaurant's reluctance to cough up the numbers behind its food has generally been a pretty good indication that it has something to hide. Last year, we were pleased to announce that both Olive Garden and Red Lobster had finally handed over the numbers that allowed customers to make smart decisions. This year, we welcome Applebee's and Outback Steakhouse to the club.

As we predicted, both restaurants carry a bevy of calorie- and sodium-heavy entrees, appetizers, and desserts. No surprise there. But a funny thing happens when restaurants start shining lights into their own nutritional caverns. They become suddenly motivated to start building healthier entrées. At Applebee's, customers now have a handful of options that fall below 550 calories, and at Outback, select items can be ordered "light style," which drops them down to 500 calories or less. And we're not talking tofu scrambles here—at Applebee's the low-cal fare includes Asiago Peppercorn Steak and Spicy Shrimp Diavolo, and at Outback there's the Grilled Chicken on the Barbie and Filet with Wild Mushroom Sauce. We've doled out plenty of (much-deserved) criticism to them over the years, but for now, we tip our calorie-conscious hats to both chains with hopes that there are more lean options to come.

The FDA cracks down on bogus label claims

Remember a few years back when companies such as Kellogg's and General Mills started taking flak for years of targeting children in campaigns for sugar-loaded cereals? Well, part of their amends-making process was to pull nutrition highlights from the back label and feature them prominently on the front of the box, right next to the mug shots of Tony the Tiger and that Toucan Sam. In theory, front-of-package labeling would allow consumers to quickly ascertain key facts like calorie and sugar counts as they buzzed hurriedly through the aisles.

By the end of last year, the FDA realized two major flaws in the plan: 1) The numbers are for impractically small serving sizes: In order to show their cereals in a more attractive light, brands such as Fruity Pebbles and Lucky Charms started listing serving sizes at just three-quarters of a cup—not more than a few spirited spoonfuls. And 2), by highlighting only positive numbers, packagers are distracting from the negative. Sure that cereal has only 130 calories, but when it's hiding 15 grams of sugar in each serving, breakfast starts to look a lot like dessert in disguise. What's more, seeing the opportunity provided by the selective front-of-package labeling, food manufacturers quickly retooled other lousy foods—chips, cookies, crunchy snacks—to don the same type of beneficial labeling.

Always the last to arrive at the dance, the FDA finally decided to crack down, sending out a flurry of letters to industry heads and joining forces with the Institute of Medicine to try to develop a new labeling system that keeps packagers honest and consumers healthy. Here's to hoping the FDA does the right thing and holds these companies accountable for peddling their dodgiest products in a positive light.

Michelle Obama takes a stand against childhood obesity

In February, Michelle Obama outlined a plan called Let's Move that aims to cut childhood obesity from 20 percent to 5 percent by 2030. The first lady's aggressive plan includes educating parents about nutrition at home, improving the standards of the school lunch program, putting heavier emphasis on physical activity, and introducing healthier foods to low-income areas.

The timing is perfect in that it taps into the momentum of another high-profile campaign, Jamie Oliver's Food Revolution, wherein British celebrity chef Jamie Oliver uses reality TV as a platform for raising awareness about the deficiencies in childhood nutrition. Other top-tier chefs and food authorities are following suit, a trend we love to see.

The high-fructose corn syrup era passes its prime

According to USDA estimates, every man, woman, and child in this country is responsible for digesting 130 pounds' worth of caloric sweeteners every year, and much of that is driven by high-fructose corn syrup. But here's the twist: In 2009 we actually consumed 20 percent less HFCS than we did in 2002. The spark behind the dramatic drop was a wave of negative publicity that hurt sales and prompted many companies to eliminate it from their recipes. And with the high-profile cuts still piling up—both Gatorade and Hunt's Ketchup nixed it earlier this year—2010 is quite likely the first year since 1990 that Americans will consume fewer than 50 pounds of the HFCS per person.

Is that good news? Sure it is. It's great news. The fewer empty calories companies slip into your diet, the better your chances of staying slim and dodging the diabetes bullet. The problem is that in most cases, high-fructose corn syrup is simply being elbowed out to make room for old-fashioned refined sugar—in effect trading one problem for another. The issue over whether high-fructose corn syrup is unhealthy was never in dispute, but whether it's significantly worse than table sugar is one that was never properly resolved. By composition, both sweeteners consist of about 50 percent fructose and 50 percent glucose, so your body probably recognizes them as the same compound. If you want to stay thin, you need to minimize all forms of sugar—that applies to evaporated cane juice just as much as high-fructose corn syrup.

What's Really in Your Food

Once upon a time, back when Ray Kroc was still pushing milk-shake machines, a hamburger and fries meant a wad of freshly ground chuck and a peeled, sliced, and fried potato. Now, these two iconic foods—like nearly everything we consume—have taken on a whole new meaning. Sadly, many of our favorite foods today (especially fast foods) weren't crafted in kitchens, but designed and perfected in laboratories. So before you mindlessly chew your way through another value meal, take these mini-mysteries (conveniently solved below) into account. Sometimes the truth is tough to swallow.

What's really in . . .
A CHICKEN MCNUGGET?

You'd think that a breaded lump of chicken would be pretty simple. Mostly, it would contain bread and chicken. But the McNugget and its peers at other fast-food restaurants are much more complicated creatures than that. The "meat" in the McNugget *alone* contains seven ingredients, some of which are made up of yet more ingredients. (Nope, it's not just chicken. It's also such nonchicken-related stuff as water, wheat starch, dextrose, safflower oil, and sodium phosphates.) The "meat" also contains something called "autolyzed yeast extract." Then add another 20 ingredients that make up the breading, and you have the industrial chemical—I mean, fast-food meal—called the McNugget.

Still, McDonald's is practically all-natural compared to Wendy's Chicken Nuggets, with 30 ingredients, and Burger King Chicken Fries, with a whopping 35 ingredients.

What's really in . . .
A WENDY'S FROSTY?

Wendy's Frosty requires 14 ingredients to create what traditional shakes achieve with only milk and ice cream. So what accounts for the double-digit ingredient list? Mostly a barrage of thickening agents that includes guar

Feeling saucy? Just know that even fast food's most unadulterated nugget takes 27 ingredients to make.

gum, cellulose gum, and carrageenan. And while that's enough to disqualify it as a milk shake in our book, it's nothing compared with the chemist's list of ingredients in the restaurant's new line of bulked-up Frankenfrosties.

Check out the Coffee Toffee Twisted Frosty, for instance. It seems harmless enough; the only additions, after all, are "coffee syrup" and "coffee toffee pieces." The problem is that those two additions collectively contain 25 extra ingredients, seven of which are sugars and three of which are oils. And get this: Rather than a classic syrup, the "coffee syrup" would more accurately be described as a blend of water, high-fructose corn syrup, and propylene glycol, a laxative chemical that's used as an emulsifier in food and a filler in electronic cigarettes. Of all 10 ingredients it takes to make the syrup, coffee doesn't show up until near the end, eight items down the list.

What's really in . . .
A FILET-O-FISH?

The world's most famous fish sandwich begins as one of the ocean's ugliest creatures. Filet-O-Fish, like many of the fish patties used by fast-food chains, is made predominantly from hoki, a gnarly, crazy-eyed fish found in the cold waters off the coast of New Zealand. In the past, McDonald's has purchased up to 15 million pounds of hoki a year, each flaky fillet destined for a coat of batter, a bath of oil, a squirt of tartar, and a final resting place in a warm, squishy bun. But it seems the world's appetite for this and other fried-fish sandwiches has proven too voracious, as New Zealand has been forced to cut the allowable catch over the years in order to keep the hoki population from collapsing. Don't expect McDonald's to scale down Filet-O-Fish output anytime soon, though; other whitefish like Alaskan pollock will likely fill in the gaps left by the hoki downturn. After all, once it's battered and fried, do you really think you'll know the difference?

What's really in . . .
MY SALAMI SANDWICH?

Salami, the mystery meat: Is it cow? Is it pig? Well, if you're talking Genoa salami, like you'd get at Subway, then it's both. Most mass-produced salami is made from slaughterhouse leftovers that are gathered using "advanced meat recovery," which sounds like a rehab center for vegans but is actually

Captain Ron will always find another fish to fry.

a mechanical process that strips the last remaining bits of muscle off the bone so nothing is wasted. It's then processed using lactic acid, the waste product produced by bacteria in the meat. It both gives the salami its tangy flavor and cures it as well, making it an inhospitable place for other bacteria to grow. Add in a bunch of salt and spices—for a total of 15 ingredients in all—and you've got salami.

But now that you know what's in there, you might need to check yourself into an advanced meat recovery center.

What's really in . . .
A FAST-FOOD HAMBURGER?

It comes from a cow, yes, but before being stuffed into the bun of a Whopper or Big Mac, fast-food hamburger patties pass through the hands of a company called Beef Products.

The company specializes in taking slaughterhouse trimmings traditionally used only in pet food and cooking oil and turning them into patties. The challenge is getting this by-product meat clean enough for human consumption, as both *E. coli* and salmonella like to concentrate themselves in the fatty deposits. So how does Beef Products go about "cleaning" the meat? With an approach similar to what you might use in your bathroom—by using ammonia.

See, the company has developed a process for killing beef-based pathogens by forcing the ground meat through pipes and exposing it to ammonia gas. And not only has the USDA approved the process, but they've also allowed those who sell the beef to keep it hidden from their customers. At Beef Products' behest, ammonia gas has been deemed a "processing agent" that need not be identified on nutrition labels. Nevermind that if ammonia gets on your skin, it can cause severe burning, and if it gets in your eyes, it can blind you. As an ingredient in one of the foods we consume most, our government doesn't even deem it important enough to inform eaters of its presence.

Disturbing? Sure, but this is even more so: Documents uncovered last year by the *New York Times* show that the cleaning might not be as effective as the fast-food titans would like us to believe. Since 2005, beef coming from Beef Products has tested positive for *E. coli* three times and salmonella 48 times. By Beef Products' own estimation, the company is producing more than 7 million pounds

Would you like a side of ammonia with your burger? Didn't think so.

of ground beef per week, and aside from fast-food joints and quick-service restaurants, they're also shipping to schools and supermarkets. That makes it tough to avoid. Add to the gross-out factor the fact that after moving through this lengthy industrial process, a single beef patty can consist of cobbled-together pieces from different cows from all over the world—a practice that only increases the odds of contamination. So if you're set on the challenge of eating fresh, single-source hamburger, pick out a nice hunk of sirloin from the meat case and have your butcher grind it up fresh. Hold the ammonia.

What's really in . . .
BETTY CROCKER'S BAC-Os BITS?

We've all been there before: A big bowl of lettuce or a steamy baked potato is set before us and the sudden desire for a bit of smoky, porky goodness pervades. We try to resist, but we grab for the bottle anyway: Mmmmm . . . bacon.

Not quite. If it's Bac-Os you grab for, just know that there's not the slightest whiff of anything pork-like to be found in the bottle. So what are those little chips you've been shaking over your salads? Well, mostly soybeans. The bulk of each Bac-O is formed by tiny clumps of soy flour bound with trans-fatty, partially hydrogenated soybean oil and laced with artificial coloring, salt, and sugar.

But here's what's really odd: Hormel makes a product called Real Bacon Bits, and as the name implies, it's made with real bacon. And gram-for-gram, the real bacon actually has fewer calories than Betty Crocker's Bac-Os. The difference is only 5 calories, but still, if Hormel can make a nutritionally superior product using real bacon, then why would you ever choose the artificial one that's loaded with partially hydrogenated soybean oil?

What's really in . . .
SUBWAY'S 9-GRAIN WHEAT?

Okay, so you're probably not in the habit of ordering a la carte hero rolls at Subway, but there's a good chance you've eaten at least a few sandwiches built on the this bread. The good news is that Subway actually delivers on the nine-grain promise. The bad news: Eight of those nine grains appear in miniscule amounts. If you look at a Subway ingredient statement, you'll find every grain except wheat listed at the bottom

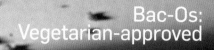
Bac-Os:
Vegetarian-approved

of the list, just beneath the qualifier "contains 2 percent or less." In fact, the primary ingredient in this bread is enriched wheat flour, which is refined wheat stripped of its better qualities then supplemented with nutrients. Plus, high-fructose corn syrup plays a more prominent role than any single whole grain.

So outside the nine grains, how many ingredients does Subway use to keep this bread together? Sixteen, among which aren't exactly items you'd find in the average baker's pantry: DATEM, sodium stearoyl lactylate, calcium sulfate, and azodiacarbonamide. But here's one that's a little unnerving: ammonium sulfate. This compound is rich with nitrogen, which is why it's most commonly used as a fertilizer. You might have used it to nourish your plants at home. And Subway does the same thing: The ammonium sulfate nourishes the yeast and helps the bread turn brown. What, did you think that dark hue was the result of whole grains? Hardly. It's a combination of the ammonium sulfate and the caramel coloring Subway adds in to darken its bread and deceive its customers. Seems like Jared might frown on that sort of subterfuge.

What's really in . . .
SKITTLES?

"Taste the rainbow?" We're not sure what rainbows are made of (light, no?), but we doubt it's the unsettling mashup of sugar, corn syrup, and hydrogenated palm kernel oil used to construct these neon orbs. That explains why every gram of fat is saturated and each package has more sugar than two twin-wrapped packages of Peanut Butter Twix.

To achieve that color spectrum, Skittles brings in a whole new list of additives. When a Skittles ad tells you to "taste the rainbow," what it's really telling you to do is taste the laboratory-constructed amalgam of nine artificial colors, many of which have been linked to behavioral and attention deficit problems in children. A few years ago the British journal *Lancet* published a study linking the artificial additives to hyperactivity and behavioral problems in children, which prompted the Center for Science in the Public Interest to petition the FDA for mandatory labels on artificially colored products. The FDA's response: We need more tests. In the meantime, there's a very large-scale test going on all across the country, and every Skittles eater is an unwilling participant.

What's really in . . .
A TACO BELL MEXICAN PIZZA?

It's Italian, it's Mexican, it's . . . well, it's got a whopping 64 different ingredients, so it's hard to tell just what exactly it is. On the face of it, this meal doesn't look too bad. There are two pizza shells, ground beef, beans, pizza sauce, tomatoes, and cheese. Even the nutritional vital signs, while high (540 calories, 30 grams of fat), compare favorably with most fast-food pizzas. It only gets scary when you zoom in on what it takes to stitch those pieces together. That's when you see all of those 64 smaller ingredients, including an astounding 24 in the ground beef alone. Yikes.

Now, some of those ingredients amount to little more than Mexican seasonings and spices, but there is a whole cluster of complex compounds such as autolyzed yeast extract, maltodextrin, xanthan gum, calcium propionate, fumaric acid, and silicon dioxide. Any of those sound familiar? That last one might if you've spent any time at the beach. But chances are you normally refer to it by its common name: sand.

That's right, sand is made from fragmented granules of rock and mineral, and the most common of

them is silicon dioxide, or silica. This is also the stuff that helps strengthen concrete and—when heated to extreme temperatures—hardens to create glass bottles and windowpanes.

So why exactly does Taco Bell put sand in the Mexican Pizza? To make it taste like spring break in Cancun? Not quite. As it turns out, Taco Bell adds silica to the beef to prevent it from clumping together during shipping and processing.

Is it unusual to add silica to food? Yes. Is it dangerous? Probably not. The mineral actually occurs naturally in all sorts of foods, including vegetables and milk. Of course, inhaling it is a different story. Construction workers who breathe in too much silica dust on the job can develop serious lung problems such as bronchitis or silicosis. Guess that's another reason to eat slowly—you don't want to make the mistake of inhaling your silica.

What's really in . . .
A BASKIN-ROBBINS OREO LAYERED SUNDAE?

Do your homemade sundaes carry swirls of vegetable oil? How about a sprinkle of thiamine mononitrate? What about a bit of nitrous oxide on top? Probably not, but that's exactly what you're in for at Baskin. Actually, it contains gluts of soybean oil, palm oil, and hydrogenated coconut oil. Plus sugar shows up a staggering 11 times on the list of ingredients. All told, this 1,330-calorie sundae is made from a carefully balanced amalgamation of 79 different ingredients. Seventy-nine ingredients! If you make a sundae at home, you're looking at 10 ingredients tops. Of course, you'd probably choose to leave out the polysorbate 80 and mono- and diglycerides—ingredients that Baskin relies on to keep other ingredients properly dissolved and certain fats from separating out. Sundae? More like a third period chemistry experiment gone awry.

What's really in . . .
NACHO CHEESE DORITOS?

To create each Dorito, the Frito-Lay food scientists draw from a well of 39 different ingredients. How many does it take to make a regular tortilla chip? About three. That means some 36 ingredients wind up in that weird cheese fuzz. Of those 36, only two are ingredients you'd use to make nachos at home: Romano and cheddar cheeses. Alongside those, processors rely on a cache of carbohydrate fillers such as maltodextrin, dextrose, flour, and corn syrup solids. Then comes a rotating cast of oils. Depending on what bag you get, you might find any combination of corn oil, soybean oil, cottonseed oil, and sunflower oil. Some of those will be partially hydrogenated, meaning they give the chip a longer shelf life and spike your cholesterol with a little shot of trans fat.

But for a brief moment before the fats and empty starches reach your stomach, your taste buds will enjoy the Doritos seasoning blend, which includes sugar, "artificial flavoring," and a rather worrisome compound called monosodium glutamate. Monosodium glutamate, or MSG, is the flavor enhancer largely responsible for the chip's addicting quality. The drawback is that it interferes with the production of an appetite-regulating hormone called leptin. That's why a study of middle-aged Chinese people found a strong correlation between MSG consumption and body fat. What's more, the FDA receives new complaints every year from people who react violently to MSG, suffering symptoms like nausea, headaches, numbness, chest pains, and dizziness—not to mention orange fingers.

Scientifically
engineered so
that you can't
eat just one

The Secret Confession of A. Donut

For years, researchers have been trying to answer the question, "What made America so fat?" Several suspects have been identified: too little exercise, too much work, too many hours behind the wheel or in front of the tube. But in a recent, shocking development, *Eat This, Not That!* has obtained secret transcripts of a police interrogation involving a leading suspect in the ongoing obesity epidemic. In this transcript, the suspect—identified by interrogators only as "A. Donut"—reveals his role in a sinister plot to force Americans to gain unnatural amounts of weight. Portions of that transcript have been presented here.

During prolonged observation by officers, A. Donut remained silent. Donut was sweated out for 2 days under standard heat-lamp interrogation methods. After repeated failures at eliciting a response, officers began preparations for Procedure 4.01.2, known as "eating A. Donut" (aka "the full Jack Bauer").

At 0600 hours on day 3, Donut gave this statement:

Yeah, sure. I did it. I made America fat.

It was a plot. It was me and a whole bunch of my buddies: Cupcake. Nacho Chip. Angel Food—oh, she's the worst, she'll break your heart! We were all in on it!

Yeah, our handlers taught us how to do it. Food marketers. Food scientists. They gave us the perfect combination of fat and sugar to make us irresistible. They took a bunch of raw, fresh-off-the-farm whole grains and they refined us, made us smoother, faster, more lethal. Took out all our good stuff and just left the evil inside.

It was hard going at first. Then, we found some secret weapons. Trans-fatty acid—fake fat, liquid grease turned solid through chemistry. Once we had that, we could stay greasy and gooey for days. Then, the sweet stuff: high-fructose corn syrup. No more plain sugar, we had artificial corn syrup that delivered carb calories like a bazooka! And you could put it in liquids, like sodas and iced teas. It was brilliant!

Now we could flood the zone. Combine HFCS with refined grains and you've got a carb rush comin' at you harder than a Miami rainshower. None of that fiber or protein to slow us down. Your bloodstream gets flooded with glucose—blood sugar—and boom! Insulin kicks in, and starts shuttling that glucose right to your belly. And guess what? An hour later, you're hungry again. And guess who you're going to come to for a quick fix? Ha! We had it all: We were greasy, gooey, sweet, and we stayed fresh for weeks.

I said to the team, "What if the American people wise up?" And my buddy Biscuit, he's from the South, he says, "Them American people won't wise up. They's square as a pool table and twice as green!"

We had you dead to rights. And we would've gotten away with it, too, if it weren't for those meddling kids from *EAT THIS, NOT THAT!*

At this point, officers proceeded to eat A. Donut, and the interrogation ended.

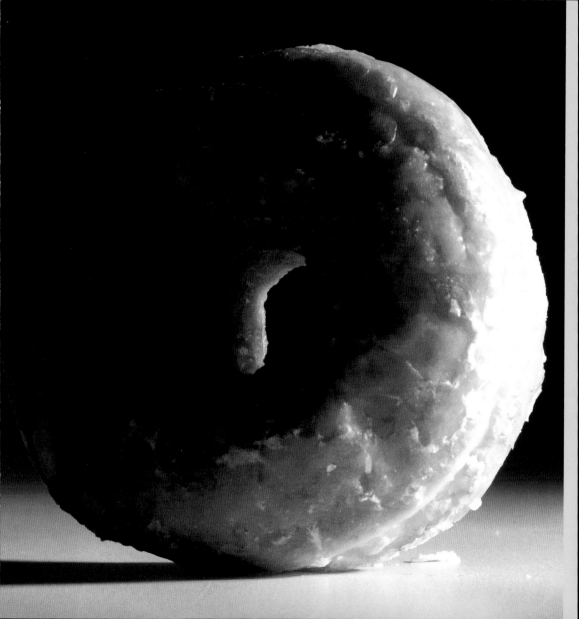

The Eat This, Not That! No-Diet Cheat Sheets

SATISFY YOUR HUNGER SMARTLY WITH THESE AT-A-GLANCE CRAVING SELECTORS

BREAKFAST SANDWICHES	CALORIES	FAT (G)	SATURATED (G)	TRANS (G)	SODIUM (MG)
1. Subway Black Forest Ham, Egg & Cheese Muffin Melt	180	7	2	0	650
2. Dunkin' Donuts Turkey Sausage Flatbread	280	6	2.5	0	820
3. McDonald's Egg McMuffin	300	12	5	0	820
4. Jack in the Box Bacon Breakfast Jack	300	13	5	0	760
5. Burger King Ham, Egg, & Cheese Croissan'wich	330	17	7	0	1,110
6. Starbucks Bacon, Gouda Cheese, & Egg Fritatta on Artisan Roll	350	18	7	0	840
7. Hardee's Frisco Breakfast Sandwich	400	18	7	N/A	1,350
8. Chick-fil-A Chicken Biscuit	440	20	8	0	1,240
9. Carl's Jr. Sourdough Breakfast Sandwich	470	25	9	0	1,090
10. Panera Bacon, Egg, and Cheese Breakfast Sandwich	510	24	10	0.5	1,060
11. Sonic Bacon, Egg, and Cheese Breakfast Toaster	530	32	10	0.5	1,440
12. Hardee's Monster Biscuit	770	55	18	N/A	2,310
13. Au Bon Pain Sausage, Egg, and Cheddar on Asiago Bagel	810	46	20	0	1,340

(Some restaurants do not disclose complete nutritional data.)

PASTA

		CALORIES	FAT (G)	SATURATED (G)	TRANS (G)	SODIUM (MG)
1.	Romano's Macaroni Grill Capellini Pomodoro	390	14	2	N/A	980
2.	Olive Garden Linguine alla Marinara	430	6	1	N/A	900
3.	Sbarro Penne alla Vodka	640	28	N/A	N/A	1,000
4.	Olive Garden Chicken Marsala	770	37	5	N/A	1,800
5.	Bob Evans Spaghetti with Meat Sauce	820	40	13	0	2,213
6.	Romano's Macaroni Grill Spaghetti & Meatballs with Bolognese Sauce	880	37	14	N/A	2,400
7.	Fazoli's Chicken Broccoli Penne Bake	920	42	24	0.5	2,310
8.	T.G.I. Friday's Bruschetta Chicken Pasta	990	N/A	N/A	N/A	N/A
9.	Red Lobster Chef's Signature Lobster and Shrimp Pasta (full portion)	1,020	50	21	N/A	2,170
10.	Applebee's Three-Cheese Chicken Penne	1,310	61	34	1.5	2,910
11.	California Pizza Kitchen Garlic Cream Fettuccine with Chicken & Shrimp	1,491	N/A	52	N/A	1,918
12.	Ruby Tuesday Chicken & Broccoli Pasta	1,513	95	N/A	N/A	3,177
13.	Cheesecake Factory Bistro Shrimp Pasta	2,819	77	N/A	N/A	1,008

FAST-FOOD BURGERS (MINIMUM ¼-LB PATTY)

		CALORIES	FAT (G)	SATURATED (G)	TRANS (G)	SODIUM (MG)
1.	McDonald's Quarter-Pounder	410	19	8	1	730
2.	Carl's Jr. Big Hamburger	460	17	8	0.5	1,090
3.	McDonald's Big N' Tasty	460	24	8	1.5	720
4.	Wendy's ¼-Pound Single	470	21	8	1	880
5.	McDonald's Big Mac	540	29	10	1.5	1,040
6.	Jack in the Box Jumbo Jack	540	32	11	1	850
7.	Dairy Queen ¼-lb Classic GrillBurger with Cheese	560	28	12	0.5	1,090
8.	Sonic Sonic Burger with ketchup	560	26	9	1	820
9.	Burger King Whopper	670	40	11	1.5	1,020
10.	A&W Papa Burger	690	39	14	1	1,350
11.	Five Guys Hamburger	700	43	19.5	0	430
12.	Hardee's Six Dollar ThickBurger	930	59	21	N/A	1,960

RESTAURANT BURGERS

	CALORIES	FAT (G)	SATURATED (G)	TRANS (G)	SODIUM (MG)
1. Red Robin Natural Burger	569	24	N/A	N/A	989
2. Cheesecake Factory The Factory Burger	737	N/A	15	N/A	1,018
3. Applebee's Hamburger	770	46	15	2	1,170
4. Uno Chicago Grill Uno Burger	1,080	72	28	4	1,620
5. Ruby Tuesday Ruby's Classic Burger	1,122	75	N/A	N/A	1,820
6. Denny's Western Burger	1,160	65	21	3	1,820
7. Chili's Oldtimer	1,260	62	16	N/A	3,140
8. Applebee's Quesadilla Burger	1,420	104	43	3	3,740
9. Cheesecake Factory The Classic Burger	1,450	N/A	28	N/A	1,638
10. Chili's Mushroom-Swiss Burger	1,460	84	24	N/A	3,570
11. Outback Bacon Cheese Burger	1,482	99	40	0	2,205
12. T.G.I. Friday's Jack Daniels Burger	1,560	N/A	N/A	N/A	N/A

FISH

	CALORIES	FAT (G)	SATURATED (G)	TRANS (G)	SODIUM (MG)
1. Red Lobster Broiled Sole	240	4	1	N/A	1,530
2. Applebee's Cajun Lime Tilapia	310	6	1.5	0	2,160
3. Ruby Tuesday Asian Glazed Salmon	370	26	N/A	N/A	971
4. Uno Chicago Grill Lemon Basil Salmon	480	34	5	0	370
5. Outback Fresh Tilapia with Pure Lump Crab Meat	504	28	12	0	702
6. Olive Garden Herb-Grilled Salmon	510	26	6	N/A	760
7. Chili's Guiltless Grill Salmon with Garlic and Herbs	530	19	6	N/A	1,640
8. Applebee's Garlic Herb Salmon	750	37	11	0.5	2,640
9. Romano's Macaroni Grill Grilled Halibut	770	34	11	N/A	1,100
10. T.G.I. Friday's Honey Pecan Salmon	810	N/A	N/A	N/A	N/A
11. P.F. Chang's Mahi Mahi	840	34	16	N/A	1,210
12. Cheesecake Factory Wasabi Crusted Ahi Tuna	1,610	N/A	49	N/A	1,075

CHICKEN SANDWICHES

		CALORIES	FAT (G)	SATURATED (G)	TRANS (G)	SODIUM (MG)
1.	Chick-fil-A Chargrilled Chicken Sandwich	300	3.5	1	0	1,120
2.	Wendy's Crispy Chicken Sandwich	350	15	3	0	830
2.	Hardee's BBQ Chicken Sandwich	400	6	1	N/A	1,370
4.	Arby's Roasted Chicken Fillet Sandwich	400	16	2.5	0	950
5.	KFC Tender Roast Sandwich	410	15	3	0	790
6.	McDonald's Premium Grilled Chicken Classic Sandwich	420	10	2	0	1,190
7.	Jack in the Box Chicken Sandwich	440	23	4	0	910
8.	Sonic Crispy Chicken Sandwich	550	32	4.5	0	1,070
9.	Dunkin' Donuts Chicken Bruschetta Sandwich	580	26	7	0	1,200
10.	Dairy Queen Grilled Flame Thrower Chicken Sandwich	590	36	9	0	1,480
11.	Burger King Original Chicken Sandwich	630	39	7	0.5	1,390
12.	Carl's Jr. Bacon Swiss Crispy Chicken	750	40	9	1.5	1,990

STEAKS

		CALORIES	FAT (G)	SATURATED (G)	TRANS (G)	SODIUM (MG)
1.	Chili's Guiltless Grill Classic Sirloin	240	8	4	N/A	1,820
2.	Applebee's 9 oz House Sirloin	310	13	5	0	970
3.	Ruby Tuesday Grilled Top Sirloin	317	16	N/A	N/A	112
4.	T.G.I. Friday's 8 oz Flat Iron Steak	340	N/A	N/A	N/A	N/A
5.	Uno Chicago Grill Brewmaster's Grill NY Sirloin	520	14	5	0	1,580
6.	Red Lobster Wood-Fire Grilled NY Strip Steak	590	33	14	N/A	1,420
7.	Outback New York Strip	713	37	17	N/A	694
8.	Denny's T-Bone Steak	740	56	25	0	740
9.	Olive Garden Steak Toscano	880	43	14	N/A	1,700
10.	IHOP T-Bone Steak	1,100	N/A	N/A	N/A	N/A
11.	P.F. Chang's Asian Marinated New York Strip	1,110	60	27	N/A	2,799
12.	Cheesecake Factory Carne Asada Skirt Steak	1,703	N/A	24	N/A	3,695

ENTRÉE SALADS (WITH DRESSING)

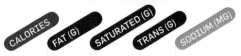

	CALORIES	FAT (G)	SATURATED (G)	TRANS (G)	SODIUM (MG)
1. **Romano's Macaroni Grill Scallops and Spinach Salad**	330	18	4	N/A	1,610
2. **Chili's Guiltless Grill Asian Salad**	360	22	3	0	930
3. **Panera Full Asian Sesame Chicken Salad**	400	20	3.5	0	910
4. **Chili's Guiltless Grill Caribbean Salad**	520	24	4	N/A	630
5. **Uno's Chicken Caesar Salad**	580	40	9	0	720
6. **Quiznos Classic Cobb Regular Chopped Salad**	800	56	17.5	0.5	1,790
7. **Outback Queensland Salad with Thousand Island**	1,075	81	28	0	1,978
8. **California Pizza Kitchen Thai Crunch Salad with Avocado**	1,279	N/A	9	N/A	1,313
9. **Applebee's Oriental Chicken Salad**	1,310	93	15	2.5	1,470
10. **Cheesecake Factory Caesar Salad with Chicken**	1,513	N/A	16	N/A	1,481
11. **T.G.I. Friday's Santa Fe Chicken Salad**	1,800	N/A	N/A	N/A	N/A
12. **IHOP Chicken and Spinach Salad**	1,840	N/A	N/A	N/A	N/A

FRIES

	CALORIES	FAT (G)	SATURATED (G)	TRANS (G)	SODIUM (MG)
1. **KFC Potato Wedges**	260	13	2.5	0	740
2. **Dairy Queen Regular Fries**	310	13	2	0	640
3. **Sonic Medium French Fries**	330	13	2.5	0	440
4. **McDonald's Medium French Fries**	380	19	2.5	0	270
5. **In-N-Out French Fries**	400	18	5	0	245
6. **Wendy's Medium Fries**	410	19	3.5	0	350
7. **Jack in the Box Medium Fries**	410	19	1.5	0	750
8. **Chick-fil-A Waffle Potato Fries**	430	23	4.5	0	210
9. **Burger King Medium Fries**	440	22	4.5	0	670
10. **Carl's Jr. Medium Natural-Cut Fries**	460	22	4.5	0	1,180
11. **Arby's Medium Curly Fries**	540	29	4	0	1,230
12. **Five Guys Regular Fries**	620	30	6	0	90

SUNDAES

		CALORIES	FAT (G)	SATURATED (G)	TRANS (G)	SUGARS (G)
1.	A&W Hot Fudge Sundae	350	11	6	0	15
2.	Uno Chicago Grill Mini Hot Chocolate Brownie Sundae	370	16	8	0	38
3.	McDonald's Hot Fudge Sundae with Peanuts	375	13.5	7.5	0	48
4.	Dairy Queen Medium Chocolate Sundae	400	10	6	0.5	59
5.	Bob Evans Strawberry Sundae	419	20	14	0	44
6.	Sonic Hot Fudge Sundae	520	27	20	0	54
7.	IHOP Hot Fudge Brownie Sundae	550	N/A	N/A	N/A	N/A
8.	Baskin-Robbins Banana Royale Sundae	620	28	19	1	73
9.	Red Robin Hot Fudge Sundae	800	36	N/A	N/A	80
10.	Baskin-Robbins Oreo Outrageous Sundae	1,330	61	31	1	146
11.	Uno Chicago Grill Uno Deep Dish Sundae	1,400	68	36	0	136
12.	Applebee's Chocolate Chip Cookie Sundae	1,660	82	51	0	N/A

KIDS' ENTRÉES

		CALORIES	FAT (G)	SATURATED (G)	TRANS (G)	SODIUM (MG)
1.	Red Lobster Popcorn Shrimp	140	7	0.5	N/A	530
2.	McDonald's 4-piece Chicken McNuggets	190	12	2	0	400
3.	Red Robin Rad Robin Burger	286	12	N/A	N/A	380
4.	Fazoli's Kids' Spaghetti with Meatballs	300	7	2.5	0	570
5.	Chili's Pepper Pals Little Mouth Burger	350	17	6	N/A	660
6.	California Pizza Kitchen Kid's Pepperoni Pizza	478	N/A	10	N/A	1,114
7.	Baja Fresh Kids' Chicken Taquitos	630	33	7	1	990
8.	Outback Kids' Kookaburra Chicken Fingers	676	41	12	0	1,942
9.	Ruby Tuesday Kids' Beef Minis	719	43	N/A	N/A	1,265
10.	Applebee's Kids' Two Mini Cheeseburgers	730	46	15	1.5	1,100
11.	On the Border Kids' Cheese Quesadilla	850	67	27	N/A	1,120
12.	Cheesecake Factory Kids' Pasta with Alfredo Sauce	1,803	N/A	87	N/A	876

Chapter

2

FOODS THAT CURE

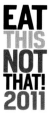

You might think,

after skimming a few chapters in this book, that we'd like nothing more than to have you stop eating food altogether. And you might think, after surveying the American dietary landscape, that that's not such a bad idea.

After all, it's hard to escape the reality of America's obesity crisis—especially after a day at the shore, when you watch a crowd of environmentally conscious children trying to save a beached whale, only to discover it's just a pale, middle-aged guy in a Speedo who's had one too many margaritas. Or after an evening on the couch watching the news, when you listen intently to the debate over national health care and realize that if our food supply weren't so tainted by calorie-laden junk, we wouldn't be spending one in every five health care dollars supporting Americans who suffer from diabetes. You might think the solution is to put the whole country on a diet and make everybody stop eating so many meals and so many snacks.

But eating too much food isn't the problem. The problem is that we're eating too many things that aren't actually food—the additives, the preservatives, the chemically enhanced foodlike substances. And when we do eat real food, those meals and snacks are often served in such calorie-laden portions that even our old-fashioned grandmothers who always told us to "eat, eat" would step back, aghast, and yell, "Take that out of your mouth!"

But in reality, food—real food—is a good thing. Real food—the kind that comes from the earth, not a science lab—is about more than just calories and carbs, salts and sugars. Real food can have nearly magical properties—amazing abilities to prevent or even heal many of our physical and emotional woes.

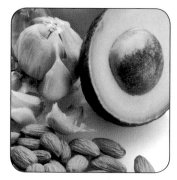 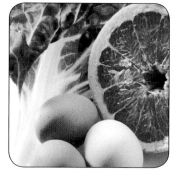 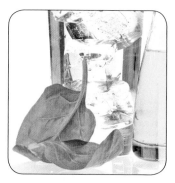

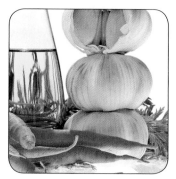 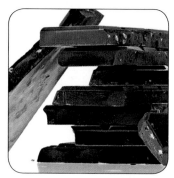 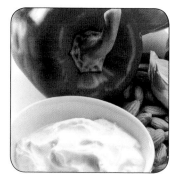

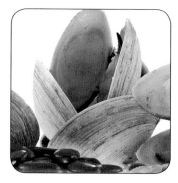 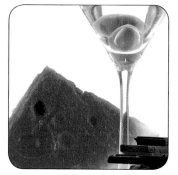 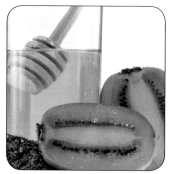

Our bodies are designed to function at their optimum levels and to look and feel lean, strong, and vibrant when they're fed the vitamins, minerals, healthy fats, and micronutrients in real food.

Imagine, if you will, a world with less stress, less insanity, and less self-loathing. It would look a lot like today's world, except for two things: (1) Lewis Black wouldn't have a job, and (2) the rest of us would be dining on salmon, washing it down with a glass of wine, and snacking on dark chocolate for dessert. Those three things have been shown in studies to brighten our moods and beat back the fatigue, depression, and anxiety so many of us labor under.

But chances are the screaming, frothing comedian will still have plenty of angst to get out in coming years, as long as he and the rest of us keep chowing down on foods that are high in carbs, high in fat, and high in preservatives. And we will continue to battle weight issues as well because all of those bad-for-you foodstuffs set us up for even more hunger and even more weight gain.

But eating lots and lots of healthy foods can help you lose weight—in fact, it's a much better way to keep off extra pounds than not eating anything at all.

That's because our bodies are designed not only to enjoy real food and to thrive on the nutrients within, but also to burn off the calories in real food and drink. Indeed, eating smart throughout the day revs up your body's metabolism—the internal fat furnace that turns calories into energy—and gives you all-day get-up-and-go energy. Stop feeding yourself good food and your body goes into starvation mode, saving calories like a Depression-era miser—except instead of saving them under a mattress, you'll be saving them in your belly, your butt, and other unsightly hiding places.

So, we're outlining the best foods for whatever ails you and explaining exactly how these mealtime miracle workers will improve your looks, your life, and even your attitude. Consider this your nutritional prescription program to cure anything—and you don't even need preapproval from your HMO!

When You're Stressed

Eat This
FRIED EGGS

Go ahead, crack under pressure: Eating fried eggs may help reduce high blood pressure. In a test-tube study, scientists in Canada discovered that the breakfast standby produced the highest levels of ACE inhibitory peptides, amino acids that dilate blood vessels and allow blood to flow more easily.

WINE

It's true: A glass of wine really does take the edge off. But you may want to stop there. Researchers from the University of Toronto discovered that one alcoholic drink caused people's blood vessels to relax, but two drinks began to reverse the benefits. That's because when your blood alcohol content reaches a certain level, your central nervous system releases noradrenaline—the same hormone released when you're in high stress.

GUM

When you find yourself feeling overwhelmed at work, reach for the Wrigley's: Chewing gum can help tame your tension, according to Australian researchers. People who chewed gum while taking multitasking tests experienced a 17 percent drop in self-reported stress. This might have to do with the fact that we associate chewing with positive social interactions, like mealtimes.

Not That!
COFFEE

A cup of joe can cut through your morning mental fog, but too much coffee may exacerbate your work anxiety, according to researchers from the University of Oklahoma. The scientists found that when people downed the caffeine equivalent of three cups of java, their symptoms of psychological stress increased. Caffeine triggers a rise in your blood level of cortisol, the hormone released when you feel threatened.

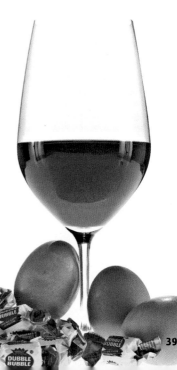

When You're Feeling Down

Eat This

SALMON

Omega-3s may calm your neurotic side, according to a study in the journal *Psychosomatic Medicine*. Researchers found that adults with the lowest blood levels of eicosapentaenoic acid (EPA) and docosahexaenoic acid (DHA) were more likely to have neuroses, which are symptoms for depression. EPA and DHA are key brain components, and higher levels of each can bolster the potent mood enhancers serotonin and dopamine. Salmon is loaded with EPA and DHA, as are walnuts, flaxseeds, and even cauliflower.

GARLIC

Tuck a few extra cloves into your next stir-fry or pasta sauce: Research has found that enzymes in garlic can help increase the release of serotonin, a neurochemical that makes you feel relaxed. Plus, garlic may have the added benefit of improving memory. Pakistani researchers found that rats fed a puree of garlic and water performed better on a memory test than rats that weren't fed the mixture.

DARK CHOCOLATE

Research shows that dark chocolate can improve heart health, lower blood pressure, reduce LDL cholesterol, and increase the flow of blood to the brain. It also boosts serotonin and endorphin levels, which are associated with improved mood and greater concentration. Look for chocolate that is 60 percent cocoa or higher.

Not That!

WHITE CHOCOLATE

White chocolate isn't technically chocolate, since it contains no cocoa solids. Instead, it's made mostly with fats and sugar, lacking any of the nutritional vigor of the real stuff. That means it also lacks the ability to stimulate the euphoria-inducing chemicals that real chocolate does, especially serotonin.

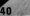

When You Want to Boost Your Metabolism

Eat This

CHILE PEPPERS

It turns out that capsaicin, the compound that gives chile peppers their mouth-searing quality, can also fire up your metabolism. Eating about 1 tablespoon of chopped red or green chiles boosts your body's production of heat and the activity of your sympathetic nervous system (responsible for our fight-or-flight response), according to a study published in the *Journal of Nutritional Science and Vitaminology*. The result is a metabolism spike 23 percent higher than in those who didn't take capsaicin.

CAFFEINATED COFFEE

A study published in the journal *Physiology & Behavior* found that the average metabolic rate of people who drank caffeinated coffee increased 16 percent over those who drank decaf. Caffeine stimulates your central nervous system by increasing your heart rate and breathing.

YOGURT

The probiotics in yogurt may speed weight loss. British scientists found that these active organisms boosted the breakdown of fat molecules in mice, preventing the rodents from gaining weight. Try the Horizon brand of yogurt—it contains the probiotic *L. casei*, the same organism used in the study.

Not That!

NOTHING

That's right: There's no better way to grind your metabolism to a halt than skipping a meal. When your body goes without food, it switches into survival mode, storing calories rather than burning them. Breakfast is most important, because your body is still in shutdown mode and your metabolism needs a strong protein- and fiber-based jump start.

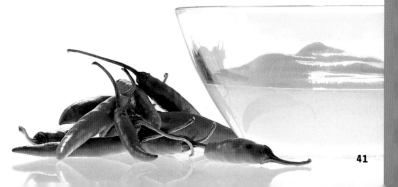

When You Need More Energy

Eat This
CLAMS

Clams stock your body with magnesium, which is important in metabolism, nerve function, and muscle function. When magnesium levels are low, your body produces more lactic acid— the same fatigue-inducing substance that you feel at the end of a long workout.

GRILLED CHICKEN BREAST

The protein in lean meat like chicken, fish, or pork loin isn't just vital in squashing hunger and boosting metabolism, it's also a top source of energy. University of Illinois researchers found that people who ate higher amounts of protein had higher energy and didn't feel as tired as people with proportionally higher amounts of carbs in their diet.

KIDNEY BEANS

These legumes are an excellent source of thiamin and riboflavin. Both vitamins help your body use energy efficiently, so you won't be nodding off mid PowerPoint.

BARLEY

Swedish researchers found that if you eat barley for breakfast, the fibrous grain cuts blood sugar response by 44 percent at lunch and 14 percent at dinner. And the less your sugar spikes, the more stable your energy levels will be.

Not That!
BAGELS

MIT researchers analyzed blood samples from people who had eaten either a high-protein or a high-carbohydrate breakfast. Two hours after eating, the carb eaters had tryptophan levels 14 percent higher than before, and the people who had eaten protein decreased their tryptophan levels by 28 percent. The higher your tryptophan level, the more likely you are to feel tired and sluggish. That means fewer waffles, pancakes, and muffins and more eggs and oatmeal.

When You're Sick

Eat This

KIWI

The vitamin C in kiwi won't prevent the onslaught of a cold, but it might decrease the duration of your symptoms. One kiwifruit provides 117 percent of your daily recommended intake of vitamin C.

HONEY

Penn State scientists have discovered that honey is a powerful cough suppressant—so next time you're hacking up a lung, head for the kitchen. When parents of 105 sick children doled out honey or dextromethorphan (the active ingredient in over-the-counter cough medicines like Robitussin), the honey was better at lessening cough frequency and severity. Try a drizzle in a cup of tea.

ROOIBOS TEA

Animal research suggests that this South African tea may provide potent immunity-boosting benefits. Large human studies have yet to be conducted, though.

OLIVES

Foods rich in healthy fats help reduce inflammation, a catalyst for migraines. One study found that the anti-inflammatory compounds in olive oil suppress the enzymes involved in inflammationin the same manner as ibuprofen. Avocados and almonds are also high in monounsaturated fats.

Not That!

CAFFEINATED BEVERAGES AND ENERGY DRINKS

Excessive caffeine screws with your sleep schedule and suppresses functions of key immunity agents. And insufficient sleep opens the door to colds, upper respiratory infections, and other ills. What's more, caffeine can dehydrate you, and hydration is vital during illness: Fluids not only transport nutrients to the illness site but also dispose of toxins.

When You Want to Get in the Mood

Eat This
DARK CHOCOLATE

Chocolate is full of anandamide and phenylethylamine, two compounds that cause the body to release the same feel-good endorphins triggered by sex and physical exertion. Cocoa also contains methylxanthines, which make skin more sensitive to touch.

WATERMELON

The summer staple contains citrulline, a nutrient that relaxes blood vessels throughout the body in the same way Viagra works below the belt, according to Texas A&M researchers.

ALCOHOL

Booze acts as a depressant in the brain's cerebral cortex, lowering inhibitions that could otherwise restrain arousal. When men consumed too much, though, their erections weren't as strong as if they'd limited themselves to one or two drinks.

Not That!
OYSTERS

Okay, they won't exactly inhibit your bedroom behavior, but these legendary "aphrodisiacs" have never been proven to actually boost libido. While zinc, abundant in oysters of all shapes and sizes, is linked to male fertility, the connections to actual arousal have never been borne out in clinical research.

44

When You Work Out

▲ *Eat This*
SPINACH

In a test-tube study, Rutgers researchers discovered that treating human muscle cells with a compound found in spinach increased protein synthesis by 20 percent. The compound allows muscle tissue to repair itself faster, the researchers say.

▲ GREEN TEA

Brazilian scientists found that participants who consumed three cups of the beverage every day for a week had fewer markers of the cell damage caused by resistance to exercise. That means that green tea can help you recover faster after an intense workout.

▲ CHOCOLATE MILK

Nothing like a little dessert after a long workout. British researchers found that chocolate milk does a better job than sports drinks at replenishing the body after a workout. Why? Because it has more electrolytes and higher fat content. And scientists at James Madison University found that the balance of fat, protein, and carbs in chocolate milk makes it nearly one-third more effective at replenishing muscles than other recovery beverages. And, of course, don't forget H_2O: Even as little as a 1 percent decrease in your body water can impair exercise performance.

▲ FISH OIL

Australian researchers found that cyclists who took fish oil for 8 weeks had lower heart rates and consumed less oxygen during intense bicycling than a control group did.

▲ *Not That!*
RED BULL

Caffeine is a proven training aid, but drinking a Red Bull won't provide enough stimulation to affect your workouts, according to Canadian studies. Seventeen fit adults who drank up to two cans of the drink an hour before a sprint workout didn't experience a performance boost. The beverage just doesn't provide enough of a jolt.

When You Need a Brain Boost

For Focus

🔖 Eat This
SARDINES

According to research published in *Nutrition Journal,* fish oil can help increase your ability to concentrate. Credit EPA and DHA, fatty acids that bolster communication among brain cells and help regulate neurotransmitters responsible for mental focus. Can't stomach sardines at your desk? Try a handful of omega-3 rich walnuts instead.

🔖 Not That!
CANDY

Sugary foods provoke sudden surges of glucose that result in energetic highs and lows. Unfortunately, the lows outlast the highs, as do the possible headaches and lack of concentration.

For Memory

🔖 Eat This
GARLIC

Researchers in Pakistan found that rats fed a puree of garlic and water performed better on a memory test than rats that weren't fed the mixture. That's because garlic increases the brain's levels of serotonin, which has been shown to enhance memory function.

🔖 BANANAS

The antioxidants in bananas, apples, and oranges may help protect you from Alzheimer's, report Korean scientists. In a test-tube study, the researchers discovered that plant chemicals known as polyphenols helped shield brain cells from oxidative stress, a key cause of the disease.

Not That!
SODA AND JUICE

Spikes in blood sugar can wreck your short-term memory, states a study in the *European Journal of Clinical Nutrition*. When scientists conducted memory tests on adults who had just downed a sugary drink, those with the highest blood glucose levels had the worst recall. Soda's an obvious offender, but even many "juice" drinks are loaded down with a rush of added sugars and high-fructose corn syrup.

ENERGY DRINKS AND VENTI LATTES

Like a politician whose smile is just a little too eager, caffeine has a dark side, too. Too much of it can make you jittery, anxious, and unsure of yourself. It can also derail your sleep schedule, meaning that extra cup of coffee today can blunt your cognitive powers tomorrow.

For Long-Lasting Brainpower

Eat This
STEAK

Vitamin B_{12}, an essential nutrient found in meat, milk, and fish, may help protect you against brain loss, say British scientists. The researchers found that older people with the highest blood levels of the vitamin were six times less likely to have brain shrinkage than those with the lowest levels.

CARROTS

Researchers from Harvard found that men who consumed more beta-carotene over 18 years had significantly delayed cognitive aging. Carrots are a tremendous source of the antioxidant, as are other orange foods like butternut squash, pumpkin, and bell peppers.

For Sharper Senses

Eat This
GROUND FLAXSEED

Flax is the best source of alpha-linolenic acid (ALA)—a healthy fat that improves the workings of the cerebral cortex, the area of the brain that processes sensory information, including that of pleasure. To meet your quota, sprinkle 1 tablespoon flaxseed on salads or oatmeal once a day, or mix it into a smoothie or shake.

Not That!
ALCOHOL

This one's obvious, but worth stressing anyway. While a drink or two can increase arousal signals, more than a few drinks will actually depress your nervous system. This will dull sensations and make you tired, not sharp—in your brain and throughout the rest of your body.

10 Foods You Should Eat Every Day

We talk a lot about the foods you can't eat in these books, foods so infused with calories, fat, and sodium they should come with Surgeon General warnings like cigarette packs. And often times the better choice for you when eating on the run still isn't textbook nutritious stuff—it's the lesser of two formimidable fast-food or sit-down evils. But these 10 foods highlighted below are as perfect as food on this planet gets, capable not just of helping you boost metabolism and melt fat, but also fight disease, lower cholesterol, stabilize blood sugar, and live a longer, better life. And did we mention that they're delicious? Make it your goal to work these edible all-stars into your diet every day.

EGGS

When it comes to breakfast, you can't beat eggs. (That was too easy, wasn't it?) Seriously though, at a cost of only 72 calories, each large egg holds 6.3 grams of high-quality protein and a powerhouse punch of vital nutrients. A study published in the *International Journal of Obesity* found that people who replace carbs with eggs for breakfast lost 65 percent more weight. Researchers in Michigan were able to determine that regular egg eaters enjoyed more vitamins and minerals in their diets than those who ate few or no eggs. By examining surveys from more than 27,000 people, the researchers found that egg eaters were about half as likely to be deficient in vitamin B_{12}, 24 percent less likely to be deficient in vitamin A, and 36 percent less likely to be deficient in vitamin E. And here's something more shocking: Those who ate at least four eggs a week had significantly lower cholesterol levels than those who ate fewer than one. Turns out the dietary cholesterol in the yolk has little impact on your serum cholesterol. **Substitutes:** Egg Beaters

SWISS CHARD
Chop the leaves and ribs into rough pieces and sauté in olive oil, garlic, and chili flakes; mix sautéed or steamed chard with golden raisins and toasted pinenuts and serve with meat or fish; or stir the green tops into minestrone or add to a pot of boiling white rice.

GRAPEFRUIT
Skip the morning OJ and have a GJ instead; chop the fruit over a leafy salad; or pop half a grapefruit underneath the broiler for 5 minutes until caramelized and juicy.

EGGS
Serve a fried egg over a whole-wheat English muffin with salsa; hard-boil a dozen eggs and keep them in the fridge to eat on their own or chopped over salads; or sauté diced vegetables and scramble them into a panful of eggs.

GREEN TEA
Start your day by making a smoothie with chilled green tea instead of juice. Then sip a cup after lunch when your eyelids start feeling like lead drapes.

QUINOA
Forget rice; make quinoa your go-to starchy staple: Toss boiled grains with wilted spinach leaves, dried cranberries, goat cheese, lemon juice, and olive oil; sub in quinoa for risottos and pilafs; or mix hot quinoa with a bit of milk, brown sugar, and sliced banana for a great oatmeal alternative.

49

BELL PEPPERS
Use sliced bell peppers in place of tortilla chips to scoop bean dip; paint with olive oil and grill them alongside your favorite meat; or sauté a mix of diced peppers with garlic and chili flakes for a side to any entrée.

AVOCADO
Stuff slices into omelets; remove the pit and fill an avocado half with tuna salad; spread some onto a sandwich in place of mayonnaise; or mash one with a few tablespoons of salsa for a quick, guacamole-like dip to use with tortilla chips.

GARLIC
Mix minced garlic with chopped parsley and fresh lemon zest for a bright topping for pasta and grilled meat; or roast an entire head in a foil packet at 350˚F and fold the sweet, soft cloves into mashed potatoes or spread on crusty bread.

GREEK YOGURT
Don't restrict your enjoyment to the morning hours. Use Greek yogurt in place of mayonnaise in your next potato salad, or combine with minced garlic, chopped parsley, olive oil, and fresh lemon juice for a versatile sauce with fish and meat.

ALMONDS
Sprinkle crushed almonds over yogurt, cereal, or salad; toss sliced almonds into your next stir-fry; or smear a spoonful of almond butter over whole-wheat toast the next time you need an out-the-door breakfast.

GREEN TEA

Literally thousands of studies have been carried out to document the health benefits of catechins, the group of antioxidants concentrated in the leaves of tea plants. Among the most startling studies was one published by the American Medical Association in 2006. The study followed more than 40,000 Japanese adults for a decade, and at the 7-year follow-up, those who had been drinking five or more cups of tea per day were 26 percent less likely to die of any cause compared with those who averaged less than a cup. Looking for more immediate results? Another Japanese study broke participants into two groups, only one of which was put on a catechin-rich green-tea diet. At the end of 12 weeks, the green-tea group had achieved significantly smaller body weights and waistlines than those in the control group. Why? Because researchers believe that catechins are effective at boosting metabolism.

Substitutes: Yerba mate, white tea, oolong tea, rooibos (red) tea

GARLIC

Allicin, an antibacterial and antifungal compound, is the steam engine pushing forward garlic's myriad health benefits. The chemical is produced by the garlic plant as a defense against pests, but inside your body it fights cancer, strengthens your cardiovascular system, decreases fat storage, and fights acne inflammation. To activate the most possible allicin, you first must crush the garlic as finely as possible. Peel the cloves, then use the side of a heavy chef's knife to crush the garlic before carefully mincing. Then be sure not to overcook it, as too much heat will render the compound completely useless (and your food totally bitter).

Substitutes: Onions, chives, leeks

GRAPEFRUIT

Just call it the better-body fruit. In a study of 100 obese people at the Scripps Clinic in California, those who ate half a grapefruit with each meal lost an average of 3.6 pounds over the course of 12 weeks. Many lost more than 10 pounds. The study's control group, in contrast, lost a paltry ½ pound. But here's something even better: Those who ate the grapefruit also exhibited a decrease in insulin levels, indicating that their bodies had improved upon the ability to metabolize sugar. If you can't stomach a grapefruit-a-day regime, try to find as many ways possible to sneak grapefruit into your diet. Even a moderate increase in grapefruit intake should yield results, not to mention earning you a massive dose of lycopene— the cancer-preventing antioxidant found most commonly in tomatoes.

Substitutes: Oranges, watermelon, tomatoes

GREEK YOGURT

Regular yogurt is more of a dessert than a meal. If you want substance, go Greek. What sets the two apart? Greek yogurt is separated from the watery whey that sits on top of regular yogurt, and the process removes excessive sugars such as lactose and increases the concentration of protein by as much as three times. That means it fills your belly more like a meal than a snack. Plus a single cup has almost a quarter of your day's calcium, and studies show that dieters on calcium-rich diets have an easier time losing body fat. In one of these studies, participants on a high-calcium dairy diet were able to lose 70 percent more body weight than those on a calorie-restricted diet alone. If only everything you ate could make a similar claim.

Substitutes: Kefir and yogurt with "live and active cultures" printed on the product label

AVOCADO

Here's what often gets lost in America's fat phobia: Some of those fats are actually good for you. More than half the calories in each creamy green fruit comes from one of the world's healthiest fats, a kind called monounsaturates. These fats differ from saturated fats in that they have one double-bonded carbon atom, but that small difference at the molecular level amounts to a dramatic improvement to your health. Numerous studies have shown that monounsaturated fats both improve your cholesterol profile and decrease the amount of triglycerides (more fats) floating around in your blood. That can lower your risk of stroke and heart disease. Worried about weight gain? Don't be. There's no causal link between monounsaturated fats and body fat.

Substitutes: Olive, canola and peanut oils, peanut butter, tahini

QUINOA

Although not yet common in American kitchens, quinoa boasts a stronger distribution of nutrients than any grain you'll ever get a fork into. It has more fiber and nearly twice as much protein as brown rice, and the proteins it has consist of a near-perfect blend of amino acids, the building blocks that your body pulls apart to reassemble into new proteins. And get this: All that protein and fiber—in conjunction with a handful of healthy fats and a comparatively small dose of carbohydrates—help ensure a low impact on your blood sugar. That's great news for pre-diabetics and anyone watching their weight. So what's the trade-off? There is none. Quinoa's soft and nutty taste is easy to handle even for picky eaters, and it cooks just like rice, ready in about 15 minutes.

Substitutes: Oats, amaranth, millet, pearl barley, bulgur wheat

BELL PEPPERS

All peppers are loaded with antioxidants, but none so much as the brightly colored reds, yellows, and oranges. These colors result from carotenoids concentrated in the flesh of the pepper, the same carotenoids that give tomatoes, carrots, and grapefruits their healthy hues. The range of benefits provided by these colorful pigments include improved immune function, better communication between cells, protection against sun damage, and a diminished risk for several types of cancer. And if you can take the heat, try cooking with chile peppers. The bell pepper cousins are still loaded with carotenoids and vitamin C but have the added benefit of capsaicins, temperature-raising phyto-chemicals that have been shown to fight headache and arthritis pain as well as boost metabolism.

Substitutes: Carrots, sweet potatoes, watermelon

ALMONDS

An ounce of almonds a day, about 23 nuts, provides nearly 9 grams of heart-healthy oleic acid, which is more than pea-nuts, walnuts, or cashews. This monounsaturated fat is known to be responsible for a flurry of health benefits, the most recent of which is improved memory. Rats in California were better able to navigate a maze the second time around if they'd been fed oleic acid, and there's no reason to assume that the same treatment won't help you navigate your day-to-day life. If nothing else, snacking on the brittle nuts will take your mind of your hunger. Nearly a quarter of an almond's calories come from belly-filling fiber and protein. That's why when researchers at Purdue fed subjects nuts or rice cakes, those who ate the nuts felt full for a full hour and a half longer than the rice cake group.

Substitutes: Walnuts, pecans, peanuts, sesame seeds, flaxseeds

SWISS CHARD

Most fruits and vegetables are role players, supplying us with a monster dose of a single nutrient. But Swiss chard is nature's multivita-min, delivering substantial amounts of 16 vitamins and vital nutrients, and it does so at a rock-bottom caloric cost. For a mere 35 calories' worth of cooked chard, you get more than 716 percent of your recommended daily intake of bone-strengthening vitamin K, 214 percent of your day's vitamin A (shown to help defend against cancer and bolster vision), and 17 percent of hard-to-get vitamin E (which studies have shown may help sharpen mental acuity). Plus, emerging research suggests that its combination of phytonutri-ents and fiber may provide an effective defense against colon cancer.

Substitutes: Spinach, mustard greens, collard greens, watercress, arugula, romaine lettuce

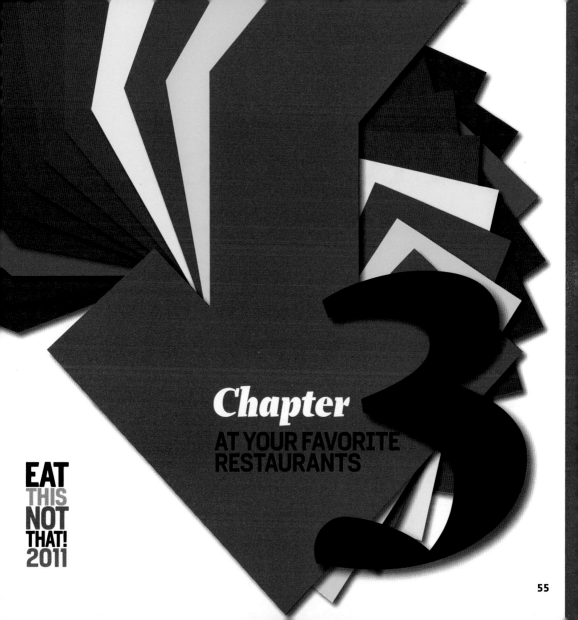

Chapter

AT YOUR FAVORITE RESTAURANTS

On television,

being a restaurant chef looks so romantic. You could go one-on-one with Gordon Ramsay on *Hell's Kitchen,* cook yourself to victory over Bobby Flay on *Iron Chef America,* find a recipe to melt Padma Lakshmi's heart on *Top Chef,* or travel the world feasting on critters like Anthony Bourdain does on *No Reservations.* Foodie television makes it seem as though anyone with a ladle and a spatula is a swashbuckling pirate prince.

The reality is very, very different. The vast majority of professional cooks in the United States don't work under wild-eyed slave drivers, whipping up ingenious new recipes out of scrod liver, bull testicles, and bok choy and wowing their customers with stunning new taste sensations. The average cook works in your local Olive Garden, or TGI Friday's, or Applebee's, and the *last* thing his boss or his customers want is for him to get *creative.* Indeed, the line cooks at the IHOP in Tucson are cooking the exact same ingredients in the exact same way as their compatriots in Tuscaloosa. Uniformity, not creativity, is the key to modern restaurant success.

So when it comes to knowing exactly what's in your restaurant meal—and how many calories you're consuming when you eat it—you'd think getting the facts would be pretty easy. After all, it's not like the Tucson chefs are hunting the desert for cactus leaves and the Tuscaloosa cooks are picking berries on the banks of the Black Warrior River. They're using the same stuff in every Bacon Temptation Omelette from Arizona to Alabama, from Connecticut to California.

Yet many restaurant chains—IHOP included—refuse to tell their customers what it is, exactly, that they're putting into their bodies, claiming that it's just too hard to figure out. And one thing we've learned is this: Nobody hesitates to tell you *good* news. As we began researching our first edition of **EAT THIS, NOT THAT!**, we asked IHOP repeatedly for nutritional information—and we were turned down time and again. It was only after New York City imposed a law forcing chain restaurants operating within the city to reveal their calorie counts that we learned the terrible truth about that Bacon Temptation Omelette: That little breakfast treat packs more than 1,400 calories, or about two-thirds of what the average adult should eat in an entire day. Indeed, IHOP is the land of 1,000-calorie crepes, 1,200-calorie breakfast combos, and 1,800-calorie chicken dishes. Put an *e* on the end of that restaurant's name and *hope* it's located close to a 24-hour fitness center.

On the other hand, many restaurants have heeded our call to action and started taking their customers' right to know seriously. A great example: Red Lobster. While the seafood purveyor at first withheld its nutritional information, they recently relented and gave **EAT THIS, NOT THAT!** an inside look at their menu. The result: We give Red Lobster an A for its array of healthy menu options.

Still, trusting a multinational corporation to put things into your body—and not let you know what exactly those things contain—sounds like a foolhardy enterprise (and maybe the plot to a Philip K. Dick novel). So for this chapter, we have dug deep and revealed the secrets that many top restaurants don't want you to know. Whether you're Outback, On the Border, or in the Subway, everything you need to know is in these pages.

The
20
Worst Foods
in America

Many of the worst offenders have vanished
since last year, but new enemies are
on the march. Protect yourself from these,
the most destructive dishes in the
restaurant galaxy.

No. 20

WORST KIDS' MEAL

Pasta robed in melted cheese will never pass muster with the nutritionist set; nevertheless, there are some versions out there you can feel good about feeding your kid. Bob Evans, TGI Friday's, and even Burger King all serve reasonable versions of the kiddie staple. CPK decidedly does not. This bowl represents about 70 percent of the calories the average 6-year-old should consume in a day. What's worse, it delivers as much saturated fat as an adult should consume over the course of 48 hours. Good news is you can dissuade them from ordering the mac by suggesting the pizza instead. We doubt they'll object.

California Pizza Kitchen Kids Curly Mac 'n' Cheese
1,038 calories
38 g saturated fat
1,651 mg sodium

SATURATED FAT EQUIVALENT:
8½ large orders of Burger King onion rings

Eat This Instead! > Kids Hawaiian Pizza
463 calories, 8 g saturated fat, 1,165 mg sodium

WORST SUPERMARKET MEAL

Of all the frozen options that fill out the supermarket aisles, none is more dubious than the pot pie. It sits in the freezer like a leaden bomb, ready to explode waistlines with a troubling mix of oil, cream, butter, and refined carbohydrates. (The package claims it serves two, but really, when have you ever split a pot pie?) The good news is that there are more than a few safe options for those looking for the rich, comforting flavors of a pot pie without the caloric consequences. This version of chicken à la king from Stouffer's is our favorite of the bunch.

Stouffer's White Meat Chicken Pot Pie (large)

1,160 calories
66 g fat
(26 g saturated)
1,780 mg sodium

FAT EQUIVALENT:
10 Reese's Peanut Butter Cups

Eat This Instead! > Stouffer's Chicken à la King

360 calories, 12 g fat (4 g saturated), 800 mg sodium

WORST "HEALTHY" SANDWICH

Goes to show the risk in trusting buzz-terms. A "vegetarian" sandwich might sound like a guaranteed lean lunch, but after Blimpie tops it with multiple layers of cheese, an onslaught of sauces, and crushed Doritos (no joke), you're left with a hunkin' hoagie that gnaws through nearly your entire day's fat allotment and more than 1½ days of sodium. You'd be better off with a towering bacon Dagwood (but really, you'd be best to opt for the vegetarian-friendly Mediterranean Ciabatta).

Blimpie Special Vegetarian
(12-inch)

1,180 calories
59 g fat
(18 g saturated)
3,540 mg sodium

SODIUM EQUIVALENT:
2½ large bags of Fritos Corn Chips

Eat This Instead! > Mediterranean Ciabatta

450 calories, 8 g fat (3 g saturated), 1,720 mg sodium

America has caught bacon fever, making way for a market flooded with bacon-infused chocolates, bacon salts, and yes, even bacon sprays (spritz yourself with the essence of pig!). This profusion of porcine is a trend Wendy's is taking full advantage of with its line of bacon-buoyed burgers. Consider the recipe here: three quarter-pound beef patties interspersed with nine strips of bacon, three slices of cheese, and a big smear of mayonnaise. It's fat on top of fat on top of fat, 10 layers in all—a tower of nutritional terror.

Wendy's Triple Baconator
1,350 calories
90 g fat
(40 g saturated,
3.5 g trans)
2,780 mg sodium

SATURATED FAT EQUIVALENT:
1 full Pizza Hut medium Supreme Pan Pizza

Americans consume more French fries than any other single vegetable. Scary stuff, especially when you see just how punishing a side of deep-fried potatoes can really be. The worst part is Five Guys offers no sensible solutions. There are no other sides on the menu, and even if you downgrade to a "regular" order, you still wind up with more calories than if you ordered one of Five Guys' little bacon burgers. You're better off ordering two "little" sandwiches and skipping the fries.

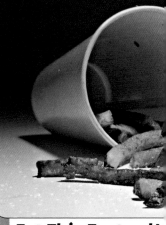

Eat This Instead!
Double Stack with Bacon
400 calories, 21 g fat (9 g saturated), 990 mg sodium

Eat This Instead!
Grilled Cheese Sandwich

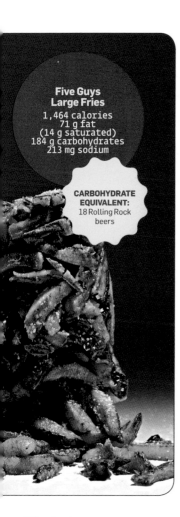

**Five Guys
Large Fries**

1,464 calories
71 g fat
(14 g saturated)
184 g carbohydrates
213 mg sodium

**CARBOHYDRATE
EQUIVALENT:**
18 Rolling Rock
beers

No. 15
WORST FOOD HYBRID

Edible bowls just might be the pinnacle of American gluttony. Next thing you know, restaurants will be serving Pepsi from cups made of chocolate. It sounds ridiculous, but the concept is exactly the same: refined carbs (pasta) served inside of refined carbs (white bread). It's kryptonite for diabetics (and anyone who values self-preservation). The result isn't just a stratospheric escalation of your blood sugar levels, but also the consumption of more than a day's worth of saturated fat, 92 percent of your sodium allotment, and a punishing glut of calories. Skip the terrifying Frankenfood and stick to what Domino's is known for: pizza.

**CALORIE
EQUIVALENT:**
9 bowls of Cocoa
Puffs cereal

**Domino's
Chicken Carbonara
Breadbowl Pasta**

1,480 calories
56 g fat
(24 g saturated)
2,220 mg sodium

470 calories
26 g fat (9 g saturated)
715 mg sodium

Eat This Instead!

Hand Tossed Pizza with grilled chicken, green peppers, and shredded parmesan cheese (2 slices, medium pie)
430 calories, 16 g fat (7 g saturated), 1,030 mg sodium

WORST FAST-FOOD BREAKFAST

Biscuits and gravy fall pretty low in the hierarchy of healthy breakfast options, and the two hockey pucks of sausage that Hardee's throws on top don't help matters (especially when you consider that the gravy is already studded with sausage). What that amounts to is a full day's worth of saturated fat before you tack on the side of spuds. If breakfast is the most important meal of the day, then this is one of the most important meals in America to avoid.

FAT EQUIVALENT:
48 Oreo Cookies

Hardee's Loaded Biscuit 'N' Gravy with Large Hash Rounds
1,530 calories
110 g fat
(26 g saturated)
3,020 mg sodium

Eat This Instead! > Frisco Breakfast Sandwich
400 calories, 18 g fat (7 g saturated), 1,350 mg sodium

No. 13 WORST SANDWICH

It's hard to imagine how a grilled-shrimp sandwich, even a triple decker with a hefty load of bacon on top, could possibly pack more calories than three Big Macs, but if the Cheesecake Factory has taught us anything, it's that its cooks are capable of defying the laws of nutritional science with the dishes they create. Your safest bet is to skip the place entirely. Failing that, pass on the sandwiches and pastas ; instead, look to split a pizza with a friend or take half home in a box.

Cheesecake Factory Grilled Shrimp & Bacon Club
1,746 calories
28 g saturated fat
2,306 mg sodium

CALORIE EQUIVALENT:
6½ Wendy's
Jr. Cheeseburgers

Eat This Instead! > Tomato, Basil, and Cheese Pizza (½ pizza)
663 calories, 12 g saturated fat, 1,210 mg sodium

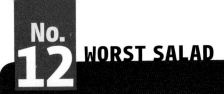

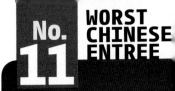

Rumor has it that Hollywood elite turn to the Friday's salad section when it comes time to gain weight for onscreen roles. Okay, that might be an exaggeration, but get too cozy with these leaves and you can expect some dire repercussions. The average entrée-size salad packs a walloping 1,216 calories, making it one of the most dangerous sections of an already-disastrous menu. It comes as no surprise that the Santa Fe emerges as the worst of this sad heap; Mexican- or Southwestern-themed salads—with their abundance of shredded cheese, greasy proteins, and tortilla chips—are the worst species of salad. If those are the flavors you're after, why not a crunchy taco from Taco Bell? You could have a dozen for the same caloric cost.

The human body needs about 1,500 milligrams of sodium each day to function properly. Anything beyond that is unnecessary, and possibly dangerous. And sure, Chinese food is notorious for its higher-than-usual salt factor, but few dishes we've seen come anywhere close to this number. It packs enough of the white stuff to meet your body's needs for more than 5 days. And the rest of Chang's menu isn't much better. Stick with the Hong Kong Beef and plan to avoid the saltshaker for the next couple meals.

TGI Friday's Santa Fe Chopped Salad
1,800 calories

CALORIE EQUIVALENT:
12 Taco Bell Fresco Crunchy Tacos

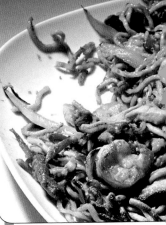

Eat This Instead!
Cobb Salad
361 calories

Eat This Instead!
Hong Kong Beef with Snow Peas

No. 10 WORST RIBS

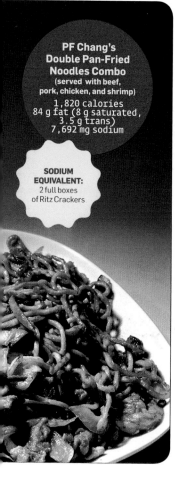

PF Chang's Double Pan-Fried Noodles Combo
(served with beef, pork, chicken, and shrimp)

1,820 calories
84 g fat (8 g saturated, 3.5 g trans)
7,692 mg sodium

SODIUM EQUIVALENT:
2 full boxes of Ritz Crackers

620 calories
28 g fat (6 g saturated)
1,852 mg sodium

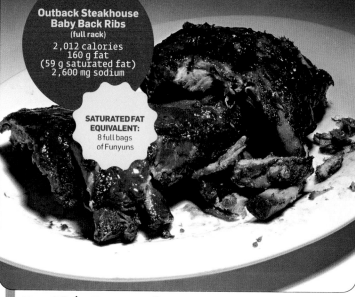

Keep in mind that this caloric heft comes without the addition of Aussie Fries, which will invariably adorn most of the plates at Outback. Nor does it take into account the free brown bread and salad that comes with every entrée order. For all that you can factor in an extra 800 calories or so, bringing the total damage dangerously close to the 3,000-calorie threshold. That much energy will add nearly a pound of fat to your body, which means if you start eating this meal once a week, one year from today you'll have 41 extra pounds of baby-back body fat hanging from your midsection.

Outback Steakhouse Baby Back Ribs
(full rack)

2,012 calories
160 g fat
(59 g saturated fat)
2,600 mg sodium

SATURATED FAT EQUIVALENT:
8 full bags of Funyuns

Eat This Instead!

Outback Special (9oz)

445 calories, 23 g fat (11.5 g saturated), 610 mg sodium

WORST BURGER

Okay, technically this is three burgers, but the idea behind the mini-burger is that the restrained vessels will help you knock off some calories from the hulking mothership burger that inspired them. Rarely, though, does it actually work out that way. In fact, after searching high and low, we still haven't found a single slider or mini-burger safe enough to order. Skip them all, but these especially, which up the caloric ante by crowning the not-so-mini patties with both bacon and onion crispers. They may look harmless, but this trio will knock out your entire day's caloric allotment.

**Denny's
Smokin' Q Three Pack**
2,020 calories
110 g fat
(22 g saturated,
3 g trans)
3,570 mg sodium

**CALORIE
EQUIVALENT:**
11 Jack in the Box
beef tacos

Eat This Instead! > Bacon, Lettuce, and Tomato Sandwich
520 calories, 35 g fat (8 g saturated, 0.5 g trans), 620 mg sodium

No. 8

WORST DRINK

A couple years ago, Baskin-Robbins' milk shake line could have easily claimed the top five worst drinks in America, but when it decided to reel in some of the caloric excesses, Cold Stone's PB&C was left exposed as the biggest bully on the block. And the damage is severe: This blended peanut-butter-cup concoction makes it possible to slurp down a day's worth of energy with a mere 10-minute straw session. We hope Cold Stone decides to follow Baskins' lead and downsize this atrocity, but if not, we're happy to keep doling out the negative publicity.

Cold Stone Creamery PB&C Shake
(Gotta Have It size, 24 fl oz)

2,030 calories
131 g fat (68 g saturated, 2.5 g trans)
153 g sugars

SUGAR EQUIVALENT:
12 Twix Bars

COLD STONE CREAMERY

MADE FRESH DAILY • ULTIMATE INDULGENCE

MADE FRESH DAILY • ULTIMATE IND

Eat This Instead! > Sinless Oh Fudge! Shake (Like It size, 16 fl oz)
490 calories, 2 g fat (2 g saturated), 44 g sugars

WORST BREAKFAST

Here's the anatomy of a breakfast disaster: Take a 12-ounce steak, bread it, fry it, and then cover it with gravy. Then, on the side, drop three eggs and three buttermilk pancakes. Does it not occur to IHOP that this is actually three full meals? And that two of those meals—all but the eggs—are the sort of indulgences that should be eaten only in extreme moderation? If this is the first thing you eat in the morning, don't even bother getting out of bed.

SODIUM EQUIVALENT:
1,076 Original Goldfish pieces

IHOP "Big" Country Breakfast

2,040 calories
55 g saturated fat
159 g carbohydrates
4,500 mg sodium

Eat This Instead! > Turkey Bacon Omelette for Me

470 calories, 25 g fat (11 g saturated), 890 mg sodium

No. 6
WORST MEXICAN ENTRÉE

If the full day of calories doesn't get you, then the 2 days of saturated fat will. If that saturated fat doesn't bring you to your knees, then the 2 days of trans fat surely will. If the trans fat doesn't wreak total havoc on your system . . . we could go on like this for days. Is it just us, or is it slightly disturbing that you could eat eight full steak tacos and still take in fewer calories than what's found in this plate of cheesy chips? Stick to two tacos and save nearly a half pound of body fat in one sitting.

Baja Fresh Charbroiled Steak Nachos
2,120 calories
118 g fat (44 g saturated, 4.5 g trans)
2,990 mg sodium

CALORIE EQUIVALENT:
An entire tray of lasagna

Eat This Instead! > 2 Original Baja Steak Tacos
460 calories, 16 g fat (4 g saturated), 520 mg sodium

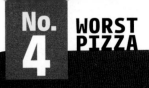

No. 5 WORST APPETIZER

Outback Steakhouse Kookaburra Wings

2,145 calories
185 g fat
(75 g saturated)
3,711 mg sodium

SATURATED FAT EQUIVALENT:
15 Applebee's
9-oz sirloin steaks

Outside of Outback, a kookaburra is an Australian bird that makes a noise like a chuckling human. Inside Outback, "kookaburra" denotes a piece of fried chicken that's been lacquered with egregious amounts of fat and sodium. Even if you have two other victims to help defray the damage, you'll still wind up with 715 calories and well over a day's worth of saturated fat. It would be easier on your gut if you just skipped the appetizer and instead wolfed down a Burger King Whopper on your way to dinner.

Eat This Instead!
Grilled Shrimp on the Barbie
315 calories, 21 g fat (9 g saturated), 561 mg sodium

No. 4 WORST PIZZA

In all the years we've been putting this list together, this pizza from Uno's is the only item to never budge from the hypercaloric countdown. While a number of burgers, salads, and pastas battle it out for the dubious distinction of being America's worst, there is simply no competition for this nightmarish creation. With a day's worth of calories, more than 2 days' worth of sodium, and nearly 3 days' worth of fat, bread, cheese, and sauce have never been stretched to such extremes.

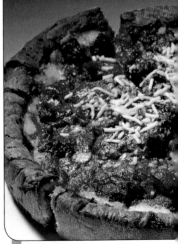

Eat This Instead!
Cheese and Tomato Flatbread Pizza

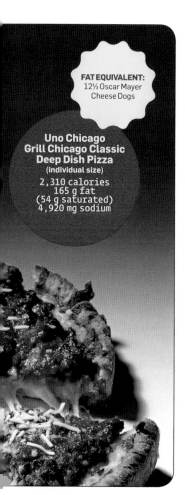

No. 3

WORST CHICKEN ENTRÉE

Here's the secret to stuffing more than a day's worth of energy—mostly from fat—into a plate of chicken and vegetables: First, pound the chicken until it's paper thin. That provides the most possible surface area on which to attach oily breading. Then, cover the whole plate with a layer of butter. In this case, Cheesecake uses what they call "lemon sauce," but don't be fooled. You don't get 4 days' worth of saturated fat from lemons. To complete the caper, toss on a few token asparagus spears to make them think they're eating healthy. Yeah, right. Nice try.

FAT EQUIVALENT:
12½ Oscar Mayer Cheese Dogs

Uno Chicago Grill Chicago Classic Deep Dish Pizza
(individual size)

2,310 calories
165 g fat
(54 g saturated)
4,920 mg sodium

Cheesecake Factory Crispy Chicken Costoletta

2,494 calories
85 g saturated fat
1,677 mg sodium

SATURATED FAT EQUIVALENT:
12 slices of Sara Lee cherry pie (or 1½ whole pies)

(½ pizza) and a house side salad

495 calories,
22 g fat (8 g saturated),
1,065 mg sodium

Eat This Instead!

The Factory Burger

737 calories, 15 g saturated fat, 1,018 mg sodium

WORST DESSERT

Uno Chicago Grill has a dangerous obsession with deep dishes. Not content merely serving the worst pizza in America from those calorie-collecting troughs, they use the same vessel to dish out the worst dessert in the country, too. The crust is replaced with an enormous cookie, the tomato sauce with a thick river of molten chocolate, and the cheese with a mountain of vanilla ice cream. The only thing keeping this from the bottom slot in our Worst Food countdown is the fact that Uno's encourages sharing, but even if you split this dessert four ways, you'll still take in more than twice as many calories as you would with a hot fudge sundae at McDonald's.

Uno Chicago Grill Mega-Sized Deep Dish Sundae

2,800 calories
136 g fat
(72 g saturated)
272 g sugars

SUGAR EQUIVALENT:
18 Breyers Smooth and Dreamy Chocolate Chip Cookie Dough Sandwiches

Eat This Instead! > Mini Hot Chocolate Brownie Sundae

370 calories, 16 g fat (8 g saturated), 38 g sugars

THE WORST FOOD IN AMERICA

CALORIE EQUIVALENT:
6 McDonald's
Quarter Pounders

**Cheesecake Factory
Bistro Shrimp Pasta**
2,727 calories
78 g saturated fat
1,737 mg sodium

The troubling truth is this entire list of America's Worst Foods could be fueled solely by the Cheesecake Factory's atrocious fare. No restaurant combines elephantine portion sizes with a heavy-handed application of cheap cooking fats more recklessly than the Factory folk, resulting in dishes like the 2,582-calorie Chicken and Biscuits and the 2,455-calorie French Toast Napoleon. But it's a relatively healthy-sounding plate of shrimp pasta that wears the tainted crown, delivering to your bloodstream more saturated fat than you'd find in three packages of Oscar Mayer Center Cut Bacon and as many carbs as you'd slurp down from 1½ cases of Amstel Light. Gross.

Eat This Instead! > Grilled Mahi Mahi
237 calories, 1 g saturated fat, 364 mg sodium

A&W

The issue with A&W isn't one of egregious calorie gouging, but rather the absence of any discernible level of true nutrition to be found anywhere on the menu. Every side is deep-fried; there is but one entrée that isn't a burger, a hot dog, or fried chicken; and more than half the menu is dedicated to shakes, floats, and sundaes. Oh, and A&W is one of the last fast-food joints still clinging to the use of trans fat.

SURVIVAL STRATEGY

The best item on the entire menu is the Grilled Chicken Sandwich. Start with that or a small burger, skip the sides and the regular root beer, and finish (if you must have something sweet) with a small sundae or a vanilla cone.

Eat This
Coney (Chili) Cheese Dog

380 calories
23 g fat
(9 g saturated,
1.5 g trans)

1,100 mg sodium

It's difficult to imagine a chili- and cheese-covered hot dog being nutritionally superior to anything, but that's what happens when the rest of the menu is populated with cheeseburgers and fried chicken. Truth is, unless it's of the nefarious foot-long variety, a chili dog is rarely as bad as it sounds.

Other Picks

Cheeseburger
420 calories
21 g fat (7 g saturated, 0.5 g trans)
1,040 mg sodium

Regular Corn Dog Nuggets
280 calories
13 g fat (3 g saturated, 0.5 g trans)
830 mg sodium

Hot Fudge Sundae
350 calories
11 g fat (6 g saturated)
15 g sugars

550 calories

25 g fat
(4.5 g saturated,
1.5 g trans)

1,130 mg sodium

Not That!
Crispy Chicken Sandwich

The word "crispy" is the restaurant's way of discreetly warning you that this piece of chicken has been covered with breading and plunged into a bucket of sizzling hot oil. Any similarity to regular chicken was completely lost in the process.

WEAPON OF MASS DESTRUCTION
Large Breaded Onion Rings

480 calories
27 g fat
(7 g saturated,
7 g trans)
990 mg sodium

A&W is proud of the fact that they use real onions for these rings (as if that's worth bragging about), but they should really start using real frying oil. By refusing to give up partially hydrogenated oil, they infuse this side with nearly four day's of cholesterol-spiking trans fat.

HIDDEN DANGER

A&W Root Beer
(medium, 14 oz)

Like all soda, root beer is a nutritionally bankrupt blend of carbonated water and high-fructose corn syrup. But A&W's namesake beverage packs nearly twice the calories and sugar of a Coke of the same size.

Other Passes

660 calories
46 g fat (7.5 g saturated, 2 g trans)
1,290 mg sodium

Chicken Strips
(3), with ranch

480 calories
27 g fat (7 g saturated, 7 g trans)
990 mg sodium

Large Breaded Onion Rings

880 calories
36 g fat (23 g saturated, 2 g trans)
75 g sugars

Chocolate Milk Shake
(medium)

290 calories
76 g sugars

Applebee's

After years of stonewalling health-conscious eaters and *ETNT* authors alike, Applebee's has finally released the nutritional numbers for its entire menu. Unfortunately, we now see why they were so reluctant to relinquish them in the first place: the 1,700-calorie Riblets Basket, the 1,310-calorie Oriental Chicken Salad, and the 2,510-calorie Appetizer Sampler. The one bright spot is the new Under 550 Calories menu.

SURVIVAL STRATEGY

Skip the meal-wrecking appetizers, pastas, and fajitas, and be very careful with salads, too; half of them pack more than 1,000 calories with dressing. Instead, concentrate on the excellent line of lean steak entrees, or anything from the laudable 550-calorie-or-less menu.

Eat This

Grilled Dijon Chicken

450 calories
16 g saturated fat (6 g saturated)
1,810 mg sodium

Want to know the blueprint for a healthy meal? Lean meat and loads of veggies, just like you see here. If only Applebee's could scale back that sodium, they might be able to lay claim to a perfectly balanced dinner.

Other Picks

Garlic Herb Chicken

370 calories
6 g fat (1 g saturated)
1,930 mg sodium

House Sirloin
(9 oz)

310 calories
13 g fat (5 g saturated)
970 mg sodium

Sweet & Spicy Buffalo Chicken Wings

690 calories
35 g fat (9 g saturated)
1670 mg sodium

1,040 calories

60 g fat
(29 g saturated,
1 g trans)

3,280 mg sodium

Not That!
Chicken Fajita Rollup

Basically this is a mass of chopped chicken insulated with a thick pad of cheese and held together with a massive flour tortilla. Sounds a lot like a quesadilla, right? To this day, we've never met a restaurant quesadilla worth eating.

Other Passes

1,230 calories
67 g fat (16 g saturated, 1 g trans)
4,390 mg sodium

Fiesta Lime Chicken

700 calories
41 g fat (10 g saturated, 1 g trans)
2,310 mg sodium

Bourbon Street Steak

1,150 calories
55 g fat (11 g saturated, 0.5 g trans)
3,400 mg sodium

Sweet and Spicy Boneless Buffalo Chicken Wings

GUILTY PLEASURE

Steak & Fried Shrimp Combo

630 calories

So they may not win the "Health Food of the Year" award, but Applebee's steak combos pair one of their leanest menu items with a small portion of their less-than-diet-friendly fare. Just make sure you swap the potato that comes alongside the meat for a helping of seasonal vegetables—it'll save you 300 calories.

MENU DECODER

● **SHOOTERS**: Tasty layered desserts served up in small whiskey glasses. Part of a (thankfully!) growing trend toward downsized desserts, they average around 390 calories.

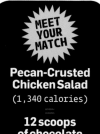

MEET YOUR MATCH

Pecan-Crusted Chicken Salad

(1,340 calories)

12 scoops of chocolate ice cream

Arby's

C+

Arby's offers a long list of sandwiches with fewer than 500 calories. Problem is, there's an even longer list of sandwiches with considerably more than 500 calories, many with warm, virtuous-sounding names. Credit Arby's for nixing the trans fat from their frying oil back in 2006, but it seems they might be just a little too proud of that fact; the restaurant doesn't offer a single side that hasn't had a hot oil bath.

SURVIVAL STRATEGY

You're not doing yourself any favors by ordering off the Market Fresh sandwich menu. You're better off with a regular roast beef or Melt Sandwich, which will save you an average of nearly 300 calories over a Market Fresh sandwich or wrap.

Eat This
Super Roast Beef

430 calories
18 g fat
(6 g saturated,
1 g trans)
1,070 mg sodium

Roast beef claims fewer fat calories than ground hamburger, yet it still delivers the same cache of energy-burning B vitamins and sleep-regulating tryptophan. Makes you wonder why Arby's is the one of the only fast food spots to cash in on the deli cut.

Other Picks

Roast Chicken Fillet Sandwich
400 calories
16 g fat (2.5 g saturated)
950 mg sodium

Chopped Farmhouse Turkey & Ham Salad
with balsamic vinaigrette
380 calories
26 g fat (9 g saturated)
1,370 mg sodium

Ham, Egg, & Cheese Croissant
360 calories
20 g fat (10 g saturated)
1,130 mg sodium

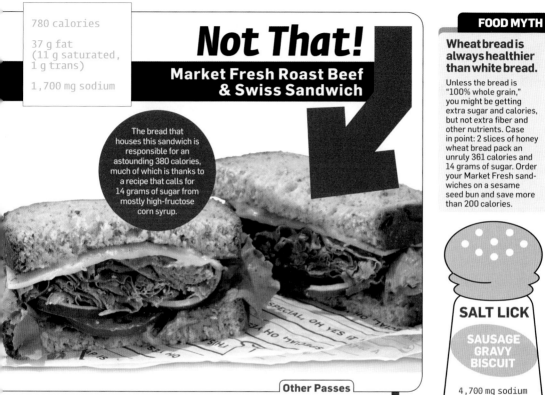

780 calories

37 g fat
(11 g saturated,
1 g trans)

1,700 mg sodium

Not That!

Market Fresh Roast Beef & Swiss Sandwich

The bread that houses this sandwich is responsible for an astounding 380 calories, much of which is thanks to a recipe that calls for 14 grams of sugar from mostly high-fructose corn syrup.

SPECIAL, OH YES IF

Other Passes

710 calories
30 g fat (7 g saturated)
2,030 mg sodium

Roast Ham & Swiss Sandwich

670 calories
48 g fat (12.5 g saturated)
1,470 mg sodium

Chopped Farmhouse Crispy Chicken Salad
with buttermilk ranch

570 calories
29 g fat (11 g saturated)
2,140 mg sodium

Ham, Egg, & Cheese Wrap

FOOD MYTH

Wheat bread is always healthier than white bread.

Unless the bread is "100% whole grain," you might be getting extra sugar and calories, but not extra fiber and other nutrients. Case in point: 2 slices of honey wheat bread pack an unruly 361 calories and 14 grams of sugar. Order your Market Fresh sandwiches on a sesame seed bun and save more than 200 calories.

SALT LICK

SAUSAGE GRAVY BISCUIT

4,700 mg sodium
1,040 calories
60 g fat
(22 g saturated,
2 g trans)

Nothing like waking up to 2 full days' worth of sodium. Sausage and gravy both carry dizzying sodium loads; nix them both from the morning routine and opt for anything on a croissant.

Atlanta Bread Company

The bad news is that the breakfast menu is riddled with unnecessary fats and refined carbohydrates, and most of the sandwiches are a little too high in calories for comfort. The good news is that there's also a robust selection of healthy soups and salads to offset these problems, so focus your appetite there and you'll escape relatively unscathed.

SURVIVAL STRATEGY

Atlanta Bread Company lets you order a half sandwich with a half salad or a cup of soup, which is the perfect compromise for those who prefer a handheld lunch. Hold the mayo on your sandwich and this is a pretty safe bet. Oh, and avoid the pizzas, pastas, and calzones at all costs.

Eat This

Honey Maple Ham on Honey Wheat

½ sandwich, with ½ Balsamic Bleu Salad

370 calories
11.5 g fat
(4 g saturated)
890 mg sodium

The low caloric price tag isn't the only impressive facet of this meal. It's also the fact that the sodium and saturated fat are kept in check, while the fiber (5 grams) and the protein (18.5 grams) are not.

Other Picks

Tomato Bacon Omelette

360 calories
27 g fat (12 g saturated)
1,000 mg sodium

Turkey on Nine Grain Sandwich

370 calories
6 g fat (2 g saturated)
1,240 mg sodium

Chopstix Chicken Salad
with Asian sesame dressing

360 calories
20 g fat (3 g saturated)
850 mg sodium

Not That!

Turkey Club Panini

½ panini, with ½ Salsa Fresca Salmon Salad

635 calories
26.5 g fat
(7 g saturated)
1,255 mg sodium

Not an altogether terrible meal, but certainly not up the standard one would expect from a collaboration between turkey and salmon—two all-star proteins with serious low-calorie potential. The problem is the sandwich comes on oversized panini bread and the salad carries an aggressive dose of sugar and oil.

Other Passes

Three Cheese Omelette

1,100 calories
85 g fat (44 g saturated)
1,990 mg sodium

California Avocado Sandwich

930 calories
55 g fat (11 g saturated)
1,120 mg sodium

Salsa Fresca Salmon Salad
with balsamic vinaigrette

740 calories
48 g fat (7.5 g saturated)
840 mg sodium

SANDWICH SELECTOR

CHICKEN SALAD ON SOURDOUGH
440 calories, 19 g fat
(2 g saturated)

VEGGIE ON NINE GRAIN
500 calories, 25 g fat
(8 g saturated)

TUNA SALAD ON FRENCH
630 calories, 33 g fat
(4.5 g saturated)

NY HOT PASTRAMI
660 calories, 29 g fat
(11 g saturated)

CHICKEN PESTO PANINI
710 calories, 26 g fat
(9 g saturated)

ABC SPECIAL
750 calories, 38 g fat
(10 g saturated)

TURKEY BACON RUSTICA
960 calories, 56 g fat
(19 g saturated)

Au Bon Pain

A-

There are plenty of ways you could go wrong here, but Au Bon Pain couples an extensive inventory of healthy items with an unrivaled standard of nutritional transparency. Each store has an on-site nutritional kiosk to help customers find a meal to meet their expectations, and the variety of ordering options provides dozens of paths to a sensible meal.

SURVIVAL STRATEGY

Many of the café sandwiches come in around 650 calories, so make a lean meal instead by combining soup with one of the many low-calorie options on the All Portions menu. And if you're in the mood to indulge, pass up the baked goods in favor of a cup of fruit and yogurt or a serving of chocolate-covered almonds.

Eat This

Bacon and Egg Melt on Ciabatta

470 calories
23 g fat
(10 g saturated)
980 mg sodium

Yes, it looks and sounds a little too decadent to count as a sound breakfast, but any dish that delivers 27 grams of protein for fewer than 500 calories and 40 grams of carbohydrates consitutes a sound start to the day in our book.

Other Picks

Thai Peanut Chicken Salad
with Thai peanut dressing

400 calories
16 g fat (1 g saturated)
1,020 mg sodium

Apple Croissant

280 calories
11 g fat (7 g saturated)
160 mg sodium

Spicy Tuna Sandwich

470 calories
16 g fat (3 g saturated)
1,180 mg sodium

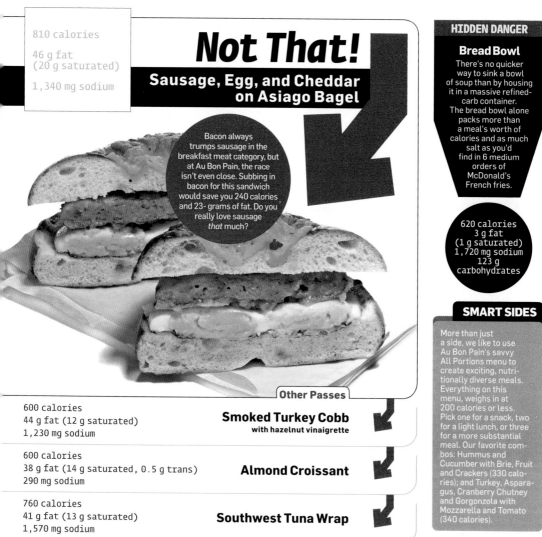

810 calories
46 g fat
(20 g saturated)
1,340 mg sodium

Not That!

Sausage, Egg, and Cheddar on Asiago Bagel

Bacon always trumps sausage in the breakfast meat category, but at Au Bon Pain, the race isn't even close. Subbing in bacon for this sandwich would save you 240 calories and 23- grams of fat. Do you really love sausage *that* much?

HIDDEN DANGER

Bread Bowl

There's no quicker way to sink a bowl of soup than by housing it in a massive refined-carb container. The bread bowl alone packs more than a meal's worth of calories and as much salt as you'd find in 6 medium orders of McDonald's French fries.

620 calories
3 g fat
(1 g saturated)
1,720 mg sodium
123 g carbohydrates

SMART SIDES

More than just a side, we like to use Au Bon Pain's savvy All Portions menu to create exciting, nutritionally diverse meals. Everything on this menu, weighs in at 200 calories or less. Pick one for a snack, two for a light lunch, or three for a more substantial meal. Our favorite combos: Hummus and Cucumber with Brie, Fruit and Crackers (330 calories); and Turkey, Asparagus, Cranberry Chutney and Gorgonzola with Mozzarella and Tomato (340 calories).

Other Passes

600 calories
44 g fat (12 g saturated)
1,230 mg sodium

Smoked Turkey Cobb
with hazelnut vinaigrette

600 calories
38 g fat (14 g saturated, 0.5 g trans)
290 mg sodium

Almond Croissant

760 calories
41 g fat (13 g saturated)
1,570 mg sodium

Southwest Tuna Wrap

85

Auntie Anne's

C+

Is there anything redeeming on Auntie Anne's menu? Not really. The average pretzel is about 360 calories of refined carbohydrates, and they supplement the twisted-bread menu with a long list of sweetened beverages and smoothies. But you can find far worse indulgences on just about any dessert menu in the country, so go here in search of relatively healthy indulgences, not genuinely nutritious food.

SURVIVAL STRATEGY

Cut most of the fat and half of the sodium by skipping the butter and salt they put on most pretzels, relying instead on a healthier dipping sauce such as marinara or sweet mustard for big flavor.

Eat This

Pretzel Dog

with ketchup and mustard

375 calories
20 g fat
(9 g saturated,
0.5 g trans)
930 mg sodium

Not only does it have fewer calories than half the regular pretzels on the menu, but it also delivers your best ratio of protein to carbohydrates. That means you can count on it to hang out in your belly a little longer, keeping your appetite at bay.

Other Picks

Raisin Pretzel
360 calories
5 g fat (3 g saturated)
16 g sugars

Strawberry Dutch Ice
(14 oz)
160 calories
0 g fat
37 g sugars

480 calories

16 g fat
(4.5 g saturated)

1,570 mg sodium

Not That!

Sesame Pretzel

with Auntie Anne's Melted Cheese Dip

The only thing worse than choosing the wrong pretzel is pairing it with the wrong dunkin' sauce. With a quarter of your day's sodium per 2-ounce serving, this dastardly dip should make you happy that Anne's not your real aunt.

DIP DECODER
(per serving)

SWEET MUSTARD
60 calories, 2 g fat
(1 g saturated),
9 g sugars

CREAM CHEESE
80 calories, 6 g fat
(4.5 g saturated)

MELTED CHEESE
80 calories, 6 g fat
(1 g saturated)

CHEESE SAUCE
100 calories, 8 g fat
(3 g saturated)

HOT SALSA CHEESE
110 calories, 8 g fat
(3.5 g saturated)

CARAMEL
130 calories, 3 g fat
(1.5 g saturated),
19 g sugars

Other Passes

470 calories
12 g fat (7 g saturated)
29 g sugars

Cinnamon Sugar Stix

300 calories
10 g fat (7 g saturated)
44 g sugars

Wild Cherry Dutch Smoothie
(14 oz)

Baja Fresh

D It's a surprise that Baja Fresh's menu has not yet collapsed under the weight of its own fatty fare. About a third of the items on the menu have more than 1,000 calories, and most are spiked with enough sodium to melt a polar ice cap. Fajitas, nachos, and burritos are all off-limits fare. First-rate tacos and the Baja Ensaladas are the only redeeming features of this otherwise troubling menu.

SURVIVAL STRATEGY

Unless you're comfortable stuffing 108 grams of fat into your arteries, avoid the nachos at all costs. In fact, avoid almost everything on this menu. The only safe options are the Baja tacos or a salad topped with salsa verde and served without the elephantine tortilla bowl.

Eat This

Chicken Torta
without chips

620 calories
23 g fat
(6 g saturated)
1,330 mg sodium

Tortas are Mexican sandwiches loaded with grilled or braised meat, avocado, salsa, and other fresh fixings. At Baja, it's one of your best bets for a decent entrée. Order this one without the side of chips, and you'll cut 240 calories off your meal.

Other Picks

Charbroiled Chicken Salad
with fat-free salsa verde dressing

325 calories
7 g fat (2 g saturated)
1,580 mg sodium

Veggie and Cheese Bare Burrito

580 calories
10 g fat (4 g saturated)
1,950 mg sodium

Corn Tortilla Chips
(1.5 oz side) and Guacamole (3 oz side)

320 calories
22 g fat (2 g saturated)
325 mg sodium

Not That!
Chicken Quesadilla

1,330 calories

80 g fat
(37 g saturated,
2.5 trans)

2,590 mg sodium

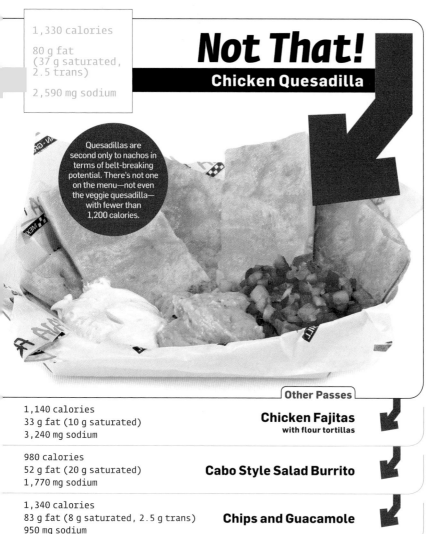

Quesadillas are second only to nachos in terms of belt-breaking potential. There's not one on the menu—not even the veggie quesadilla— with fewer than 1,200 calories.

Other Passes

1,140 calories
33 g fat (10 g saturated)
3,240 mg sodium

Chicken Fajitas
with flour tortillas

---

980 calories
52 g fat (20 g saturated)
1,770 mg sodium

Cabo Style Salad Burrito

1,340 calories
83 g fat (8 g saturated, 2.5 g trans)
950 mg sodium

Chips and Guacamole

HIDDEN DANGER

Tostada Salad with Chicken

Chicken salad isn't so bad—until you drown it in cheese and sour cream and serve it up in a deep-fried tortilla shell. (And that's without dressing!) Stick to a Baja Ensalada and save 830 calories.

1,140 calories
55 g fat
(14 g saturated,
1 g trans)
2,370 mg sodium

BAD BREED

Nachos

A mere 5 ounces of Baja's tortilla chips contain a whopping 740 calories, so it's no surprise that a mountain of them smothered in melted cheese, guacamole, and sour cream will cost you big: at least 1,890 calories (for the plain cheese variety). Add meat and you'll cross the dreaded 2,000-calorie threshold. Unless you've got a crew of six to split 'em, nix the nachos.

Baskin-Robbins

C-

Baskin-Robbins did health-conscious consumers a solid by nixing their line of Premium Sundaes and Shakes. But the reality is that it would take more than just a little pruning to really clean up this menu; its soft serve is among the most caloric in the country, the smoothies and shakes contain a glut of added sugars, and anything that BR turns into a sundae winds up with more fat than a steakhouse buffet.

SURVIVAL STRATEGY

With choices like frozen yogurt, sherbet, and no-sugar-added ice cream, Baskin's lighter menu is the one bright spot in this otherwise darkly caloric place. Just be sure to ask for a sugar or cake cone—the waffle cone will swaddle your treat in an extra 160 calories.

Eat This

Double Header Cone

(cake cone with one scoop Jamoca Almond Fudge ice cream topped with a swirl of soft serve)

335 calories
15 g fat
(8 g saturated)
36 g sugars

What could be better than a vanilla-chocolate one-two punch? How about the fact that it actually has fewer calories than some of BR's single scoops? If you want to go overboard, here's how you do it.

Other Picks

Oreo Cookies 'n Cream Ice Cream
(2 scoops) in a cake cone

365 calories
18 g fat (10 g saturated)
34 g sugars

Peach Passion Fruit Blast
(small, 16 oz)

270 calories
0 g fat
65 g sugars

Rainbow Sherbet
(4-oz scoop)

160 calories
2 g fat (1.5 g saturated)
34 g sugars

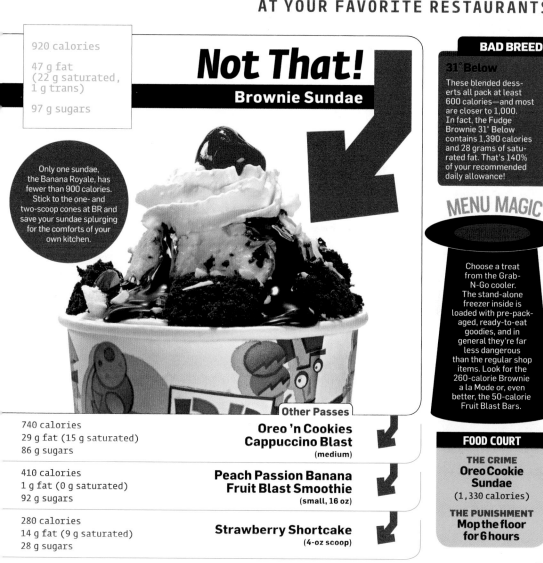

920 calories

47 g fat
(22 g saturated,
1 g trans)

97 g sugars

Not That!
Brownie Sundae

Only one sundae,
the Banana Royale, has
fewer than 900 calories.
Stick to the one- and
two-scoop cones at BR and
save your sundae splurging
for the comforts of your
own kitchen.

BAD BREED

31° Below

These blended dess-
erts all pack at least
600 calories—and most
are closer to 1,000.
In fact, the Fudge
Brownie 31° Below
contains 1,390 calories
and 28 grams of satu-
rated fat. That's 140%
of your recommended
daily allowance!

MENU MAGIC

Choose a treat
from the Grab-
N-Go cooler.
The stand-alone
freezer inside is
loaded with pre-pack-
aged, ready-to-eat
goodies, and in
general they're far
less dangerous
than the regular shop
items. Look for the
260-calorie Brownie
a la Mode or, even
better, the 50-calorie
Fruit Blast Bars.

Other Passes

740 calories
29 g fat (15 g saturated)
86 g sugars

Oreo 'n Cookies
Cappuccino Blast
(medium)

410 calories
1 g fat (0 g saturated)
92 g sugars

Peach Passion Banana
Fruit Blast Smoothie
(small, 16 oz)

280 calories
14 g fat (9 g saturated)
28 g sugars

Strawberry Shortcake
(4-oz scoop)

FOOD COURT

THE CRIME
Oreo Cookie
Sundae
(1,330 calories)

THE PUNISHMENT
Mop the floor
for 6 hours

Ben & Jerry's

C What sets B&J's apart from the competition amounts to more than just an affinity for jam bands and green pastures. The shop also adheres to a lofty commitment to the quality and sources of its ingredients. All dairy is free from rBGH (recombinant bovine growth hormone) and the chocolate, vanilla, and coffee ingredients are all Fair Trade Certified. From a strictly nutritional standpoint, though, it's still just an ice cream shop.

SURVIVAL STRATEGY

With half of the calories of the ice cream, sorbet makes the healthiest choice on the menu. If you demand dairy, the frozen yogurt can still save you up to 100 calories per scoop.

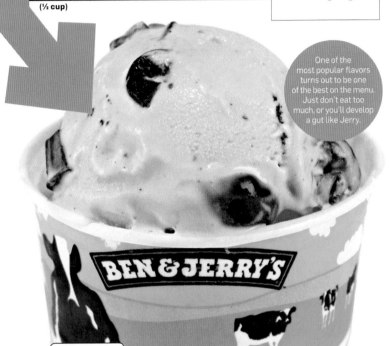

Eat This

Cherry Garcia Ice Cream
(½ cup)

200 calories
11 g fat
(8 g saturated)
20 g sugars

One of the most popular flavors turns out to be one of the best on the menu. Just don't eat too much, or you'll develop a gut like Jerry.

Other Picks

Strawberry Cheesecake Ice Cream
(½ cup)

210 calories
11 g fat (6 g saturated)
20 g sugars

Half Baked Frozen Yogurt
(½ cup)

180 calories
3 g fat (1.5 g saturated)
23 g sugars

340 calories

24 g fat
(12 g saturated)

24 g sugars

Not That!

Peanut Butter Cup Ice Cream

(½ cup)

There's only one peanut butter ice cream in the country with more calories than this one, and that's Häagen-Dazs Chocolate Peanut Butter. But as far as saturated fat goes, this one is the national loser.

BEN & JERRY'S

Other Passes

276 calories
17 g fat (11 g saturated, 0.5 g trans)
20 g sugars

Coconut Seven Layer Bar Ice Cream
(½ cup)

260 calories
20 g fat (8 g saturated)
24 g sugars

Butter Pecan Original Ice Cream
(½ cup)

ICE CREAM EQUATIONS

SORBET
Water + sugar + fruit puree = *100 calories per serving for any and all flavors*

FROZEN YOGURT
Skim milk + water + sugar + flavorings (cookie dough, raspberry puree, and so on) = *130 to 160 calories per serving*

NO SUGAR ADDED
[Ice cream]— sugar + artificial sweetener = *About 180 calories per serving*

ICE CREAM
Cream + skim milk + sugar + ingredients = *152 to 276 calories per serving (from Orange and Cream and Coconut Seven Layer Bar, respectively)*

MENU DECODER

● **GUAR GUM AND CARRAGEENAN:** These two industrial thickening agents, found in nearly every pint of Ben & Jerry's, are used to give commercial ice cream a richer texture.

Blimpie

B In the past, we admonished Blimpie for its love of trans fat. Since then, the chain has quietly removed all the dangerous oils from its menu and earned itself a place of honor in our book. But that doesn't mean the menu is free from danger. Blimpie likes to splash oil on just about everything containing deli meat, and there are a handful of sinful subs that top the 1,000-calorie mark.

SURVIVAL STRATEGY

A ham Bluffin makes a decent breakfast, and the Grilled Chicken Teriyaki Sandwich is one of the best in the sandwich business. But skip the wraps and most of the hot sandwiches. And no matter which sandwich you choose, swap out mayo and oil for mustard or light dressing.

Eat This

Turkey and Cranberry
(6-inch sub)

350 calories
4 g fat
(0.5 g saturated)
1,220 mg sodium

Kudos to Blimpie for harnessing the most under-utilized spread in the sandwich-builder's arsenal. By displacing mayonnaise and other high-calorie dressings, the antioxidant-rich cranberries help make this the leanest creation on Blimpie's menu.

Other Picks

BLT
(6-inch regular)

430 calories
22 g fat (5 g saturated)
960 mg sodium

Ham, Egg & Cheese Bluffin

280 calories
10 g fat (5 g saturated)
1,049 mg sodium

Hot Pastrami
(6-inch regular)

435 calories
16 g fat (7 g saturated)
1,354 mg sodium

580 calories

20 g fat
(5 g saturated)

1,480 mg sodium

Not That!

Grilled Chicken Caesar Ciabatta

The emperor has no clothes! Nine times out of 10, when you see the word Caesar, expect trouble. Consider this in the same nutritional red zone as mayo-bloated chicken salad. Ciabatta sounds fancy, but it's essentially no different from white bread. Switch to 6-inch wheat and you'll gain an immediate 3 grams of belly-filling fiber.

Other Passes

642 calories
29 g fat (10 g saturated)
1,570 mg sodium

Chicken Cheddar Bacon Ranch
(6-inch regular)

773 calories
24 g fat (9 g saturated)
2,368 mg sodium

Breakfast Panini
(6-inch regular)

607 calories
24 g fat (9 g saturated)
2,072 mg sodium

Meatball
(6-inch regular)

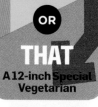

For 1,180 calories, you can have

ALL THIS
A 6-inch Turkey and Avocado, Blimpie Burger, Chicken Gumbo and a Brownie

OR

THAT
A 12-inch Special Vegetarian

CONDIMENT CATASTROPHE

Oil Blend
(0.5 oz)

130 calories
14 g fat
(2 g saturated)
0 mg sodium

There's nothing more dangerous than an apathetic sandwich maker with a bottle of oil in his hand, and many of Blimpie's subs get this treatment whether you ask for it or not. With 130 calories in each ½ ounce, you can imagine how fast that adds up when poured on with careless indifference. Save yourself the needless fat by asking them to skip the oil treatment.

95

Bob Evans

Bob offers up an array of healthy entrée and side options on the menu, making it easy to cobble together a well-balanced meal. Still, too much of the food here still suffers from an overdose of dangerous trans fat—even a side of "garden" vegetables comes with a gram of the cholesterol-spiking stuff. Bob, isn't it time to follow the lead of nearly every other restaurant and drop the nasty stuff?

SURVIVAL STRATEGY

Remember this: If it sounds unhealthy (chicken fried steak, potpie, stuffed hotcakes), it is. Breakfast should consist of staples like oatmeal, eggs, fruit, and yogurt; for lunch and dinner, stick with grilled chicken or fish paired with one of the fruit and vegetable sides that avoid the fry treatment.

Eat This

Strawberry Stuffed French Toast

685 calories
19 g fat
(9 g saturated)
49 g sugars

French toast is far from an ideal breakfast, but you'll have a hard time finding one for fewer calories. Even with vanilla cream cheese, whipped cream, powdered sugar, and strawberry compote, this plate still manages to squeeze by with 40% fewer calories than Bob's Stacked & Stuffed Hotcakes.

Other Picks

Bob-B-Q Pulled Pork Sandwich

596 calories
24 g fat (7 g saturated)
927 mg sodium

Savor Size Heritage Chef Salad
with vinegar & oil dressing

294 calories
18 g fat (9 g saturated)
926 mg sodium

Steak Tips
with Glazed Carrots and Green Beans

388 calories
20 g fat (6 g saturated)
1,428 mg sodium

1,168 calories

36 g fat
(16 g saturated,
6 g trans)

103 g sugars

Not That!

Stacked & Stuffed Strawberry Banana Cream Hotcakes

It's with great dishonor that we present to you America's trans-fattiest breakfast. Each serving has 3 times as much artery-narrowing sludge as you should consume in an entire day, according to recommendations from the American Heart Association.

Other Passes

856 calories
30 g fat (12 g saturated)
1,362 mg sodium

Knife & Fork Bob-B-Q Pulled Pork Sandwich

861 calories
63g fat (14 g saturated)
1,658 mg sodium

Country Spinach Salad
with Colonial Dressing

1,008 calories
43 g fat (11 g saturated)
3,686 mg sodium

Steak Tip Stir-Fry

MEET YOUR MATCH

Knife and Fork Meatloaf Sandwich

(3,182 mg sodium)

=

18 small tubs of Pringles

Boston Market

SURVIVAL STRATEGY

Pair roasted turkey, ham, white-meat chicken, or even sirloin with a vegetable side or two, and you've got a solid dinner. But avoid calorie-laden dark-meat chicken, meat loaf, potpie, and hot Carver Sandwiches.

Eat This

Beef Brisket, Green Beans, and Dill Potatoes

480 calories
27 g fat
(4 g saturated)
560 mg sodium

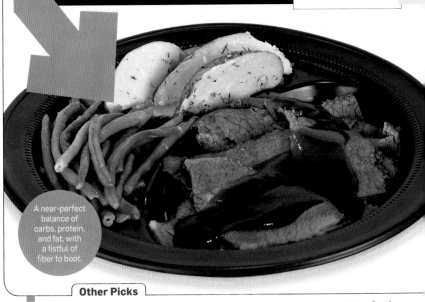

A near-perfect balance of carbs, protein, and fat, with a fistful of fiber to boot.

Other Picks

Roast Turkey
with Baked Beans

450 calories
4.5 g fat (1 g saturated)
1,635 mg sodium

Beef Brisket

230 calories
13 g fat (3.5 g saturated)
570 mg sodium

Chocolate Chip Fudge Brownie

320 calories
13 g fat (3 g saturated)
36 g sugars

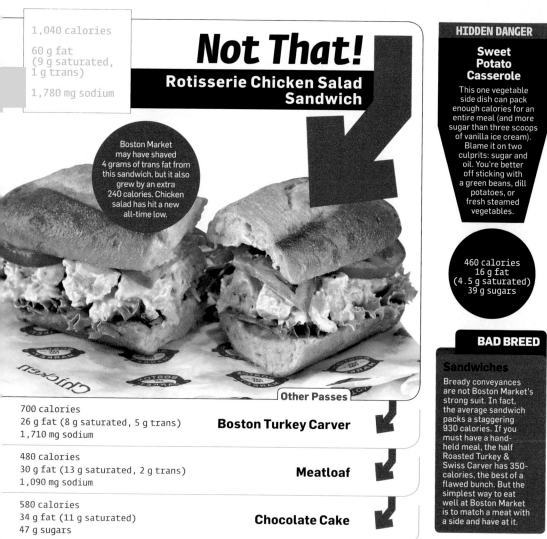

1,040 calories

60 g fat
(9 g saturated,
1 g trans)

1,780 mg sodium

Not That!

Rotisserie Chicken Salad Sandwich

Boston Market may have shaved 4 grams of trans fat from this sandwich, but it also grew by an extra 240 calories. Chicken salad has hit a new all-time low.

Other Passes

700 calories
26 g fat (8 g saturated, 5 g trans)
1,710 mg sodium

Boston Turkey Carver

480 calories
30 g fat (13 g saturated, 2 g trans)
1,090 mg sodium

Meatloaf

580 calories
34 g fat (11 g saturated)
47 g sugars

Chocolate Cake

HIDDEN DANGER

Sweet Potato Casserole

This one vegetable side dish can pack enough calories for an entire meal (and more sugar than three scoops of vanilla ice cream). Blame it on two culprits: sugar and oil. You're better off sticking with a green beans, dill potatoes, or fresh steamed vegetables.

460 calories
16 g fat
(4.5 g saturated)
39 g sugars

BAD BREED

Sandwiches

Bready conveyances are not Boston Market's strong suit. In fact, the average sandwich packs a staggering 930 calories. If you must have a hand-held meal, the half Roasted Turkey & Swiss Carver has 350-calories, the best of a flawed bunch. But the simplest way to eat well at Boston Market is to match a meat with a side and have at it.

Burger King

C We got word from Burger King in October 2008 that they were finally removing the trans fat from their deep fryer. Excellent news, but the burgers are still sullied with the dangerous oils. Although the King holds the dubious distinction of being the unhealthiest of the Big Three burger joints, the trans fat transition and the introduction of healthy sides like Apple Fries signal that Burger King is finally trying to move in the right nutritional direction.

SURVIVAL STRATEGY

For breakfast, pick the Ham Omelet Sandwich. For lunch, match the regular hamburger, the Whopper Jr., or the Tendergrill Sandwich with Apple Fries and water, and you'll escape for under 600 calories.

Eat This

Whopper Jr., and Crown-Shaped Chicken Tenders

(without mayonnaise; 4-piece chicken)

440 calories
22 g fat
(6 g saturated)
770 mg sodium

Nix the mayo and the Whopper Jr. becomes one of the most reliable burgers in the fast-food kingdom. And the Chicken Tenders? They have about half as many calories as a small order of fries.

Other Picks

Flame Broiled Double Cheeseburger
510 calories
29 g fat (14 g saturated, 1.5 g trans)
1,020 mg sodium

Cheesy Tots Potatoes
(6 pieces)
220 calories
12 g fat (4 g saturated)
630 mg sodium

Ham Omelet Sandwich
290 calories
12 g fat (4 g saturated)
870 mg sodium

670 calories

40 g fat
(11 g saturated,
1.5 g trans)

1,020 mg sodium

Not That!

Whopper

It's only a quarter-pound burger, yet somehow the infamous Whopper manages to eat up nearly two-thirds of your day's fat recommendation before you even get to the side. The same-size burger at Wendy's will cost you 200 fewer calories.

Other Passes

770 calories
48 g fat (16 g saturated, 1.5 g trans)
1,450 mg sodium

Whopper Sandwich
with cheese

340 calories
17 g fat (3.5 g saturated)
530 mg sodium

French Fries
(small)

420 calories
31 g fat (10 g saturated, 0.5 g trans)
910 mg sodium

Sausage and Cheese
Breakfast Shots
(2 sandwiches)

FOOD COURT

THE CRIME:
Triple Whopper
with Cheese
(1,250 calories)

THE PUNISHMENT:
Pedal
vigorously
on a stationary
bike for 1 hour
and 40 minutes

LITTLE TRICK

Ask to 86 the mayo on your burger or sandwich. You'll save about 150 calories and 18 grams of fat.

GUILTY PLEASURE

Chicken Tenders
(8 pieces)

360 calories
21 g fat
(4 g saturated)

Even BK's largest serving of chicken tenders isn't half bad—it contains about the same amount of calories as the relatively harmless Whopper Jr., plus it packs in 18 grams of protein. Pair them with barbecue sauce or sweet and sour sauce, rather than high-cal ranch or honey mustard.

California Pizza Kitchen

D+

Like Applebee's and Outback, CPK has finally decided to give up the nutritional goods for its entire menu. There is some reason to rejoice: The pizzas are relatively low in calories and the Thai Crunch Salad, which used to be the worst salad in America, has shrunk by nearly 1,000 calories. We like the fact that CPK is showing a willingness to improve its fare, but the pastas, salads, and entrees still have a long way to go.

SURVIVAL STRATEGY

Either turn a healthier appetizer (like the chicken dumplings, crab cakes, or spring rolls) into an entrée, or stick with pizza—thin crust, preferably.

Eat This

Chicken Milanese

618 calories
11 g saturated
1,209 mg sodium

The fact that this one is breaded and lightly fried and still has fewer than half the calories of the marsala goes to show you just how much butter goes into your average restaurant sauce. Here, that butter is replaced with arugula and fresh tomatoes.

Other Picks

Portobello Mushroom Ravioli
with tomato basil sauce

718 calories
10 g saturated
1,550 mg sodium

Tricolore Salad Pizza with Grilled Chicken Breast
(3 slices)

618 calories
8 g saturated
1,098 mg sodium

Cabo Crab Cakes

511 calories
5 g saturated
1,533 mg sodium

1,412 calories
15 g saturated
3,038 mg sodium

Not That!
Chicken Marsala

The anatomy of a restaurant disaster: You're in the mood for chicken so you glance over the CPK chicken section and end up picking marsala without giving it much thought. You might have just as easily picked milanese, but instead you end up with nearly 70 percent of your day's calories and a day and a half of sodium.

Other Passes

1,287 calories
14 g saturated
2,368 mg sodium

Broccoli Sundried Tomato Fusilli

1,485 calories
25 g saturated
1,864 mg sodium

Waldorf Chicken Salad
with dijon balsamic

895 calories
1 g saturated fat
2,790 mg sodium

Lettuce Wraps with Shrimp

Ginger Salmon

Salmon and ginger, on their own, are paragons of nutritious eating. So how does CPK manage to mutilate them so severely? Step one is the employment of a high-calorie Sweet Ginger Sauce, and step two is piling the plate high with a profusion of oily Mandarin noodles.

1,345 calories

Small Cravings Menu

Give credit to CPK for introducing this new portion-controlled concept to their menu. The offerings are pretty decadent (Sweet Corn Tamale Ravioli, Buffalo Chicken), but thanks to the restrained serving sizes, nothing on the menu tops the 500 calorie mark—a minor miracle at this place. The salads and the Crispy Artichoke Hearts are the best of the bunch.

Carl's Jr.

C-

After years of thumbing their noses at health-conscious eaters, Carl's Jr. is beginning to understand the value of a few sound alternatives to an otherwise dizzying cluster of ultra-caloric menu items. Grilled chicken sandwiches and salads offer a respite from the burgers and sides, the worst in the fast-food industry. But the breakfast menu, with no entrée under 450 calories, is in desperate need of a decent option or two.

SURVIVAL STRATEGY

Fast-food chains tend to group in clusters, so your first strategy should be to find another place to grab lunch. Failing that, settle on either the Original Grilled Chicken Salad with low-fat balsamic dressing or the Charbroiled BBQ Chicken Sandwich.

Eat This

Charbroiled BBQ Chicken Sandwich

380 calories
7 g fat
(0.5 g saturated)
1,010 mg sodium

Not all chicken is created equal. Case in point: This tasty grilled rendition qualifies as one of the healthiest options on Carl's menu, while the Santa Fe brings 250 extra calories and five times the fat to the table.

Other Picks

Single Teriyaki Burger
610 calories
29 g fat (11 g saturated)
1,020 mg sodium

Sourdough Breakfast Sandwich
475 calories
25 g fat (9 g saturated)
1,090 mg sodium

Chicken Stars
(4 pieces)
210 calories
16 g fat (4 g saturated)
310 mg sodium

630 calories

35 g fat
(8 g saturated)

1,410 mg sodium

Not That!

Charbroiled Santa Fe Chicken Sandwich

Triple Whoppers are supposedly charbroiled, but that doesn't make them healthy. Here, the addition of cheese and a mayo-based sauce ups the fat ante by a factor of five.

Other Passes

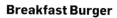

920 calories
59 g fat (23 g saturated, 1.5 g trans)
2,040 mg sodium

The Big Carl

780 calories
41 g fat (15 g saturated)
1,460 mg sodium

Breakfast Burger

330 calories
18 g fat (3 g saturated)
610 mg sodium

Fried Zucchini

MENU MAGIC

"Veg It." At Carl's Jr., you put a vegetarian spin on a Six Dollar Burger by ordering it sans meat. The option works best for the big-flavor guacamole and portobello varieties, both of which offer plenty more than just a hamburger between the buns. The best part about going meatless? You drop about 300 calories.

Cheesecake Factory

Food blogs and nutrition chat rooms were abuzz when California law forced Cheesecake Factory to reveal calorie, saturated fat, and sodium counts for all menu items. The response from commenters: "shocking," "disgusting," and "CF should be ashamed." It's tough not to agree, especially when you consider this fat Factory serves up an outstounding 90 dishes with more than 1,500 calories.

SURVIVAL STRATEGY

Your best survival strategy is to turn your car around and head home for a meal cooked in your own kitchen. Failing that, skip Pasta, Specialties, Combos, and Sandwiches at all cost. Split a pizza or a salad, or opt for the surprisingly decent Factory Burger.

Eat This

The Factory Burger

737 calories
15 g saturated
1,018 mg sodium

Amid the scads of nutritional belly flops on Cheesecake Factory's menu, this burger actually emerges as one of the all-out best entrees. It's true—even a seemingly innocuous dish like Miso Salmon has more than 1,700 calories. Just be sure you pair this burger with something beside fries—a small side salad, green beans, or broccoli will all keep you around the 800-calorie figure, which is a minor miracle at this troubled establishment.

Other Picks

Seared Tuna Tataki Salad
442 calories
3 g saturated fat
1,386 mg sodium

Chicken Pot Stickers (½ order)
192 calories
1 g saturated fat
1,174 mg sodium

Energy Breakfast
714 calories
4 g saturated fat
1,304 mg sodium

Not That!

Grilled Turkey Burger

1,331 calories
31 g saturated
1,674 mg sodium

Terms like "grilled" and "turkey" are intended to temper your nutritional worries, but a quick look behind the buzz terms reveals that you could stuff nearly four Wendy's Double Stack Burgers into the vast caloric trench created by this "healthy" alternative.

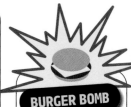

BURGER BOMB

Ranch House Burger

1,941 calories
48 g saturated fat
2,877 mg sodium

Please welcome our newest inductee to the list of Worst Burgers in America. It has nearly a full day's worth of calories, more than a day's worth of sodium, and 2½ days' worth of saturated fat.

BAD BREED

Factory Combinations

Here's a dangerous fact: Not one of the gourmet-sounding, two-meat dishes on this part of the menu has less than 2,000 calories or 50 grams of saturated fat. The best of them (or, "least terrible," anyway) is the Chicken Madeira and Herb Crusted Salmon. But even if you split it, you're still looking at more calories than a Chili Cheese Dog and large fries from Dairy Queen. Pass on this combo meal.

Other Passes

1,610 calories
49 g saturated fat
1,075 mg sodium
Wasabi Crusted Ahi Tuna

565 calories
10.5 g saturated fat
490 mg sodium
Fire-Roasted Fresh Artichoke
(½ order)

1,876 calories
40 g saturated fat
4,777 mg sodium
Sunrise Fiesta Burrito

107

Chevys Fresh Mex

D+

The taco trader earns its dismal grade by offering dozens of dishes with more than 1,000 calories, by cramming a consistently dangerous amount of fat into its entrées, and by having salt levels that make it difficult to find a meal with fewer than 2,000 milligrams of sodium. A new nutrition tool online shows some promise, though: Ordering tacos and enchiladas à la carte can make for a reasonable meal.

SURVIVAL STRATEGY

Forget the combo meals and specials that Chevy's designs. The tamalitos, rice and beans that come with those plates will ruin your dinner, no matter how healthy the rest of the meal is. Construct your own meal by pairing a taco or two with an enchilada or tamale. Just skip the sides!

Eat This

Grilled Chicken Tacos
(no tamalito or rice)

590 calories
24 g fat
(6 g saturated)
1,140 mg sodium

Warning: This is not healthy food. On a menu dominated by nutritional black holes, these tacos are the lesser of many evils. Drop the cheese and the chipotle aioli, and you'll skim off another 130 calories and 13 grams of fat.

Other Picks	
Red Chili Pork Taquitos without tamalito or rice	610 calories 37 g fat (12 g saturated) 870 mg sodium
Salsa Chicken Enchiladas (2) without sides	460 calories 22 g fat (10 g saturated) 860 mg sodium

1,551 calories

94 g fat
(37 g saturated)

2,480 mg sodium

Not That!

Tostada Salad with Chicken

Containing nearly a day's worth of calories and as much fat as 19 Twinkies, this bowl of leaves qualifies as one of the worst salads in America. (Only On the Border's Grande Taco Salad and CPK's Thai Crunch Salad are worse.)

Other Passes

1,650 calories
107 g fat (48 g saturated)
3,100 mg sodium

Carnitas Quesadilla

1,070 calories
64 g fat (30 g saturated)
2,000 mg sodium

Chipotle Chicken Enchiladas

HIDDEN DANGER

Rice and Beans

Many of the entrees themselves at Chevys are perfectly fine, but when you tack on this ubiquitous Tex-Mex duo, things take a turn south of the border. Skip the rice and opt for the Beans a la Charra and you'll save an easy 250 calories.

460 calories
19 g fat
(6 g saturated)
1,270 mg sodium

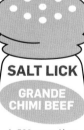

SALT LICK

GRANDE CHIMI BEEF

4,590 mg sodium
1,730 calories
90 g fat
(44 g saturated)

No one should mistake a deep-fried burrito for health food, but this one packs as much salt as you'd find in nearly 14 Taco Bell Crunchy Beef Tacos.

Chick-fil-A

A-

Chick-fil-A ranks among the best of the country's major fast-food establishments, thanks to a line of low-calorie chicken sandwiches and an impressive roster of healthy sides like fruit cups and various salads. But a recent revision to their nutritional information revealed a menu inching ever-upward in the calorie and sodium department. Any more movement and this A- becomes a B.

SURVIVAL STRATEGY

Instead of nuggets or strips, look to the Chargrilled Chicken Sandwiches, which average only 355 calories apiece. And sub in a healthy side—fruit or soup—for the standard fried fare. Just don't supplement your meal with a shake—none has fewer than 500 calories.

Eat This

Chargrilled Chicken Sandwich

with small waffle fries

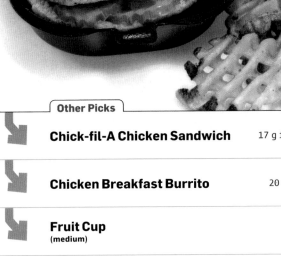

590 calories
19.5 g fat
(4 g saturated)
1,260 mg sodium

The fries are far from the best side on the menu—that distinction belongs to the 100-calorie fruit cup—but with Chick-fil-A's Chargrilled Chicken Sandwich weighing in at a mere 300 calories, you have a little room to splurge.

Other Picks

Chick-fil-A Chicken Sandwich	430 calories 17 g fat (3.5 g saturated) 1,370 mg sodium
Chicken Breakfast Burrito	450 calories 20 g fat (8 g saturated) 990 mg sodium
Fruit Cup (medium)	70 calories 0 g fat 14 g sugars

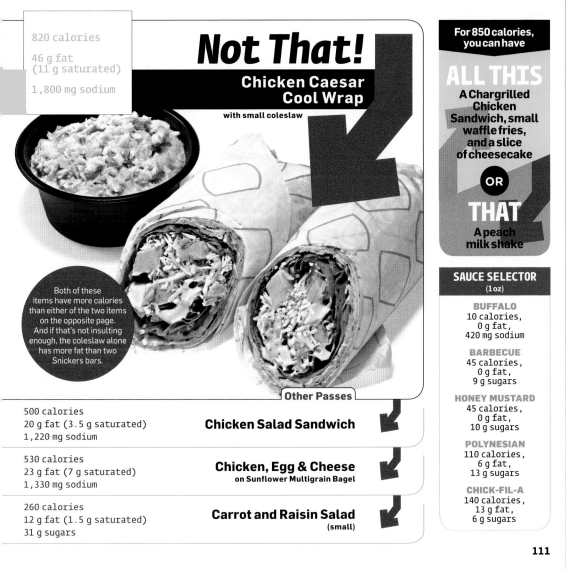

820 calories

46 g fat
(11 g saturated)

1,800 mg sodium

Not That!

Chicken Caesar Cool Wrap

with small coleslaw

Both of these items have more calories than either of the two items on the opposite page. And if that's not insulting enough, the coleslaw alone has more fat than two Snickers bars.

Other Passes

500 calories
20 g fat (3.5 g saturated)
1,220 mg sodium

Chicken Salad Sandwich

530 calories
23 g fat (7 g saturated)
1,330 mg sodium

Chicken, Egg & Cheese
on Sunflower Multigrain Bagel

260 calories
12 g fat (1.5 g saturated)
31 g sugars

Carrot and Raisin Salad
(small)

For 850 calories, you can have

ALL THIS

A Chargrilled Chicken Sandwich, small waffle fries, and a slice of cheesecake

OR

THAT

A peach milk shake

SAUCE SELECTOR
(1 oz)

BUFFALO
10 calories,
0 g fat,
420 mg sodium

BARBECUE
45 calories,
0 g fat,
9 g sugars

HONEY MUSTARD
45 calories,
0 g fat,
10 g sugars

POLYNESIAN
110 calories,
6 g fat,
13 g sugars

CHICK-FIL-A
140 calories,
13 g fat,
6 g sugars

Chili's

D From burgers to baby back ribs, Chili's serves up some of the country's saltiest, fattiest fare. Worst among the offenders are the burgers, fajitas, and appetizers, including the 1,690-calorie Loaded Beef Nachos. The Guiltless Grill menu is Chili's attempt to offer healthier options, but with only seven items and an average sodium content of 1,234 milligrams, it's a meager attempt at nutritional salvation.

SURVIVAL STRATEGY

There's not too much to choose from after you eliminate the ribs, burgers, fajitas, starters, and salads. You're best bet is the Create Your Own Combo section. Pair a spicy shrimp skewer with Margarita Chicken or sirloin and a side of black beans and salsa.

Eat This

Margarita Grilled Chicken

(served with rice, black beans, and pico de gallo)

530 calories
8 g fat
(2 g saturated)
1,650 mg sodium

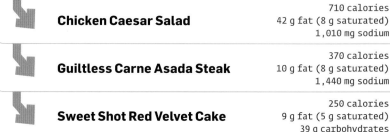

A third of the calories in this meal come from belly-filling protein, and on top of that, it delivers an impressive 17 grams of fiber. Plus research shows the anthocyanins in black beans can improve your brain's ability to process information.

Other Picks

Chicken Caesar Salad

710 calories
42 g fat (8 g saturated)
1,010 mg sodium

Guiltless Carne Asada Steak

370 calories
10 g fat (8 g saturated)
1,440 mg sodium

Sweet Shot Red Velvet Cake

250 calories
9 g fat (5 g saturated)
39 g carbohydrates

Not That!
Monterey Chicken

870 calories

47 g fat
(18 g saturated)

2,720 mg sodium

If there were ever any question about what happens when you wrap chicken and bacon together inside a cocoon of cheese, now you know: You get stuck with 90 percent of your day's saturated fat and more than a full day's worth of sodium. And that's before you add the sides.

Other Passes

1,150 calories
84 g fat (17 g saturated)
4,410 mg sodium
Boneless Buffalo Chicken Salad

610 calories
11 g fat (2 g saturated)
1,790 mg sodium
Guiltless Black Bean Burger

1,290 calories
68 g fat (33 g saturated)
163 g carbohydrates
Chocolate Chip Paradise Pie

WEAPON OF MASS DESTRUCTION
Texas Cheese Fries
with Jalapeño Ranch

1,930 calories
135 g fat
(62 g saturated)
5,530 mg sodium

Everytime Chili's gets rid of one outrageous dish, they simply replace it with another. Hence the disappearance of the Awesome Blossom and the arrival of this ticking time bomb. It's tough to decide what's worst about this plate: Is it the full day's worth of calories? The three days of saturated fat? The days of sodium? Consider each a strong enough reason to skip this nutritional nightmare.

FOOD COURT

THE CRIME
Crispy Honey-Chipotle Chicken Crispers
(1,650 calories)

THE PUNISHMENT
Swim freestyle laps for 3 hours and 45 minutes

Chipotle

Chipotle's nutritional pitfalls can be blamed on three main ingredients: the vinaigrette, white rice, and, of course, the dreaded flour tortilla. Without realizing it, the careless customer can easily construct a 1,000-calorie entrée with a combination of these staples. Still, Chipotle gets bonus points for using responsible, sustainable purveyors such as Niman Ranch to fill its fridges.

SURVIVAL STRATEGY

Chipotle assures us that they'll make anything a customer wants, as long as they have the ingredients. With fresh salsa, beans, lettuce, and grilled vegetables, you can do plenty of good. Skip the 13-inch tortillas, white rice, cheese, and sour cream and you'll do well.

Eat This

Steak Burrito Bowl
with rice, black beans, cheese, and tomato salsa

560 calories
19 g fat
(8 g saturated)
1,370 mg sodium

Whether it be by salad or burrito bowl, anything you can do to free yourself from the constraints of Chipotle's 290-calorie tortilla is well worth the sacrifice.

Other Picks

Crispy Chicken Tacos
with cheese, tomato salsa, and lettuce

495 calories
21 g fat (8.5 g saturated)
1,050 mg sodium

Fajita Chicken Salad
with fajita vegetables, black beans, cheese, and medium salsa

450 calories
17 g fat (7 g saturated)
1,200 mg sodium

Guacamole
with crispy taco shells (3)

330 calories
19 g fat (3.5 g saturated)
220 mg sodium

760 calories

42 g fat
(11 g saturated)

1,945 mg sodium

Not That!

Steak Salad

with pinto beans, cheese, corn salsa,
and Chipotle Honey Vinaigrette

Salsa is arguably the world's leanest and healthiest condiment, and thanks to the deliciously complex union of onions, peppers, and tomatoes, it's more than equipped to double as dressing. Nix the honey vinaigrette and your salad will instantly shed 260 calories.

STEALTH HEALTH FOOD
Cilantro

Found in several of Chipotle's sauces and dips (including the fresh tomato salsa, green tomatillo salsa, and guacamole), cilantro can help control blood sugar, fight bacteria, and cleanse your body of heavy metals.

HIDDEN DANGER

Chips

Hard to resist, maybe, but the chips are the single most dangerous item on the menu. Switch them out for 3 or 4 crunchy taco shells, and you'll save 410 calories and 20 grams of fat.

610 calories
27 g fat
(3.5 g saturated)

Other Passes

760 calories
34 g fat (17 g saturated)
1,590 mg sodium

Chicken Soft Tacos
with cheese, corn salsa, and sour cream

675 calories
41 g fat (11 g saturated)
1,500 mg sodium

Chicken Salad
with black beans, cheese, and
Chipotle Vinaigrette

610 calories
28 g fat (3.5 g saturated)
930 mg sodium

Chips
with red salsa

FOOD COURT

THE CRIME
Carnitas Burrito
with Black Beans, Cheese,
Sour Cream, and Corn Salsa
(1,030 calories)

THE PUNISHMENT
**5 hours of
house cleaning**

Cold Stone Creamery

"Overindulge" is the silent message emanating from every menu board in every ice-cream shop in the country, and Cold Stone is no different. In fact, its largest-size ice cream bears the spurious name "Gotta Have It." Small milk shakes weigh in at more than 1,000 calories, and troublesome toppings add up fast. On the other hand, Cold Stone offers a nice variety of sorbet, frozen yogurt, and Sinless Sans Fat ice cream.

SURVIVAL STRATEGY

Keep your intake under 400 calories by filling a 6-ounce Like It–size cup with one of the lighter scoops, and then sprinkle fresh fruit on top. Or opt for one of the creamery's 16-ounce real-fruit smoothies, which average only 252 calories apiece.

Eat This

Oreo Crème Ice Cream Sandwich

320 calories
18 g fat
(7 g saturated)
25 g sugars

Look to Cold Stone's premade frozen treats—they're almost always a better choice than straight ice cream.

Other Picks

Cake Batter Ice Cream
(Like It size)
340 calories
19 g fat (12 g saturated, 0.5 g trans)
32 g sugars

Sinless Sans Fat Sweet Cream
with York Peppermint Patties in a sugar cone
(Like It size)
310 calories
2 g fat (1.5 g saturated)
30 g sugars

Strawberry Bananza Low-Cal Smoothie
(Like It size)
140 calories
1 g fat
24 g sugars

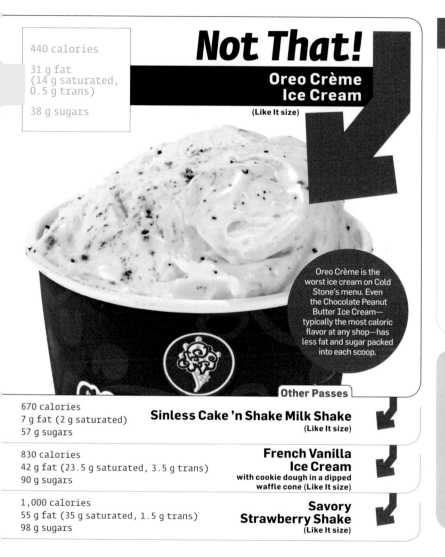

440 calories

31 g fat
(14 g saturated,
0.5 g trans)

38 g sugars

Not That!

Oreo Crème Ice Cream

(Like It size)

Oreo Crème is the worst ice cream on Cold Stone's menu. Even the Chocolate Peanut Butter Ice Cream—typically the most caloric flavor at any shop—has less fat and sugar packed into each scoop.

Other Passes

670 calories
7 g fat (2 g saturated)
57 g sugars

Sinless Cake 'n Shake Milk Shake
(Like It size)

830 calories
42 g fat (23.5 g saturated, 3.5 g trans)
90 g sugars

French Vanilla Ice Cream
with cookie dough in a dipped waffle cone **(Like It size)**

1,000 calories
55 g fat (35 g saturated, 1.5 g trans)
98 g sugars

Savory Strawberry Shake
(Like It size)

THE TOPPING TOTEM POLE

BLUEBERRIES
10 calories, 0 g fat, 2 g sugars

CHOCOLATE SPRINKLES
25 calories, 0 g fat, 6 g sugars

CHERRY PIE FILLING
50 calories, 0 g fat, 0 g sugars

KIT KAT CANDY BAR
110 calories, 5 g fat, 10 g sugars

COOKIE DOUGH
180 calories, 8 g fat, 26 g sugars

REESE'S PEANUT BUTTER CUP
190 calories, 11 g fat, 17 g sugars

PEANUTS
210 calories, 18 g fat, 0 g sugars

STEALTH HEALTH FOOD
Cinnamon

Ground cinnamon has been shown to be effective in preventing insulin resistance, which means it may help prevent the sugar in your ice cream from passing through your stomach too quickly, suppressing the post–Cold Stone blood-sugar spike. Have some sprinkled atop your next cone or cup.

117

Così

Answering the call for healthier options, Così recently unveiled the Our Lighter Side menu, which relies on light dressings, low-fat mayo, and modest cheese servings to turn some of the more egregious menu items into some decent nosh. That's a step in the right direction, to be sure, but it does little to blunt the breakfast menu's oversize muffins or bagel sandwich belt-busters, not to mention the long lineup of deleterious desserts, including the 1,594-calorie Double Trouble Brownie Sundae.

SURVIVAL STRATEGY

Get cozy with Così's Our Lighter Side menu. Only two items top the 500-calorie mark: the Cosi Cobb Light Salad and the Chicken TBM Light.

Eat This

Shrimp Remoulade Sandwich

456 calories
20 g fat
(6 g saturated)
825 mg sodium

Tuna and shrimp share a lot in common. They're both high in protein, low in fat, and make a great canvas for supporting flavors. Here, that support cast keeps the calories down below 500—exactly where they should be.

Other Picks

Così Club Sandwich
497 calories
10 g fat (4 g saturated)
677 mg sodium

Shanghai Chicken Salad
313 calories
13 g fat (2 g saturated)
839 mg sodium

Spinach Florentine Breakfast Wrap
334 calories
21 g fat (8 g saturated)
516 mg sodium

874 calories

40 g fat
(11 g saturated)

1,154 mg sodium

Not That!
Tuna Melt

Another complete waste of one of the world's healthiest proteins. What is it about tuna that drives sandwich makers to turn to an ocean of mayo and a sea of melted cheese? This is one of the worst items in the entire store.

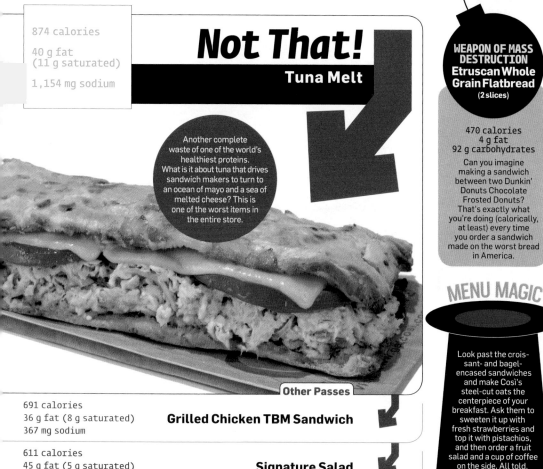

WEAPON OF MASS DESTRUCTION
Etruscan Whole Grain Flatbread
(2 slices)

470 calories
4 g fat
92 g carbohydrates

Can you imagine making a sandwich between two Dunkin' Donuts Chocolate Frosted Donuts? That's exactly what you're doing (calorically, at least) every time you order a sandwich made on the worst bread in America.

MENU MAGIC

Look past the croissant- and bagel-encased sandwiches and make Cosi's steel-cut oats the centerpiece of your breakfast. Ask them to sweeten it up with fresh strawberries and top it with pistachios, and then order a fruit salad and a cup of coffee on the side. All told, your damage will come in under 250 calories—that's about 400 fewer than any breakfast sandwich on the menu.

Other Passes

691 calories
36 g fat (8 g saturated)
367 mg sodium

Grilled Chicken TBM Sandwich

611 calories
45 g fat (5 g saturated)
664 mg sodium

Signature Salad

740 calories
45 g fat (20 g saturated)
1,491 mg sodium

Garden Pesto Omelette Croissant

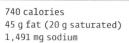

Dairy Queen

With the addition of the new 7-ounce Mini Blizzard—a perfect size for killing cravings—Dairy Queen earns its first C ever. Still, a wide array of bad burgers, horrendous chicken baskets, and cripplingly sweet concoctions leave plenty of room for error. Here's a look at one hypothetical meal: a Mushroom Swiss Burger with regular onion rings and a small Snickers Blizzard—a shocking 1,650-calorie meal with 78 grams of fat.

SURVIVAL STRATEGY

Your best offense is a solid defense: Skip elaborate burgers, fried sides, and specialty ice cream concoctions. Order a Grilled Chicken Sandwich or an Original Burger, and if you must have a treat, stick to soft serve cone or a small sundae.

Eat This

All-Beef Chili Cheese Dog and Grilled Chicken Wrap

490 calories
29 g fat
(9 g saturated)
1,380 mg sodium

Another example of a hot dog rising to the top of the nutritional heap on a burger-heavy menu. Just watch out for the fries. Opt for a Grilled Chicken Wrap instead and get a more substantial, protein-stuffed package for just 200 calories.

Other Picks

Original Double Hamburger
540 calories
26 g fat (13 g saturated, 1 g trans)
1,130 mg sodium

Pancake Platter
with bacon
400 calories
13 g fat (3.5 g saturated)
1,030 mg sodium

Hot Fudge Sundae
(small)
300 calories
10 g fat (7 g saturated)
37 g sugars

1,200 calories

60 g fat
(27 g saturated,
0.5 g trans)

2,740 mg sodium

Not That!

Iron Grilled Chicken Quesadilla Basket

A word to the wise: Anything that comes billed as a basket is never going to be a smart option. Basket means a delivery system for 400-calories of fries and hundreds of calories worth of condiments. Even without the hulking quesadilla this is trouble.

Other Passes

780 calories
52 g fat (16 g saturated, 1 g trans)
1,450 mg sodium

¼-lb FlameThrower Grillburger

750 calories
49 g fat (17 g saturated, 2.5 g trans)
1,470 mg sodium

Ultimate Hash Browns
with Bacon

700 calories
23 g fat (16 g saturated, 1 g trans)
85 g sugars

Hot Fudge Malt
(small)

BURGER BOMB

½ lb FlameThrower

1,060 calories
75 g fat, (26 g saturated)

Laced with jalapeño bacon and Tabasco mayo, this novelty burger will torch any efforts at sustaining a healthy diet. If you want the heat, ask for the Flame-Thrower treatment on a grilled chicken breast.

1,216

The average number of calories in one of Dairy Queen's Basket Meals.

GUILTY PLEASURE

Small Sundaes

230 to 300 calories

The DQ universe is awash in one dangerous dessert after the next. A good rule of thumb here and everywhere is if you can drink it, it's likely horrendous for you. If a spoon is necessary, then you're on safer ground. Spoonable sundaes are the very best of the DQ sweets parade.

121

Denny's

Too bad the adult menu at Denny's doesn't adhere to the same standard as the kids' menu, which is loaded with low-calorie entrées and sides. The famous Slam breakfasts all top 800 calories, and the burgers are even worse. Unfortunately, the new $2, $4, $6, $8 Value Menu offers up low-quality, low-nutrient meals that are cheap for Denny's to produce and easy to cram with calories.

SURVIVAL STRATEGY

Look for the Fit Fare menu, which gathers together all the best options on the menu. Outside of that, stick to the shrimp skewers, grilled chicken, or soups. For breakfast, order a Veggie Cheese Omelette or create your own meal from à la carte options such as fruit, oatmeal, toast, and eggs.

Eat This

2 Fried Eggs with Honey Ham and Hash Browns

560 calories
41 g fat
(11.5 g saturated)
1,150 mg sodium

A good approach to any breakfast diner: Ignore the house specialties and piece together your own meal from the a la carte menu. Focus primarily on lean proteins like eggs and ham and you'll end up with a meal that will defend you from hunger pangs until well past lunchtime (even if it is a touch high in fat).

Other Picks

Grilled Deluxe Chicken Salad
with fat-free ranch dressing

315 calories
10 g fat (5 g saturated)
1,000 mg sodium

Buffalo Wings
(9)

300 calories
21 g fat (5 g saturated)
1,940 mg sodium

Cheesecake
no sugar added

290 calories
23 g fat (14 g saturated)
2 g sugars

1,320 calories

90 g fat
(42 g saturated,
1 g trans)

3,070 mg sodium

Not That!

Grand Slamwich

Bacon, sausage, ham, eggs, cheese, and mayo conspire to create the worst breakfast sandwich in America. Start your day with this and you'll need to wait 48 hours before consuming another gram of saturated fat. And that's before you get to the hash browns that come on the side.

BURGER BOMB

Double Cheeseburger

1,540 calories
116 g fat
(52 g saturated,
7 g trans)
3,880 mg sodium

Care for a side of elevated blood pressure? This double stack has more than 1½ days' worth of sodium, 2½ days' worth of saturated fat, and 3 days' worth of trans fat.

ATTACK OF THE APPETIZER

Cheesy Three Pack

1,940 calories
125 g fat
(23 g saturated,
2 g trans)
3,850 mg sodium

Even split three ways, this trans-fatty triumvirate will cost you 650 calories, more than 1,000 milligrams of sodium, and 40 grams of fat... before dinner even arrives!

Other Passes

880 calories
51 g fat (10 g saturated)
1,940 mg sodium

Grilled Chicken Sandwich
with honey mustard dressing

730 calories
32 g fat (0 g saturated)
2,940 mg sodium

Buffalo Chicken Strips
(5)

770 calories
57 g fat (30 g saturated, 1.5 g trans)
38 g sugars

French Silk Pie

123

Domino's Pizza

B Sales have been great for Domino's since the company decided to roll out bolder sauce and better-seasoned dough, but from a nutritional standpoint, the concerns are exactly the same: fatty meats and oversized pies. But Domino's Crunchy Thin Crust cheese pizza is still one of the lowest-calorie pies in America. Just avoid the breadsticks and Domino's appalling line of pasta bread bowls and oven-baked sandwiches.

SURVIVAL STRATEGY

Domino's thin crust has fewer calories than any other national pizza chain's. Show your appreciation by making it your go-to order. Want toppings? Stick to ham and pineapple or just veggies.

Eat This

Chicken, Bacon, and Roasted Red Pepper Pizza
(2 slices; large, Brooklyn crust)

670 calories

16 g fat
(6.5 g saturated)

925 mg sodium

The Brooklyn crust is made with folding in mind, which means it's thin and soft by necessity. Consider it the thin-crust pizza for people who don't like crispy pies.

Other Picks

Deluxe Feast Pizza
(2 slices; medium, hand-tossed crust)

440 calories
17 g fat (7 g saturated)
1,050 mg sodium

Buffalo Chicken Kickers
(6 pieces)

300 calories
13.5 g fat (3 g saturated)
840 mg sodium

Chicken and Green Pepper Pizza
(2 slices; medium, thin crust)

300 calories
14 g fat (5 g saturated)
610 mg sodium

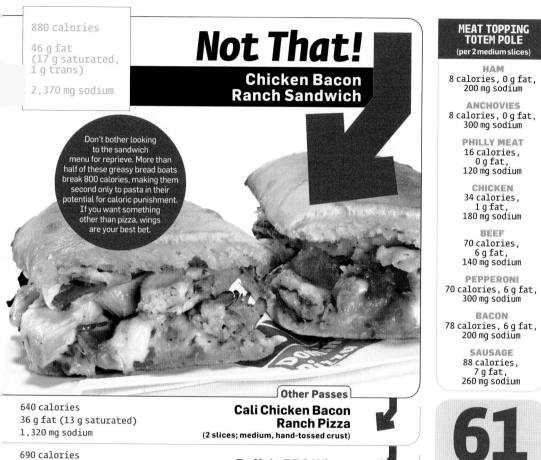

Not That!

Chicken Bacon Ranch Sandwich

880 calories

46 g fat
(17 g saturated,
1 g trans)

2,370 mg sodium

Don't bother looking to the sandwich menu for reprieve. More than half of these greasy bread boats break 800 calories, making them second only to pasta in their potential for caloric punishment. If you want something other than pizza, wings are your best bet.

Other Passes

640 calories
36 g fat (13 g saturated)
1,320 mg sodium

Cali Chicken Bacon Ranch Pizza
(2 slices; medium, hand-tossed crust)

690 calories
42 g fat (10.5 g saturated)
1,230 mg sodium

Buffalo BBQ Wings
(6 pieces)

430 calories
33 g fat (9 g saturated)
1,070 mg sodium

Grilled Chicken Caesar Salad
with blue cheese

MEAT TOPPING TOTEM POLE
(per 2 medium slices)

HAM
8 calories, 0 g fat,
200 mg sodium

ANCHOVIES
8 calories, 0 g fat,
300 mg sodium

PHILLY MEAT
16 calories,
0 g fat,
120 mg sodium

CHICKEN
34 calories,
1 g fat,
180 mg sodium

BEEF
70 calories,
6 g fat,
140 mg sodium

PEPPERONI
70 calories, 6 g fat,
300 mg sodium

BACON
78 calories, 6 g fat,
200 mg sodium

SAUSAGE
88 calories,
7 g fat,
260 mg sodium

61

The number
of ingredients
in Domino's
Cheesy Bread.

125

Dunkin' Donuts

B-

The improvements from the Dunkin' camp continue in 2010. The doughnut king cast out the trans fat in 2007, and they've been pushing the menu toward healthier options ever since—including the DDSmart Menu, which emphasizes the menu's nutritional champions and introduces the low-fat and protein-packed flatbread sandwiches. Now there's no excuse to settle for bagels, muffins, or doughnuts, which are as bad as ever.

SURVIVAL STRATEGY

Use the DDSmart Menu as a starting point, then stick to the sandwiches served on flatbread or English muffins. If you must order doughnuts, always opt for yeast doughnuts over their cakey counterparts.

Eat This

Egg & Cheese Wake-Up Wraps (2)

360 calories
20 g fat (8 g saturated)
1,020 mg sodium

Move outside the menu's concentration of doughnuts and pastries and Dunkin' Donuts proves itself to be one of the better on-the-go breakfast joints in the country. Pair a couple of these Wake-Up Wraps with a zero-calorie cup of coffee to switch your metabolism from sleep mode to high gear.

Other Picks

Chocolate Frosted Donut
230 calories
10 g fat (4 g saturated)
13 g sugars

Turkey, Cheddar, & Bacon Flatbread
410 calories
20 g fat (7 g saturated)
1,110 mg sodium

Cappuccino (small)
80 calories
4 g fat (2.5 g saturated)
7 g sugars

510 calories
16 g fat
(6.5 g saturated)
860 mg sodium

Not That!

Sesame Bagel

with reduced fat strawberry cream cheese

Remember, bagels are shaped like zeros for a reason. You'd be better off with two glazed doughnuts.

Other Passes

450 calories
10 g fat (1.5 g saturated)
45 g sugars

Reduced Fat Blueberry Muffin

770 calories
30 g fat (7 g saturated)
1,560 mg sodium

Tuna Melt Sandwich

230 calories
11 g fat (9 g saturated)
24 g sugars

Dunkaccino
(small)

WEAPON OF MASS DESTRUCTION
Vanilla Bean Coolatta
(large)

860 calories
11 g fat
(7 g saturated)
172 g sugars

This ranks up there among the very worst of the liquid-calorie offenders. Sip this and you'll be slurping up 6 Snickers bars' worth of sugar through a straw.

BAD BREED

Cake Doughnuts

Cake doughnuts are made without yeast, so they end up as dense as the most decadent pastries and levy a significantly heftier caloric toll than yeast doughnuts. A glazed cake doughnut, for example, has 100 more calories than a regular glazed does.

543

The average number of calories in a muffin from Dunkin' Donuts.

Five Guys

C Without much more than burgers, hot dogs, and French fries on the menu, it's difficult to find anything nutritionally redeeming about Five Guys. The only option geared toward health-conscious consumers is the Veggie Sandwich. The burgers range from 480 to 920 calories, so how you order can make a big difference to your waistline. Keep your burgers small, choose your topping wisely, and skip the fries.

SURVIVAL STRATEGY

The regular hamburger is actually a double, so order a Little Hamburger and load up on the vegetation. And if you must indulge somewhere, don't do it with the fries—a regular order will set you back 620 calories.

Eat This

Little Cheeseburger
with sautéed mushrooms, green peppers, and A1 Steak Sauce

580 calories

32 g fat
(15 g saturated)

1,071 mg sodium

The best way to handle the high-calorie, low-option Five Guys menu is to stick to the Little Burgers and get creative with the toppings. All veggies are fair game, and when it comes to cheese and bacon, choose one or the other—not both.

Other Picks

Little Hamburger
with mushrooms, grilled onions, and A1 Steak Sauce

515 calories
26 g fat (11.5 g saturated)
761 mg sodium

BLT
4 slices of bacon, lettuce, tomato, and mustard

434 calories
23 g fat (9 g saturated)
915 mg sodium

855 calories

55 g fat
(26.5 g saturated)

1,240 mg sodium

Not That!

Cheeseburger

with ketchup

What Five Guys calls a "cheeseburger," the healthy world calls a "double cheeseburger." Yes, even without embellishments this bulky hunk of beef has more calories than two McDonald's Quarter Pounders.

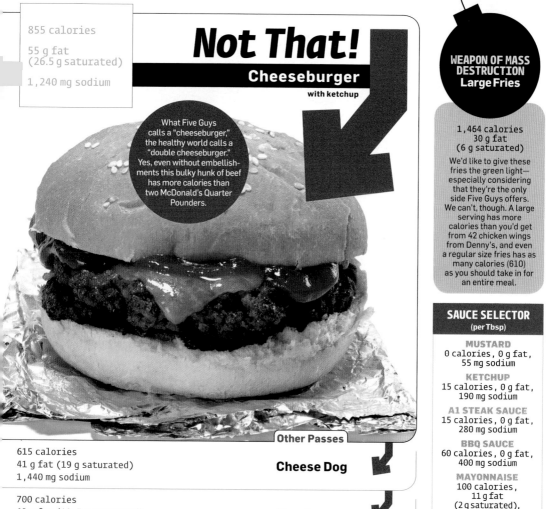

WEAPON OF MASS DESTRUCTION
Large Fries

1,464 calories
30 g fat
(6 g saturated)

We'd like to give these fries the green light—especially considering that they're the only side Five Guys offers. We can't, though. A large serving has more calories than you'd get from 42 chicken wings from Denny's, and even a regular size fries has as many calories (610) as you should take in for an entire meal.

SAUCE SELECTOR
(per Tbsp)

MUSTARD
0 calories, 0 g fat,
55 mg sodium

KETCHUP
15 calories, 0 g fat,
190 mg sodium

A1 STEAK SAUCE
15 calories, 0 g fat,
280 mg sodium

BBQ SAUCE
60 calories, 0 g fat,
400 mg sodium

MAYONNAISE
100 calories,
11 g fat
(2 g saturated),
75 mg sodium

Other Passes

615 calories
41 g fat (19 g saturated)
1,440 mg sodium

Cheese Dog

700 calories
43 g fat (19.5 g saturated)
430 mg sodium

Hamburger

129

Hardee's

C-

A 1997 purchase by CKE Restaurants put Hardee's under the same parent company as Carl's Jr., and the adopted brothers are slowly coming to look like identical twins. Hardee's penchant for oversize eats plays out most potently in the line of Monster Thickburgers. But while the Hardee's menu tips toward the heavy side, it also serves up a few more modest choices, which helps it earn a slightly less dismal grade than its big brother.

SURVIVAL STRATEGY

Choose a breakfast sandwich topped with ham or jelly, and avoid anything served in a bowl or on a platter. For lunch, stick to single-patty burgers or go for the roast beef or BBQ Chicken Sandwich.

Eat This

Little Thick Cheeseburger

450 calories
23 g fat
(9 g saturated)
1,180 mg sodium

With this burger, Hardee's has achieved what so many other restaurants fail to do: Create a ¼-pound cheeseburger with fewer than 500 calories. Remember this the next time you have a hankering for red meat.

Other Picks

2 Roast Beef and Cheddar

480 calories
20 g fat (6 g saturated)
1,640 mg sodium

Frisco Breakfast Sandwich

400 calories
18 g fat (7 g saturated)
1,350 mg sodium

Mashed Potatoes

90 calories
15 g fat (2 g saturated)
410 mg sodium

560 calories
30 g fat
(8 g saturated)
1,430 mg sodium

Not That!
Charbroiled Chicken Club Sandwich

What goes into a club at Hardee's? Cheese, bacon, and mayonnaise—the unholy trinity of sandwich toppings.

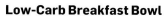
Other Passes

650 calories
36 g fat (14 g saturated)
1,620 mg sodium

⅓ lb Mushroom 'N' Swiss Thickburger

620 calories
50 g fat (21 g saturated)
1,380 mg sodium

Low-Carb Breakfast Bowl

430 calories
19 g fat (4 g saturated)
960 mg sodium

Natural-Cut French Fries
(medium)

BURGER BOMB

⅔ lb Monster Thickburger

1,320 calories
95 g fat
(36 g saturated)
3,020 mg sodium

Hardee's claims this burger has shrunk by 100 calories in the past year, but the consituents are still the same: two massive ⅓-pound patties, three slices of American cheese, and four strips of bacon.

GUILTY PLEASURE

Hand-Breaded Chicken Tenders
(5 piece)

440 calories
21 g fat
(4.5 g saturated)
1,290 mg sodium

The newest addition to the Hardee's menu is a promising one: all-white chicken meat battered in buttermilk and fried for a very reasonable caloric toll, especially when you consider these babies pack a 41-gram protein punch. The one issue is the dipping sauces: At 110 calories, the Creamy Buffalo Sauce is the best, but even with that, be sure to dunk lightly.

IHOP

F

We knew IHOP was up to no good when it refused to reveal its nutritional information back when we first asked in 2007. But we were shocked when a New York City law forced them to post calorie counts: 1,000-calorie crepes, 1,200-calorie breakfast combos, and 1,700-calorie burgers. The F is for its closed-door policy, but IHOP might not score much better even if we ran the numbers.

SURVIVAL STRATEGY

You'll have a hard time finding a regular breakfast with fewer than 700 calories and a lunch or dinner with fewer than 1,000 calories. Your only safe bet is to stick to the IHOP For Me menu, where you'll find the nutritional content for a small selection of healthier items.

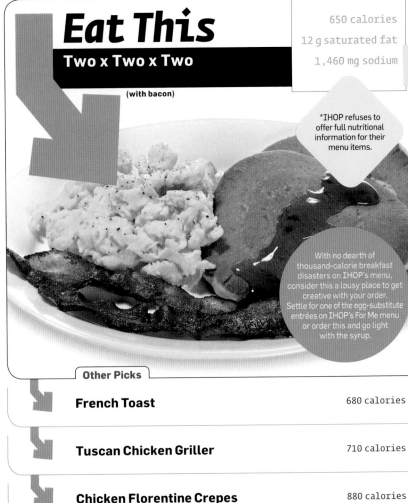

Eat This

Two x Two x Two

(with bacon)

650 calories
12 g saturated fat
1,460 mg sodium

*IHOP refuses to offer full nutritional information for their menu items.

With no dearth of thousand-calorie breakfast disasters on IHOP's menu, consider this a lousy place to get creative with your order. Settle for one of the egg-substitute entrées on IHOP's For Me menu or order this and go light with the syrup.

Other Picks

French Toast	680 calories
Tuscan Chicken Griller	710 calories
Chicken Florentine Crepes	880 calories

980 calories

30 g saturated fat

1,180 mg sodium

Not That!

Spinach and Mushroom Omelette

(no pancakes on the side)

You can make this same omelet at home for roughly 300 calories. What sets IHOP's apart? The absurd amount of cheap fats being tossed around the kitchen. This thing has more saturated fat than a half stick of butter, and if you opt for the pancakes on the side, you can tack another 450 calories onto your nutritional debt.

Other Passes

940 calories	**Harvest Grain 'N Nut Pancakes**
1,840 calories	**Chicken and Spinach Salad**
1,280 calories	**Herb Roasted Chicken**

ATTACK OF THE APPETIZER

Appetizer Sampler

1,380 calories
16 g saturated fat
2,880 mg sodium

IHOP's entire appetizer menu is a dreadful sea of beige; there's not a single option that isn't cooked in a vat of burbling oil. Skip all of them, but above all, pass on this most abominal collection of them all.

133

In-N-Out Burger

C+

In-N-Out has the most pared down menu in America. Wander in and you'll find nothing more than burgers, fries, shakes, and sodas. While that's certainly nothing to build a healthy diet on, In-N-Out earns points for offering plenty of calorie-saving menu tweaks, like the Protein-Style Burger, which replaces the bun with lettuce and saves you 150 calories.

SURVIVAL STRATEGY

A single cheeseburger and a glass of iced tea or H₂O make for a reasonable lunch, while the formidable Double-Double should be reserved for an occasional splurge (especially if you use a few of the calorie-lowering secret menu options). But flirt with the fries or the milk shake at your own peril.

Eat This

Double-Double
with grilled onion, ketchup, and mustard

590 calories
32 g fat
(17 g saturated)
1,520 mg sodium

This is more fat and sodium than you should consume in a meal, but a similar size burger down the road at Carl's Jr. or BK will pack more than 1,000 calories. Save it for the occasional answer to a raging hunger.

Other Picks

Hamburger
with grilled onion, ketchup, and mustard

310 calories
10 g fat (4 g saturated)
730 mg sodium

Tea-Ade
(half lemonade, half iced tea, 16 oz)

90 calories
0 g fat
19 g sugars

880 calories

45 g fat
(15 g saturated)

1,245 mg sodium

Not That!

Cheeseburger with Fries

Want fries with that? The answer should be a definite "no." Though these spuds may be peeled and cut in front of your eyes, a single order still carries a hefty 400-calorie tariff.

Other Passes

400 calories
18 g fat (5 g saturated)
245 mg sodium

French Fries

198 calories
0 g fat
54 g sugars

Coca-Cola Classic
(16 oz)

(SECRET) MENU DECODER

These are the most popular of In-N-Outs many off-menu items.

● **FLYING DUTCH-MAN:** Beef patty (or patties) with double cheese served with no vegetables or bun.

● **VEGGIE BURGER:** All the veggie toppings on a bun, without meat or cheese.

● **A x B:** As many beef patties (A) with as many cheese slices (B) as you want.

● **ANIMAL STYLE:** Mustard-slathered patty, topped with grilled onions, plus extra pickles and secret sauce. Also offered on fries.

● **PROTEIN STYLE:** A regular burger wrapped in lettuce, instead of on a bun.

● **WELL-DONE FRIES:** Fries cooked for an additional minute for extra crispiness.

Jack in the Box

After years of being America's Trans-Fattiest Restaurant, Jack finally threw in the towel and found himself some new frying oil. That means nearly all those cholesterol-spiking lipids are gone, and what's left at Jack's isn't nearly as bad as its previous D marks would indicate: a solid line of breakfast sandwiches, a few respectable salads, and the always-excellent Chicken Fajita Pita. Only real problem is the menu full of lousy burgers.

SURVIVAL STRATEGY

Keep your burger small, or order a Whole Grain Chicken Fajita Pita with a fruit cup on the side. For breakfast, order any Breakfast Jack without sausage. Whatever you do, don't touch the fried foods.

Eat This

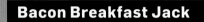

Bacon Breakfast Jack

300 calories
14 g fat
(5 g saturated)
730 mg sodium

The Breakfast Jacks are a bright spot on the menu, made even brighter by the fact that they're available all day. Take advantage.

Other Picks

Hamburger Deluxe
360 calories
19 g fat (6 g saturated, 1 g trans)
580 mg sodium

Southwest Chicken Salad
with grilled chicken strips and low-fat balsamic vinaigrette
375 calories
15.5 g fat (6 g saturated)
1,480 mg sodium

Chocolate Overload Cake
300 calories
7 g fat (1.5 g saturated)
34 g sugars

580 calories

39 g fat
(13 g saturated,
4 g trans)

770 mg sodium

Not That!
Sausage Croissant

Two simple but immutable rules are at play here: 1) Bacon always beats sausage, and 2) buns always beat croissants.

SUPREME CROISSANT
SAUSAGE CROISSANT

Other Passes

900 calories
60 g fat (19 g saturated, 1.5 g trans)
1,870 mg sodium

Sirloin Cheeseburger

770 calories
53 g fat (12 g saturated, 0.5 g trans)
1,400 mg sodium

Chicken Club Salad
with crispy chicken strips and bacon ranch dressing

800 calories
38 g fat (26 g saturated, 1.5 g trans)
88 g sugars

Chocolate Shake
with whipped topping (16 oz)

For 1,170 calories, you can have

ALL THIS

A Hamburger with Cheese, a Chicken Fajita Pita, a Regular Beef Taco, and a slice of Chocolate Overload Cake

OR

THAT

A Large Oreo Shake with Whipped Topping

GUILTY PLEASURE

Regular Beef Taco

180 calories
10 g fat
(2.5 g saturated)
270 mg sodium

Many a late-night munchie-driven diner has professed a love for the ultra-cheap tacos at Jack's. We're here to tell you that if you end up with 1 or 2 of these instead of a burger, a chicken sandwich, or anything from the fryer, you've done yourself a favor.

137

Jamba Juice

A-

There's no doubt that smoothies can be part of a healthy diet, but there's an erroneous halo of health that seems to hang over all things smoothie-related. Make this your rule: If it includes added sugar, it ceases to be a smoothie. Jamba Juice makes more than a few faux-fruit blends, but their menu has a ton of real-deal smoothies, as well. Just as exciting is Jamba's new line of satisfying, low-calorie eats.

SURVIVAL STRATEGY

For a perfectly guilt-free treat, opt for a Jamba Light or an All Fruit Smoothie in a 16-ounce cup. And unless you're looking to put on weight for your latest movie role, don't touch the Peanut Butter Moo'd or any of the other Creamy Treats.

Eat This

Fresh Banana Oatmeal
(oatmeal, bananas, brown sugar crumble)

370 calories
5 g fat
(1 g saturated)
41 g sugars

Jamba has been making a big push into the food space, and this represents one of the best new additions to their menu.

Other Picks

Strawberry Nirvana
(22 oz)

230 calories
0 g fat
43 g sugars

Berry Yumberry
(22 oz)

320 calories
1 g fat (0 g saturated)
60 g sugars

Smokehouse Chicken Flatbread

390 calories
10 g fat (4 g saturated)
690 mg sodium

590 calories

18 g fat
(3 g saturated)

55 g sugars

Not That!

Ideal Meal Chunky Strawberry

(16 oz)

Similar approaches to breakfast with very different results. Replacing an oatmeal base with sugars and granola is never a good swap.

Other Passes

430 calories
1.5 g fat (0.5 g saturated)
105 g sugars

Strawberry Surf Rider
(22 oz)

400 calories
1.5 g fat (0.5 g saturated)
82 g sugars

Banana Berry
(22 oz)

640 calories
14 g fat (1.5 g trans)
650 mg sodium

Greens and Grains Wrap

STEALTH HEALTH FOOD

Mediterranean YUM California Flatbread

250 calories
8 g fat (2.5 g saturated)
620 mg sodium

Jamba's new flatbreads all hover around 300 calories, which is just enough to turn a small smoothie into a great full meal. Plus, unlike so many flatbreads, these are actually healthy. They rely on flaxseed and olive oil to provide a tidy dose of healthy fats.

BAD BREED

Jamba Classics

Call us old-fashioned, but we just can't get behind a beverage that is made from anything but fruit. That's just what you'll find in Jamba's "classic" options, though—milk shakes in disguise.

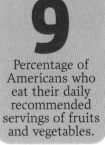

9

Percentage of Americans who eat their daily recommended servings of fruits and vegetables.

KFC

Hold on a second! KFC gets a B+? Surprisingly enough, KFC has more than a few things going for it. The menu's crispy bird bits are offset by skinless chicken pieces, low-calorie sandwich options, and a host of sides that come from beyond the fryer. Plus, they recently introduced grilled chicken to the menu, which shows that they're determined to cast aside the Kentucky fried nutritional demons of their past.

SURVIVAL STRATEGY

Avoid the bowls, pot pies, and fried chicken combos. Look instead to the grilled chicken, Toasted Wrapper, or Snackers. Then adorn your plate with one of the Colonel's healthy sides. If you want fried chicken, make sure you order the strips.

Eat This

Grilled Double Down Sandwich

460 calories
23 g fat
(9 g saturated)
1,430 mg sodium

KFC received a lot of flack for this sandwich, but the truth is it's not nearly as bad as half the burgers shooting through drive-thru windows every day. And if you get the grilled version? Well, it still has its flaws, but compared with say, a BK Whopper, it has 210 fewer calories and more than twice as much protein.

Other Picks

Original Crispy Strips
(3)

330 calories
22 g fat (5 g saturated)
720 mg sodium

Honey BBQ Sandwich

310 calories
4 g fat (1 g saturated)
810 mg sodium

Lil' Bucket Strawberry Shortcake Parfait Cup

230 calories
8 g fat (4 g saturated)
20 g sugars

660 calories

38 g fat
(7 g saturated,
0.5 g trans)

1,900 mg sodium

Not That!

Popcorn Chicken Value Box

The chicken hardly factors in to this meal. Basically you've got crunchy little balls made from oil-soaked breading and served with fried potatoes on the side. Not even the fried version of the Double Down has this much fat.

Other Passes

490 calories
31 g fat (7 g saturated)
1,080 mg sodium

Extra Crispy Chicken Breast

590 calories
31 g fat (7 g saturated)
1,220 mg sodium

Crispy Twister with Crispy Strip

390 calories
14 g fat (8 g saturated)
47 g sugars

Lil' Bucket Lemon Crème Parfait Cup

DRUMSTICK TOTEM POLE

GRILLED
70 calories, 4 g fat
(1 g saturated)

ORIGINAL RECIPE
110 calories, 7 g fat
(1.5 g saturated)

EXTRA CRISPY
150 calories, 9 g fat
(2 g saturated)

HOT & SPICY
160 calories, 10 g fat
(2 g saturated)

Krispy Kreme

While Dunkin' Donuts expands its menu to include more legitimate options, Krispy Kreme is stuck in the carb-heavy world of glazed, powdered, and jelly-filled doughnuts. Its one expansion move was to introduce Chillers, frozen beverages that can pack more than 1,000 calories into a 20-ounce cup. The good news is that Krispy Kreme has finally cut trans fat from its doughnuts. The bad news is that a single doughnut can still carry half a day's saturated fat.

SURVIVAL STRATEGY

To stay under 500 calories, you'll need to cap your sweet tooth at one filled or specialty doughnut or, worst-case scenario, two original glazed doughnuts.

Eat This

Sugar Doughnut

200 calories
12 g fat (6 g saturated)
10 g sugars

Along with the Original Glazed, this is the best of all doughnuts on the Krispy Kreme menu. In this case, "best" means "least evil," since doughnuts are pure empty carbs and added fat; proceed with caution.

Other Picks

Glazed Chocolate Cake Doughnut Holes
210 calories
10 g fat (4.5 g saturated)
17 g sugars

Very Berry Chiller
(12 oz)
170 calories
0 g fat
43 g sugars

Glazed Cruller
240 calories
14 g fat (7 g saturated)
14 g sugars

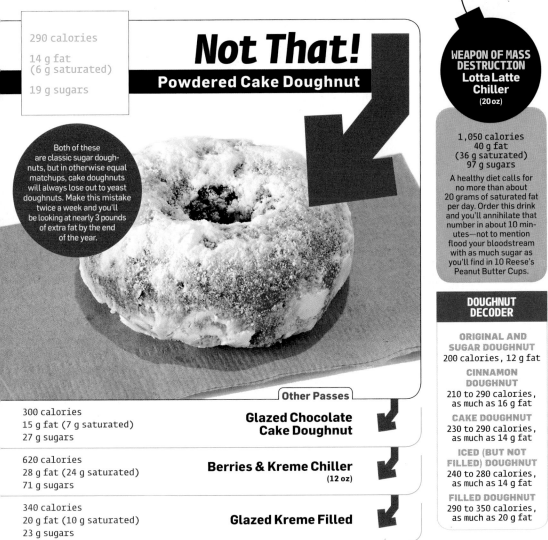

290 calories

14 g fat
(6 g saturated)

19 g sugars

Not That!
Powdered Cake Doughnut

Both of these are classic sugar doughnuts, but in otherwise equal matchups, cake doughnuts will always lose out to yeast doughnuts. Make this mistake twice a week and you'll be looking at nearly 3 pounds of extra fat by the end of the year.

WEAPON OF MASS DESTRUCTION
Lotta Latte Chiller
(20 oz)

1,050 calories
40 g fat
(36 g saturated)
97 g sugars

A healthy diet calls for no more than about 20 grams of saturated fat per day. Order this drink and you'll annihilate that number in about 10 minutes—not to mention flood your bloodstream with as much sugar as you'll find in 10 Reese's Peanut Butter Cups.

DOUGHNUT DECODER

ORIGINAL AND SUGAR DOUGHNUT
200 calories, 12 g fat

CINNAMON DOUGHNUT
210 to 290 calories, as much as 16 g fat

CAKE DOUGHNUT
230 to 290 calories, as much as 14 g fat

ICED (BUT NOT FILLED) DOUGHNUT
240 to 280 calories, as much as 14 g fat

FILLED DOUGHNUT
290 to 350 calories, as much as 20 g fat

Other Passes

300 calories
15 g fat (7 g saturated)
27 g sugars

Glazed Chocolate Cake Doughnut

620 calories
28 g fat (24 g saturated)
71 g sugars

Berries & Kreme Chiller
(12 oz)

340 calories
20 g fat (10 g saturated)
23 g sugars

Glazed Kreme Filled

143

Long John Silver's

D+ When we first started handing out grades, many major restaurants still featured trans fats prominently on their menus. But as food scientists uncovered healthier alternatives, most of those establishments switched to trans fat-free frying oils. Now, if only LJS followed suit, it would instantly be one of the healthiest fast food chains in the country, but until it does, it's one of the absolute worst.

SURVIVAL STRATEGY

The only fish that avoid the trans fat oils are those that are grilled or baked. Pair one of those options with a healthy side. If you need some extra flavor, choose cocktail sauce or malt vinegar instead of tartar sauce.

Eat This

Grilled Pacific Salmon
(2 fillets) with Langostino Lobster Stuffed Crab Cake

470 calories

19 g fat
(4 g saturated)

1,270 mg sodium

No fish competes with salmon for the crown of Omega-3 King. These fats are the most under-consumed macronutrient in the American diet, and they can improve your metabolic, nervous, and cardiovascular systems. That means you stand to lose weight, think better, and live longer.

Other Picks

Shrimp Scampi

110 calories
5 g fat (1 g saturated)
610 mg sodium

Shrimp Bowl with Sauce

380 calories
4.5 g fat (1.5 g saturated)
1,580 mg sodium

Corn Cobbette
(without butter oil)

90 calories
3 g fat (0.5 g saturated)
0 mg sodium

830 calories

46 g fat
(11.5 g saturated,
12.5 g trans)

2,040 mg sodium

Not That!

2 Fish Plank Combo
with fries

Thanks to a reluctance to part with partially hydro-genated oils, everything that gets the fryer treatment at Long John's comes out dripping with trans fat. That's what happens when restaurants put their profits above your health.

Other Passes

270 calories
16 g fat (4 g saturated, 4.5 g trans)
570 mg sodium

Popcorn Shrimp

700 calories
44 g fat (10 g saturated, 7 g trans)
1,680 mg sodium

Baja Fish Tacos
(2)

200 calories
15 g fat (2.5 g saturated)
340 mg sodium

Cole Slaw

SAUCE DECODER
(Per 1 oz)

MALT VINEGAR
0 calories, 0 g fat

COCKTAIL SAUCE
25 calories, 0 g fat

GINGER TERIYAKI SAUCE
80 calories,
10 g sugars

TARTAR SAUCE
100 calories,
9 g fat
(1.5 g saturated)

MENU DECODER

● **CRUMBLIES:**
Crunchy bits of batter thrown in with your fish—at a cost of 170-calories and 4 grams of trans fat a pop.

● **FRESHSIDE GRILLE:** LJS's new (much-needed!) healthier menu section.

4

The amount of trans fat, in grams, in the average fried fish dish at LJS.

McDonald's

The world-famous burger baron has come a long way since the publication of *Fast Food Nation*—at least nutritionally speaking. The trans fat is mostly gone, the number of calorie bombs reduced, and there are more healthy options, such as salads and yogurt parfaits, than ever. Still, too many of the breakfast and lunch items still top the 500-calorie mark, and the dessert menu is a total mess.

SURVIVAL STRATEGY

At breakfast, look no further than the Egg McMuffin—it remains one of the best ways to start your day in the fast-food world. Grilled chicken and Snack Wraps make for a sound lunch. Splurge on a Big Mac or Quarter Pounder, but only if you skip the fries and soda.

Eat This

Big Mac

540 calories
29 g fat
(10 g saturated,
1.5 g trans)

1,040 mg sodium

The Big Mac is actually far less threatening than the flagship burgers at other fast-food joints, but if you're going to order it, you should order it with a zero-calorie drink such as water or unsweetened tea and skip the fries. Instead, go for a side salad with light dressing to round out your meal.

Other Picks

Filet-O-Fish

380 calories
18 g fat (3.5 g saturated)
640 mg sodium

Chicken McNuggets
(10 piece) with sweet and sour (0.5 oz)

510 calories
29 g fat (5 g saturated)
1,150 mg sodium

Egg McMuffin
with hash browns and coffee

450 calories
21 g fat (6.5 g saturated)
1,130 mg sodium

Not That!

Angus Deluxe

750 calories

39 g fat
(16 g saturated,
2 g trans)

1,700 mg sodium

Burger purveyors like Angus because it sounds somehow superior to regular beef, but don't believe the hype. With the exception of the other Angus Burgers, no sandwich on McDonald's menu has more calories than this one.

special

deluxe

Other Passes

Premium Crispy Chicken Classic Sandwich

530 calories
20 g fat (3.5 g saturated)
1,150 mg sodium

Chicken Selects
(5 piece) with barbecue sauce

710 calories
40 g fat (6 g saturated)
1,940 mg sodium

McSkillet Burrito with Sausage

610 calories
36 g fat (14 g saturated, 0.5 g trans)
1,390 mg sodium

WEAPON OF MASS DESTRUCTION
Chocolate Triple Thick Shake
(32 oz)

1,160 calories
27 g fat (16 g saturated, 2 g trans)
168 g sugars

With as many calories as 20 doughnut holes and as much sugar as 14 bowls of Froot Loops, this is one of the worst foods in the fast food universe.

SMART SIDES
Fruit 'n Yogurt Parfait

160 calories
2 g fat
21 g sugars

Consider this a guilt-free way to indulge your sweet tooth on the go. Or sub it in for French fries with your next meal. The swap will save you 220 calories and 17 grams of fat.

FOOD COURT

THE CRIME
Crispy Chicken Sandwich and medium fries
(910 calories)

THE PUNISHMENT
Mow the lawn for 2 hours and 20 minutes

Olive Garden

D+

We initially gave the Garden an F for failing to disclose its nutritional content, and we really appreciate its effort to increase transparency since then. But when a typical entrée packs an average of 905 calories (and that's before you factor in appetizers, sides, drinks, and desserts), it's not time to celebrate just yet.

SURVIVAL STRATEGY

Most pasta dishes are packed with at least a day's worth of sodium and more than 1,000- calories, so choose either the Linguine alla Marinara or the Ravioli di Portobello; they're both reasonable options. As for chicken and seafood, stick with the Herb-Grilled Salmon, or Parmesan Crusted Tilapia.

Eat This

Cheese Ravioli

with marinara sauce

660 calories

22 g fat
(11 g saturated)

1,440 mg sodium

Besides the name and the general shape, these two dishes are identical: cheese-stuffed pasta topped with marinara and more cheese. The only other differences, of course, are 280 calories and 24 grams of fat.

Other Picks

Linguine alla Marinara
430 calories
6 g fat (1 g saturated)
900 mg sodium

Grilled Chicken Spiedini
460 calories
13 g fat (2.5 g saturated)
1,180 mg sodium

Mussels di Napoli
180 calories
8 g fat (4 g saturated)
1,770 mg sodium

940 calories

46 g fat
(25 g saturated)

2,530 mg sodium

Not That!
Manicotti Formaggio

If this book exists to do one thing, it's to expose simple swaps like this. The restaurant world is crawling with nearly-identical dishes with drastically different calorie counts. Make a swap like this once a day and you'll save 25 pounds in a year.

Other Passes

840 calories
17 g fat (3 g saturated)
1,250 mg sodium

Capellini Pomodoro

1,020 calories
53 g fat (22 g saturated)
1,880 mg sodium

Chicken Scampi

1,190 calories
84 g fat (10 g saturated)
2,680 mg sodium

Calamari
with Parmesan Peppercorn Sauce

2,220

Milligrams of sodium in the average chicken dinner entrée at the Olive Garden. That's nearly a full day's worth of salt.

On the Border

D On the Border is a subsidiary of Brinker International, the same parent company that owns Chili's. It should come as no surprise then that its food is potentially as detrimental as its corporate cousin's foods are. The massive menu suffers from appetizers with 134 grams of fat, salads with a full day's worth of sodium, and fish taco entrées with up to 2,240 calories. À la carte items, sans sides, offer the only real hope here.

SURVIVAL STRATEGY

The Border Smart Menu highlights just three items with fewer than 600 calories and 25 grams of fat each (and an average of 1,490 milligrams of sodium a piece). Create your own combo plate with two individual items, but be sure to pass on the sides.

Eat This

Chicken Al Carbon Fajitas
with tortillas, guacamole, and pico de gallo

390 calories
14.5 g fat
(2 g saturated)
1,610 mg sodium

The secret to ordering fajitas: Skip the rice, go easy with the cheese and sour cream, and make sure your meats are lean and grilled. Order this dish exactly as it appears here and you'll net the leanest plate of fajitas you've ever eaten at a restaurant.

Other Picks

Jalapeno BBQ Salmon
590 calories
21 g fat (6 g saturated)
1,220 mg sodium

Beef Enchiladas
(2) with Chile Con Carne
520 calories
30 g fat (12 g saturated)
1,300 mg sodium

Chicken Tortilla Soup
(cup) and house salad with Fat-Free Mango Citrus Vinaigrette
575 calories
30 g fat (11 g saturated)
1,230 mg sodium

940 calories

69 g fat
(24 g saturated)

2,690 mg sodium

Not That!

Sizzling Fajita Chicken Salad

with Smoked Jalapeño Vinaigrette Dressing

Basic logic would suggest that the basic fajita combination applied to a bed of lettuce would yield lower calories than when applied to a pile of tortillas. Not even close. Even before dressing, this plate of greens has more than 700 calories and an entire day's worth of saturated fat.

ATTACK OF THE APPETIZER
Firecracker Stuffed Jalapeños

1,950 calories
134 g fat
(36 g saturated)
6,540 mg sodium

What exactly are they stuffing in these chilies? Sticks of butter and bags of salt? After all, they carry 2 days' worth of fat and nearly 3 full days' of sodium.

Other Passes

1,170 calories
82 g fat (24 g saturated)
3,565 mg sodium

Shrimp Fajitas
with Classic Veggies, Tequila Lime Chile Sauce, and condiments

1,110 calories
43 g fat (19 g saturated)
2,490 mg sodium

Classic Beef Burrito
with Chili Con Carne

1,680 calories
124 g fat (38 g saturated)
2,610 mg sodium

Grande Taco Salad
with Seasoned Ground Beef and Chipotle Honey Mustard Dressing

Outback Steakhouse

Rejoice! Outback.com is now home to one of the finest nutritional tools we've seen. Go online and take a spin, but be prepared, because the numbers are bound to shock. Appetizers lurk in the 1,000 to 2,000 range, steaks and other cuts of meat routinely carry more than 800 calories, and the average side dish has more than 350 calories. Trouble abounds.

SURVIVAL STRATEGY

Curb your desire to order the 14-ounce ribeye (1,193 calories) by starting with the protein-rich Seared Ahi Tuna. Then move on to one of the leaner cuts of beef: the petite filet or the prime rib. Assuming you skip the bread and house salad (590 calories) and choose steamed vegetables as your side, you might have a shot at escaping dinner for less than 1,000 calories.

152

Eat This

Filet with Wild Mushroom Sauce
with fresh seasonal veggies

487 calories
29 g fat
(17 g saturated)
1,390 mg sodium

Want a hint on how to make everything leaner at Outback? Ask them to skip the usual butter-bath treatment. That will save you 11 grams of fat on the veggies alone.

Other Picks

Grilled Shrimp on the Barbie
(small)

315 calories
21 g fat (8 g saturated)
657 mg sodium

Teriyaki Marinated Sirloin

418 calories
12 g fat (4 g saturated)
1,815 mg sodium

Classic Roasted Filet Wedge Salad

563 calories
30 g fat (10 g saturated)
2,084 mg sodium

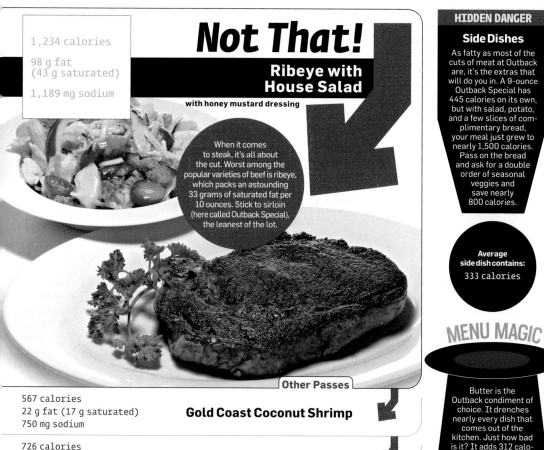

1,234 calories

98 g fat
(43 g saturated)

1,189 mg sodium

Not That!

Ribeye with House Salad

with honey mustard dressing

When it comes to steak, it's all about the cut. Worst among the popular varieties of beef is ribeye, which packs an astounding 33 grams of saturated fat per 10 ounces. Stick to sirloin (here called Outback Special), the leanest of the lot.

Other Passes

567 calories
22 g fat (17 g saturated)
750 mg sodium

Gold Coast Coconut Shrimp

726 calories
56 g fat (26 g saturated)
593 mg sodium

Victoria's 9 oz Filet

1,117 calories
76 g fat (27 g saturated)
1,767 mg sodium

Queensland Salad
with honey mustard dressing

MENU MAGIC

Butter is the Outback condiment of choice. It drenches nearly every dish that comes out of the kitchen. Just how bad is it? It adds 312 calories and 34 grams of fat to a plate of salmon and veggies. Ask for your meal sans butter and you'll save that much or more on your next order.

Panda Express

C Oddly enough, it's not the wok-fried meat or the viscous sauces that do this menu the most harm—it's the more than 400 calories of rice and noodles that form the foundation of each meal. Scrape these starches from the plate, and Panda Express starts to look a lot healthier. Only one entrée item has more than 500 calories, and there's hardly a trans fat on the menu. Gut-bloating problems arise when multiple entrées and sides start piling up on one plate, though, so bring your self-restraint.

SURVIVAL STRATEGY

Avoid these entrées: Orange Chicken, Sweet & Sour Chicken, Beijing Beef, and anything with pork. Then swap in Mixed Veggies for the scoop of rice.

Eat This

Pineapple Chicken and Broccoli Beef

380 calories
16 g fat
(3.5 g saturated)
1,430 mg sodium

With an excellent balance of protein and fresh produce, these two items are among the healthiest on the entire Panda menu. And by cutting the rice, you'll save nearly 400 calories.

Other Picks

Mongolian Beef

200 calories
09 g fat (2 g saturated)
690 mg sodium

Mixed Veggies
(entrée)

35 calories
0 g fat
260 mg sodium

820 calories

20 g fat
(3.5 g saturated)

640 mg sodium

Not That!

Orange Chicken

with Steamed Rice

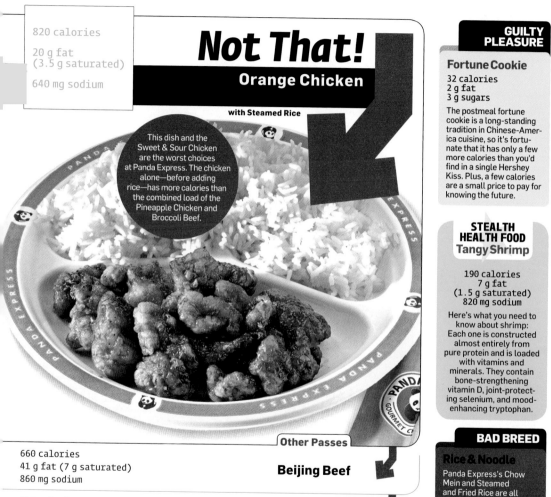

This dish and the Sweet & Sour Chicken are the worst choices at Panda Express. The chicken alone—before adding rice—has more calories than the combined load of the Pineapple Chicken and Broccoli Beef.

Other Passes

660 calories
41 g fat (7 g saturated)
860 mg sodium

Beijing Beef

310 calories
24 g fat (3 g saturated)
680 mg sodium

Eggplant and Tofu

GUILTY PLEASURE

Fortune Cookie

32 calories
2 g fat
3 g sugars

The postmeal fortune cookie is a long-standing tradition in Chinese-America cuisine, so it's fortunate that it has only a few more calories than you'd find in a single Hershey Kiss. Plus, a few calories are a small price to pay for knowing the future.

STEALTH HEALTH FOOD
Tangy Shrimp

190 calories
7 g fat
(1.5 g saturated)
820 mg sodium

Here's what you need to know about shrimp: Each one is constructed almost entirely from pure protein and is loaded with vitamins and minerals. They contain bone-strengthening vitamin D, joint-protecting selenium, and mood-enhancing tryptophan.

BAD BREED
Rice & Noodle

Panda Express's Chow Mein and Steamed and Fried Rice are all higher in calories and carbs than almost any entrée on the menu.

Panera Bread

Artisan they may be, but some of the sandwiches push into quadruple digits, and a long list of brownies, pastries, and cookies almost qualifies Panera as a dessert shop. Breakfast, limited to carb-driven confections, fatty sandwiches and souffles, doesn't improve matters. But the healthy selection of soups and salads, plus the much-needed half sandwich option, really does. (Oh, and free Wi-Fi doesn't hurt, either.)

SURVIVAL STRATEGY

For breakfast, choose between the Egg & Cheese breakfast sandwich and 280-calorie granola parfait. Skip the stand-alone sandwich lunch. Instead, pair soup and a salad, or order the soup and half-sandwich combo.

Eat This

Breakfast Power Sandwich

360 calories
14 g fat
(6 g saturated)
860 mg sodium

Ham, egg, and cheese: the best breakfast-sandwich combo known to man. This small package loads your belly with 4 grams of fiber and 23 grams of protein—enough to keep you feeling well fed until your lunch break.

Other Picks

Smoked Turkey Breast Sandwich on Sourdough

580 calories
18 g fat (2.5 g saturated)
1,910 mg sodium

Strawberry Poppyseed Salad
with Cherry Balsamic Vinaigrette

300 calories
18 g fat (2 g saturated)
470 mg sodium

Caffe Latte
(8.5 oz)

120 calories
4.5 g fat (3 g saturated)
11 g sugars

510 calories

24 g fat
(10 g saturated,
0.5 g trans)

1,060 mg sodium

Not That!

Grilled Bacon,
Egg, & Cheese Sandwich

There are two differences between these sandwiches. First, this one is built on ciabatta, which provides 50 more calories and half as much fiber. And second, it replaces the ham with bacon, which means an extra 100 calories of mostly fat.

SOUP SELECTOR
(12 oz)

● **CHICKEN NOODLE:** 140 calories, 2.5 g fat, 1,350 mg sodium

● **VEGETARIAN BLACK BEAN:** 170 calories, 4 g fat, 1,590 mg sodium

● **FOREST MUSHROOM:** 250 calories, 18 g fat, 1,150 mg sodium

● **BROCCOLI CHEDDAR:** 290 calories, 16 g fat, 1,540 mg sodium

● **NEW ENGLND CLAM CHOWDER:** 450 calories, 34 g fat, 1,190 mg sodium

Other Passes

990 calories
56 g fat (15 g saturated, 1 g trans)
2,370 mg sodium

Chipotle Chicken Sandwich on Artisan French Bread

920 calories
47 g fat (19 g saturated, 1.5 g trans)
1,750 mg sodium

Tomato & Mozzarella Salad
with Fat-Free Raspberry Dressing

380 calories
17 g fat (11 g saturated)
41 g sugars

Caffe Mocha
(11.5 oz)

BAD BREED

Signature Sandwiches

Sadly, not one of Panera's delicious signature sandwiches contains fewer than 690 calories and 27 grams of fat. The worst by far is the 1,040-calorie Italian Combo. Stick with a lower-cal café sandwich, or get half a sandwich with a cup of soup.

157

Papa John's

C Give Papa John's credit for being the only pizza franchise to offer a whole-wheat crust, thus providing a viable, fiber-rich option to pizza lovers the country over. Combine that with an innovative list of healthy toppings—including the surprisingly lean Spinach Alfredo—and you start to see hope for Papa John's devotees. The chain loses big points for its line of treacherous dipping sauces, its belly-building bread sticks, and its 400-calorie-a-slice pan-crust pizza, though.

SURVIVAL STRATEGY

There are only two crust options to consider: thin and wheat. Ask for light cheese, and cover it with anything other than sausage, pepperoni, or bacon.

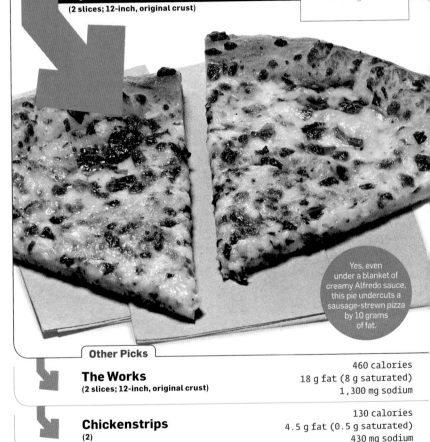

Eat This ◆

Spinach Alfredo Pizza
(2 slices; 12-inch, original crust)

420 calories

16 g fat
(8 g saturated)

940 mg sodium

Yes, even under a blanket of creamy Alfredo sauce, this pie undercuts a sausage-strewn pizza by 10 grams of fat.

Other Picks

The Works
(2 slices; 12-inch, original crust)

460 calories
18 g fat (8 g saturated)
1,300 mg sodium

Chickenstrips
(2)

130 calories
4.5 g fat (0.5 g saturated)
430 mg sodium

540 calories

26 g fat
(10 g saturated)

1,380 mg sodium

Not That!

Spicy Italian Pizza

(2 slices; 12-inch, original crust)

How bad do you really need the pepperoni and sausage? Not only are they the least creative of all pizza toppings, they're also the most detrimental to your waist line.

Other Passes

580 calories
26 g fat (10 g saturated)
1,560 mg sodium

Hawaiian BBQ Chicken Pizza
(2 slices; 14-inch, thin crust)

330 calories
10 g fat (1.5 g saturated)
720 mg sodium

Garlic Parmesan Breadsticks
(2)

P.F. Chang's

D+

A plague of quadruple-digit entrées turns Chang's menu into a nutritional minefield. Noodle dishes and foods from the grill all come with dangerously high fat and calorie counts, while traditional stir-fries are sinking in a sea of excess sodium. Chang's does have a great variety of low-cal appetizers and an ordering flexibility that allows for easy substitutions and tweaks, like the great low-fat "wok velveted" option.

SURVIVAL STRATEGY

Order a lean appetizer like an order of dumplings or the Seared Ahi Tuna for the table, and resolve to split one of the more reasonable entrées between two people. Earn bonus points by tailoring your dish to be light on the oil and sauce.

Eat This

Asian Marinated NY Strip Steak

558 calories
30 g fat
(12 g saturated)
864 mg sodium

It's shocking that one of Chang's leanest dishes is a huge strip steak, normally a heavy hunk of beef. It's also abnormally low in sodium—at least for a restaurant whose entire menu is awash in salt.

Other Picks

Wild Alaskan Salmon
steamed with ginger

330 calories
19 g fat (3 g saturated)
605 mg sodium

Almond & Cashew Chicken
with Brown Rice Lunch Bowl

535 calories
22 g fat (4 g saturated)
2,085 mg sodium

Pan-Fried Peking Dumplings

372 calories
20 g fat (4 g saturated)
860 mg sodium

850 calories

30 g fat
(15 g saturated)

10,045 mg sodium

Not That!

Wok Charred Beef

Here are a few things with *less* salt than this sodium-sunk beef blowout: 244 Saltine crackers, 40 bags of Funyuns, 175 cups of Newman's Butter popcorn, and 28 orders of McDonald's large French fries.

Other Passes

734 calories
32 g fat (14 g saturated)
1,306 mg sodium

Wild Alaskan Citrus Soy Salmon

1,020 calories
32 g fat (6 g saturated)
2,640 mg sodium

Sesame Chicken
with Brown Rice Lunch Bowl

1,288 calories
24 g fat (4 g saturated)
1,388 mg sodium

Chang's Chicken Lettuce Wrap

FOOD COURT

THE CRIME
Double Pan Fried Combo Noodles
(1,820 calories)

THE PUNISHMENT
Climb 5,824 stairs

LITTLE TRICK

Ask for your next entree "wok velveted", a cooking technique that replaces oil—the main source of Chang's high calorie counts—with stock. You'll shave hundreds of calories per dish in most cases.

MEET YOUR MATCH

1 bowl of hot & sour soup
(5,000 mg sodium)

152 Saltine crackers

161

Pizza Hut

C In an attempt to push the menu beyond the ill-reputed pizza, Pizza Hut expanded into pastas, salads, and something called a P'Zone. Sound like an improvement? Think again. Calzone-like P'Zones all pack more than 1,200 calories a piece. The salads aren't much better, and the pastas are actually worse. The thin crust pizzas and the Fit 'N Delicious offer redemption with sub-200-calorie slices. Eat a couple of those, and you'll do just fine.

SURVIVAL STRATEGY

Start with a few Baked Hot Wings, then turn to a ham or vegetable Thin 'N Crispy pie or anything on the Fit 'N Delicious menu for slices with as little as 150 calories.

Eat This

Ham & Pineapple Personal Pan Pizza

550 calories
20 g fat
(8 g saturated)
1,260 mg sodium

The ham-and-pineapple combo is one of the best you'll find at any pizza parlor. Ham traditionally has about a third of the calories of sausage and pepperoni, and the pineapple brings a jolt of inflammation-reducing antioxidants.

Other Picks

Thin 'N Crispy Pepperoni & Mushroom
(2 slices; 12-inch)

380 calories
16 g fat (7 g saturated)
1,080 mg sodium

Fit 'N Delicious Green Pepper, Red Onion, and Diced Red Tomato (3 slices)

450 calories
12 g fat (4.5 g saturated)
1,260 mg sodium

Mild Wings
(2)

110 calories
7 g fat (2 g saturated)
390 mg sodium

760 calories

38 g fat
(14 g saturated)

1,680 mg sodium

Not That!

Pepperoni Pizza

(2 slices; large, pan crust)

Ditch the little fat wheels and move to a thinner pie and you can actually get away with an entire personal pizza and still save huge calories. Plus you don't risk overeating—that third slice will shoot you up past 1,000 calories.

WEAPON OF MASS DESTRUCTION
Meaty P'Zone

1,420 calories
62 g fat
(30 g saturated,
2 g trans)
3,600 mg sodium

In July 2009, master competitive eater Takero Kobayashi avenged an earlier loss to Joey Chestnut by downing 5¾ Pizza Hut P'Zones in 6 minutes. By our calculations, Kobayashi ate his way through 7,245 calories' worth of P'Zones in those 360 seconds. We doubt you have the intestinal fortitude to tussle with Kobayashi, but put down just one of these massive meat pockets and you'll be taking in more calories than you'd find in 7 Krispy Kreme original glazed doughnuts.

Other Passes

540 calories
26 g fat (9 g saturated)
1,120 mg sodium

Italian Sausage and Red Onion
(2 slices; 12-inch)

550 calories
20 g fat (8 g saturated)
1,190 mg sodium

Veggie Lover's Personal Pan Pizza

200 calories
10 g fat (3 g saturated)
370 mg sodium

Cheese Breadstick
(1)

FOOD COURT

THE CRIME
2 slices
(14-inch) Meat Lover's Stuffed Crust Pizza
(960 calories)

THE PUNISHMENT
1,590 sit-ups at a rate of one sit-up every 4 seconds

163

Quiznos

C-

Submarine sandwiches can only be so bad, right? We thought so, too, until we saw some of the outrageous offerings on the Quiznos menu. The bigger subs can easily supply a full day's worth of saturated fat and close to 2 days' worth of sodium, and the oversize salads aren't much better. Good thing Quiznos also provides an alternative. The sub shop's Sammies are served on flatbreads and all fall between 200 and 300 calories apiece.

SURVIVAL STRATEGY

Avoid the salads, large subs, and soups that come in bread bowls. Stick with a small sub (at 310 calories, the Honey Bourbon Chicken is easily the best), or pair a Sammie with a cup of soup.

Eat This

Pesto Turkey Bullet and Tomato Basil Soup
(cup)

455 calories
18 g fat
(7 g saturated)
1,800 mg sodium

Pairing soup with a smaller sandwich—either a Sammie or a Bullet—makes for a reliably lean lunch. The possible combinations range from 305 on the low end to 700 on the high.

Other Picks

Roadhouse Steak Sammies
(2)

390 calories
8 g fat (2 g saturated)
1,150 mg sodium

Honey Bourbon Chicken Sandwich
(small)

300 calories
5 g fat (2 g saturated)
920 mg sodium

The Traditional Sandwich
(small)

410 calories
18.5 g fat (6 g saturated)
1,200 mg sodium

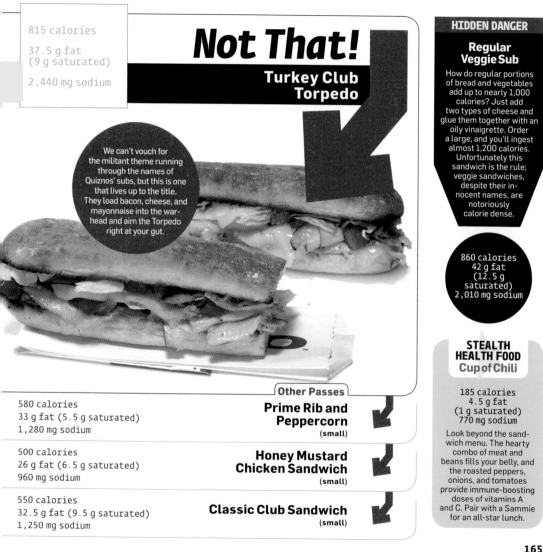

815 calories

37.5 g fat
(9 g saturated)

2,440 mg sodium

Not That!

Turkey Club Torpedo

We can't vouch for the militant theme running through the names of Quiznos' subs, but this is one that lives up to the title. They load bacon, cheese, and mayonnaise into the warhead and aim the Torpedo right at your gut.

Other Passes

580 calories
33 g fat (5.5 g saturated)
1,280 mg sodium

Prime Rib and Peppercorn
(small)

500 calories
26 g fat (6.5 g saturated)
960 mg sodium

Honey Mustard Chicken Sandwich
(small)

550 calories
32.5 g fat (9.5 g saturated)
1,250 mg sodium

Classic Club Sandwich
(small)

Red Lobster

A-

Compared with the other major sit-down chains and their four-digit fare, Red Lobster looks like a paradigm of sound nutrition. The daily rotating fish specials, ordered either blackened or grilled, are the centerpiece of a menu long on low-calorie, high-protein entrées and reasonable sides. For that, Red Lobster earns the distinction of being America's healthiest chain restaurant. The only real trouble you'll find is when the fryer is involved.

SURVIVAL STRATEGY

Avoid calorie-heavy Cajun sauces, combo dishes, and anything labeled "crispy." And tell the waiter to keep those biscuits for himself. You'll never go wrong with simple broiled or grilled fish and a vegetable side.

Eat This

Peach-Bourbon BBQ Shrimp and Scallops
with broccoli

585 calories
27.5 g fat (4.5 g saturated)
1,640 mg sodium

Shrimp and scallops are two of the most commonly abused seafood dishes in America, but with Red Lobster's light approach to this dish, you can expect lean doses of protein, omega-3 fats, and selenium, a powerful antioxidant that helps keep your immune system strong.

Other Picks

Wood-Grilled Peppercorn Sirloin and Shrimp

560 calories
21 g fat (9 g saturated)
2,210 mg sodium

Live Maine Lobster
(1¼ lb, steamed)

45 calories
0 g fat
350 mg sodium

Lobster, Crab, and Seafood Stuffed Mushrooms

380 calories
21 g fat (11 g saturated)
1,050 mg sodium

1,160 calories

58 g fat
(12.5 g saturated)

2,600 mg sodium

Not That!

Parrot Isle
Jumbo Coconut Shrimp

with rice pilaf

How is it that the pairing of shrimp and coconut—two relatively safe foods—results in such dismal nutritional numbers? Blame the bubbling fat which these crustaceans are cooked. Tack on a creamy dipping sauce and a pile of low-nutrient, high-calorie rice, and dinner at one of the safest sit-down restaurants turns into a dangerous affair.

For 890 calories, you can have

ALL THIS

Two Live Maine Lobsters, Peach Bourbon BBQ Scallops, Baked Potato and a Caramel Appletini

OR

THAT

A Traditional Lobsterita

HIDDEN DANGER

Cheddar Bay Biscuits

Just because Red Lobster gives them away doesn't mean they're free; these biscuits have a caloric price that can bankrupt an otherwise decent meal. Do your table a favor and ask your server to cut you off after one round.

150 calories
8 g fat
(2.5 g saturated)
350 mg sodium

Other Passes

1,170 calories
77 g fat (33 g saturated)
2,770 mg sodium

Steak Lobster-and-Shrimp Oscar

390 calories
3.5 g fat (1 g saturated)
3,520 mg sodium

North Pacific King Crab Legs
(steamed)

720 calories
30 g fat (13 g saturated)
1,390 mg sodium

Lobster Pizza

Romano's Macaroni Grill

B+

Before now, Macaroni Grill had never done better than a D on its report card, but an aggressive campaign to overhaul its entire menu has resulted in the most dramatic nutritional about-face we've ever witnessed. A handful of duds remain, but the majority of pastas, salads, and entrees have shed hundreds of calories or more, making Mac Grill one of the country's best sit-down restaurants.

SURVIVAL STRATEGY

Besides a few outliers (pizza, pork chops, Mama's Trio, cheesecake), this menu is relatively safe. Choose a spiedini, grilled salmon or chicken, or a pasta sans sausage or cream sauce and you'll have enough caloric wiggle room to end the meal with a bowl of vanilla gelato.

Eat This

Aged Beef Tenderloin Spiedini
with roasted vegetables

410 calories
12 g fat
(4 g saturated)
620 mg sodium

A spiedini is essentially the Italian version of a kebob. That means skewered meat and veggies cooked over an open flame—one of the most reliable cooking methods on the planet.

Other Picks

Veal Chop
520 calories
17 g fat (8 g saturated)
860 mg sodium

Spaghetti Bolognese
570 calories
19 g fat (6 g saturated)
1,480 mg sodium

Mozzarella Alla Caprese
330 calories
16 g fat (9 g saturated)
550 mg sodium

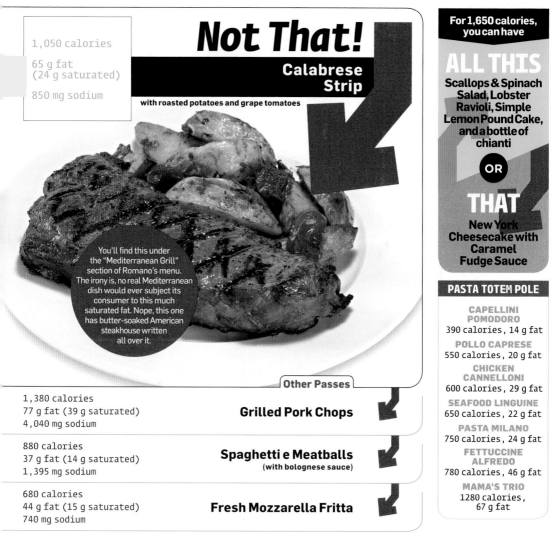

1,050 calories

65 g fat
(24 g saturated)

850 mg sodium

Not That!

Calabrese Strip

with roasted potatoes and grape tomatoes

You'll find this under the "Mediterranean Grill" section of Romano's menu. The irony is, no real Mediterranean dish would ever subject its consumer to this much saturated fat. Nope, this one has butter-soaked American steakhouse written all over it.

Other Passes

1,380 calories
77 g fat (39 g saturated)
4,040 mg sodium

Grilled Pork Chops

880 calories
37 g fat (14 g saturated)
1,395 mg sodium

Spaghetti e Meatballs
(with bolognese sauce)

680 calories
44 g fat (15 g saturated)
740 mg sodium

Fresh Mozzarella Fritta

For 1,650 calories, you can have

ALL THIS

Scallops & Spinach Salad, Lobster Ravioli, Simple Lemon Pound Cake, and a bottle of chianti

OR

THAT

New York Cheesecake with Caramel Fudge Sauce

PASTA TOTEM POLE

CAPELLINI POMODORO
390 calories, 14 g fat

POLLO CAPRESE
550 calories, 20 g fat

CHICKEN CANNELLONI
600 calories, 29 g fat

SEAFOOD LINGUINE
650 calories, 22 g fat

PASTA MILANO
750 calories, 24 g fat

FETTUCCINE ALFREDO
780 calories, 46 g fat

MAMA'S TRIO
1280 calories, 67 g fat

Ruby Tuesday

D+

The chain earned its infamy off a hearty selection of hamburgers. The problem is, they average 91 grams of fat apiece—more than enough to exceed your recommended daily limit. And now that Ruby Tuesday has finally released full sodium counts, it's apparent it's been harboring one of the saltiest menus in America for all these years. The lone bright spot is the Smart Eating Choices menu, which houses a few solid escape routes.

SURVIVAL STRATEGY

Solace lies in the 3 S's: sirloin, salmon, and shrimp all make for relatively innocuous eating, especially when paired with one of Ruby Tuesday's half-dozen healthy sides, such as mashed cauliflower and sautéed portabellas.

Eat This

New Orleans Seafood with Sautéed Baby Portabellas

487 calories
26 g fat
1,218 mg sodium

At just under 100 calories, Ruby's richly sautéed portabellas are a simple way to bring big flavor to any dish. And when the rest of your plate is covered with steamed vegetables and lean tilapia and shrimp, you can afford the extra calories.

Other Picks

Chicken Bella
417 calories
14 g fat
1,601 mg sodium

Peppercorn Mushroom Sirloin
578 calories
31 g fat
1,873 mg sodium

Jumbo Lump Crab Cakes
272 calories
16 g fat
804 mg sodium

1,465 calories
89 g fat
3,528 mg sodium

Not That!

Buffalo Shrimp Quesadilla

Shrimp is one thing, but shrimp swaddled in cheese and pressed between tortilla shells is another. Despite the healthy fillings—roasted chicken, black beans, and avocados—not one of Ruby Tuesday's quesadillas has fewer than 1,000 calories or 70 grams of fat.

Other Passes

1,153 calories 95 g fat 3,177 mg sodium	**Chicken & Broccoli Pasta**
1,141 calories 99 g fat 1,232 mg sodium	**Ribeye**
1,244 calories 68 g fat 3,456 mg sodium	**Four-Way Sampler**

Sbarro

F

Please welcome Sbarro to the list of restaurants that refuse to disclose their food facts. As of this writing, the nutritional information on Sbarro's has been "under construction" for nearly 3 years. Sounds like a pizza pie to the face of anyone who cares about healthy eating. We'll be happy to revise that grade once Sbarro cleans up the scaffolding and jackhammers and reveals a site notable for its nutritional transparency. For now, proceed with caution.

SURVIVAL STRATEGY

Sbarro serves up massive New York–style slices, so keep it to one and be sure to make it of the thin-crust variety. Round out the meal with a side of fruit or a tomato and cucumber salad.

Eat This

Meat Lasagna

650 calories
37 g fat
1,130 mg sodium

*Sbarro refuses to offer full nutritional information for its menu items.

Believe it or not, this lasagna is lighter than half the individual pizza slices on Sbarro's menu. And thanks to a generous helping of meat sauce, it also has 41 grams of protein. It's not a meal you should indulge in on a regular basis, but every once in a while, feel free to treat yourself to this Italian classic.

Other Picks

Eggplant Rollatini with Cheese

580 calories
38 g fat
900 mg sodium

New York Thin-Crust Cheese Pizza
(1 slice)

460 calories
13 g fat
1,078 mg sodium

Chicken Parmigiana

520 calories
22 g fat
750 mg sodium

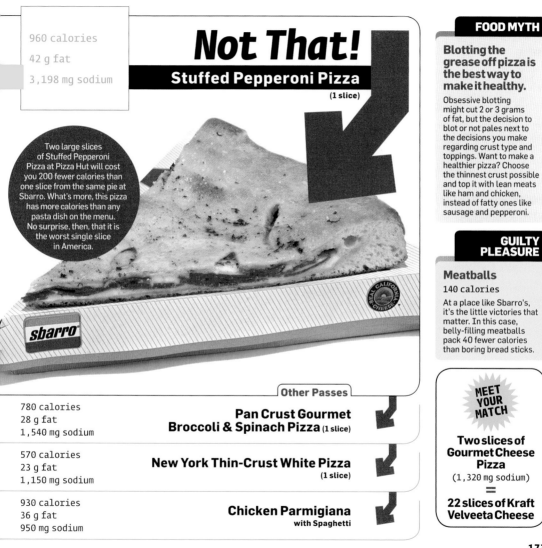

960 calories
42 g fat
3,198 mg sodium

Not That!
Stuffed Pepperoni Pizza
(1 slice)

Two large slices of Stuffed Pepperoni Pizza at Pizza Hut will cost you 200 fewer calories than one slice from the same pie at Sbarro. What's more, this pizza has more calories than any pasta dish on the menu. No surprise, then, that it is the worst single slice in America.

sbarro

REAL CALIFORNIA CHEESE

Other Passes

780 calories
28 g fat
1,540 mg sodium

Pan Crust Gourmet Broccoli & Spinach Pizza (1 slice)

570 calories
23 g fat
1,150 mg sodium

New York Thin-Crust White Pizza
(1 slice)

930 calories
36 g fat
950 mg sodium

Chicken Parmigiana
with Spaghetti

Smoothie King

Smoothie King, the older and smaller of the two smoothie titans, suffers from portion problems. The smallest adult option is 20 ounces, which makes it that much harder to keep the calories from sugar remotely reasonable. Added sugars and honey don't make things any better. (Isn't fruit sweet enough?) That being said, the menu boasts a number of great all-fruit smoothies, light options, and an excellent portfolio of smoothie enhancers.

SURVIVAL STRATEGY

Favor the Stay Healthy and Trim Down portions of the menu, and be sure to stick to 20-ounce smoothies made from nothing but real fruit. No matter what you do, avoid anything listed under the Indulge section—it's pure trouble.

Drink This

Pineapple Pleasure
(20 fl oz)

280 calories
0 g fat
62 g sugars

Or, ask the smoothie maestro to make yours "skinny," meaning without added sugar, and you'll get one of the planet's best smoothies: a 180 calorie puree of antioxidant-rich pineapple, banana, and papaya.

Other Picks

Blueberry Heaven

325 calories
1 g fat
64 g sugars

High Protein Smoothie—Pineapple

320 calories
9 g fat (1 g saturated)
23 g sugars

Youth Fountain
(20 oz)

253 calories
0 g fat
54 g sugars

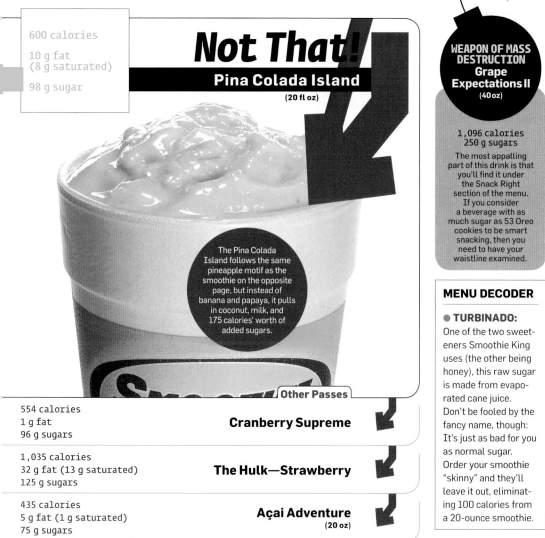

600 calories

10 g fat
(8 g saturated)

98 g sugar

Not That!
Pina Colada Island
(20 fl oz)

The Pina Colada Island follows the same pineapple motif as the smoothie on the opposite page, but instead of banana and papaya, it pulls in coconut, milk, and 175 calories' worth of added sugars.

Other Passes

554 calories
1 g fat
96 g sugars

Cranberry Supreme

1,035 calories
32 g fat (13 g saturated)
125 g sugars

The Hulk—Strawberry

435 calories
5 g fat (1 g saturated)
75 g sugars

Açai Adventure
(20 oz)

WEAPON OF MASS DESTRUCTION
Grape Expectations II
(40oz)

1,096 calories
250 g sugars

The most appalling part of this drink is that you'll find it under the Snack Right section of the menu. If you consider a beverage with as much sugar as 53 Oreo cookies to be smart snacking, then you need to have your waistline examined.

MENU DECODER

● **TURBINADO:**
One of the two sweeteners Smoothie King uses (the other being honey), this raw sugar is made from evaporated cane juice. Don't be fooled by the fancy name, though: It's just as bad for you as normal sugar. Order your smoothie "skinny" and they'll leave it out, eliminating 100 calories from a 20-ounce smoothie.

Starbucks

B+

Starbucks' signature line of drinks typically involves injecting massive loads of sugary syrup and milk into espresso, making 500-calorie concoctions too common for comfort. Plus, its baked good selection is a vortex of refined carbs. That said, Starbucks has bolstered its food program with oatmeal, healthy snacks, and better sandwiches and wraps and now make specialty drinks with fat-free milk.

SURVIVAL STRATEGY

There's no beating a regular cup of joe or unsweetened tea, but if you need a specialty fix, stick with fat-free milk, sugar-free syrup, and no whipped cream. As for food, go with the Perfect Oatmeal or an Egg White, Spinach, and Feta Wrap.

Eat This

Roma Tomato and Mozzarella Sandwich

with Grande Black Shaken Iced Tea

460 calories
18 g fat
(7 g saturated)
590 mg sodium

The new free Wi-Fi means you may be sticking around the store more, so you'll need solid sustenance. This well-balanced sandwich delivers a good shot of protein for just 380 calories, and the Shaken Tea packs in the antioxidants and a good caffeine jolt for a mere 80 calories.

Other Picks

Strawberry Banana Vivanno
(2%)

280 calories
2 g fat (1 g saturated)
39 g sugars

Nonfat Caramel Macchiato
Grande

190 calories
1 g fat (0.5 g saturated)
32 g sugars

Ham, Egg Frittata, Cheddar Cheese on Artisan Roll

370 calories
16 g fat (6 g saturated)
730 mg sodium

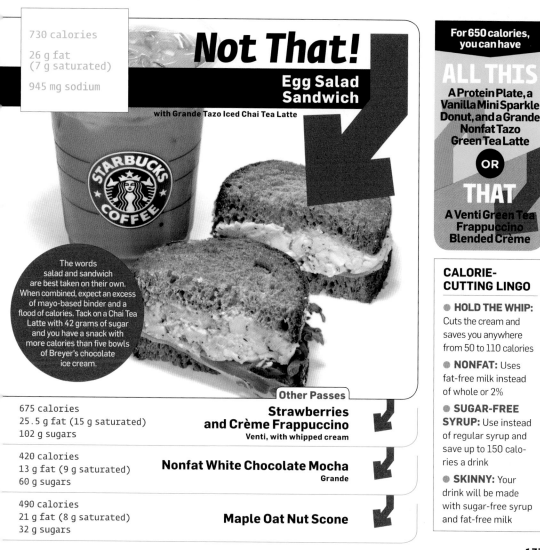

730 calories

26 g fat
(7 g saturated)

945 mg sodium

Not That!

Egg Salad Sandwich

with Grande Tazo Iced Chai Tea Latte

The words salad and sandwich are best taken on their own. When combined, expect an excess of mayo-based binder and a flood of calories. Tack on a Chai Tea Latte with 42 grams of sugar and you have a snack with more calories than five bowls of Breyer's chocolate ice cream.

For 650 calories, you can have

ALL THIS

A Protein Plate, a Vanilla Mini Sparkle Donut, and a Grande Nonfat Tazo Green Tea Latte

OR

THAT

A Venti Green Tea Frappuccino Blended Crème

CALORIE-CUTTING LINGO

● **HOLD THE WHIP:** Cuts the cream and saves you anywhere from 50 to 110 calories

● **NONFAT:** Uses fat-free milk instead of whole or 2%

● **SUGAR-FREE SYRUP:** Use instead of regular syrup and save up to 150 calories a drink

● **SKINNY:** Your drink will be made with sugar-free syrup and fat-free milk

Other Passes

675 calories
25.5 g fat (15 g saturated)
102 g sugars

Strawberries and Crème Frappuccino
Venti, with whipped cream

420 calories
13 g fat (9 g saturated)
60 g sugars

Nonfat White Chocolate Mocha
Grande

490 calories
21 g fat (8 g saturated)
32 g sugars

Maple Oat Nut Scone

177

Subway

If Jared was able to shed 245 pounds on his own Subway diet, then surely you can find a decent meal here to keep your gut in check. After all, Subway's menu houses more excellent sub-400-calorie meal options than any other menu in America. And now, with the introduction of a very respectable breakfast program, the world's largest chain eatery (yes, even larger than the Golden Arches) is seriously on a roll.

SURVIVAL STRATEGY

Trouble lurks in 3 areas at Subway: 1) hot subs, 2) footlongs, 3) chips and soda. Stick to 6-inch cold subs made with ham, turkey, roast beef, or chicken. Load up on veggies, and be extra careful about your condiment choices.

Eat This

Steak, Egg, and Cheese Muffin Melts

(2 sandwiches)

380 calories

14 g fat (5 g saturated)

1,200 mg sodium

There's no single breakfast nutrient more important than protein, and with two of these sandwiches, you'll get 32 stomach-filling, metabolism-boosting grams. Maybe that's why Subway calls it a Muffin Melt—because it's the perfect way to begin melting away that muffin swelling out above your belt line.

Other Picks

Subway Melt
(6-inch)

390 calories
11 g fat (5 g saturated, 0.5 g trans)
1,670 mg sodium

Steak & Cheese
(6-inch)

390 calories
10 g fat (4 g saturated)
1,410 mg sodium

Rosemary Chicken and Dumpling Soup

90 calories
1.5 g fat (0.5 g saturated)
810 mg sodium

490 calories

20 g fat
(8 g saturated,
0.5 g trans)

1,430 mg sodium

Not That!

Steak, Egg, and Cheese Omelet Sandwich

Subway's Omelet Sandwiches, albeit better than most fast-food breakfasts in the country, are still a big step down from the Muffin Melts. Make sure you choose accordingly.

Other Passes

520 calories
28 g fat (11 g saturated, 0.5 g trans)
1,960 mg sodium

Spicy Italian
(6-inch)

630 calories
27 g fat (11 g saturated, 1 g trans)
1,655 mg sodium

Meatball Marinara
with provolone (6-inch)

230 calories
11 g fat (3.5 g saturated)
900 mg sodium

Wild Rice with Chicken Soup

179

T.G.I. Friday's

F We salute Friday's for its smaller-portions menu; the option to order reduced-size servings ought to be the new model, dethroning the bigger-is-better principle that dominates chain restaurants. But Friday's still refuses to provide nutritional info, and our research shows why: The menu is awash in atrocious appetizers, frightening salads, and entrées with embarrassingly high calorie counts.

SURVIVAL STRATEGY

Danger is waiting in every crack and corner of Friday's menu. In fact, there are only 4 entrées with fewer than 800 calories on the menu. Your best bets? The 400-calorie Shrimp Key West, the 480-calorie Dragonfire Chicken, or finding another restaurant entirely.

Eat This

Flat Iron Steak
with chef's vegetables and mashed potatoes

820 calories*

*T.G.I. Friday's refuses to offer full nutritional information for its menu items.

Flat iron is a tasty but overlooked cut of beef. It's slightly fattier than sirloin, but you can offset the extra calories by bringing a couple lean sides to your plate. A side of vegetables, especially broccoli, is always a great choice.

Other Picks

Shrimp Key West	400 calories
Mediterranean Salad with Chicken	730 calories
Chocolate Peanut Butter Pie	780 calories

1,005 calories*

Not That!

California Turkey Burger

with sweet potato fries

This sounds like the healthy rebuttal to a plain burger and fries, but the calories tell another story entirely. When will a chain restaurant finally make a turkey burger worth eating?

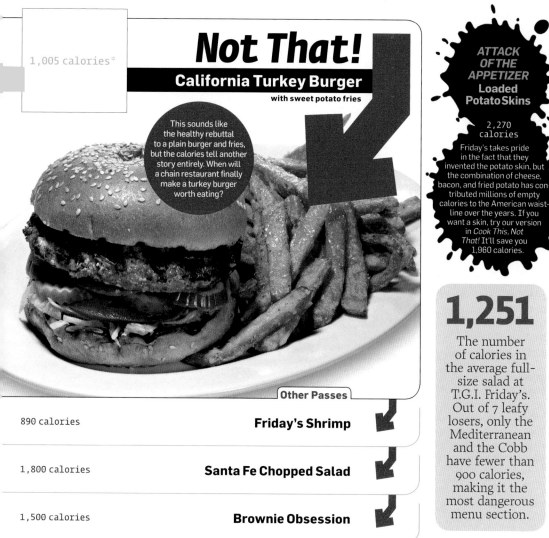

Other Passes

890 calories	**Friday's Shrimp**
1,800 calories	**Santa Fe Chopped Salad**
1,500 calories	**Brownie Obsession**

ATTACK OF THE APPETIZER

Loaded Potato Skins

2,270 calories

Friday's takes pride in the fact that they invented the potato skin, but the combination of cheese, bacon, and fried potato has contributed millions of empty calories to the American waistline over the years. If you want a skin, try our version in *Cook This, Not That!* It'll save you 1,960 calories.

1,251

The number of calories in the average full-size salad at T.G.I. Friday's. Out of 7 leafy losers, only the Mediterranean and the Cobb have fewer than 900 calories, making it the most dangerous menu section.

181

Taco Bell

The Bell made a bold play in 2010 when they began to play up their menu as a potentially healthy dieting option. A bit far-fetched, but can you blame them? Taco Bell combines two things with bad nutritional reputations—Mexican food and fast food—but provides dozens of ways for you to keep your meal under 500 calories. Stick to the Fresco Menu, where no single item exceeds 350 calories. Not a diet, but close.

SURVIVAL STRATEGY

Stay away from Grilled Stuft Burritos, food served in a bowl, and anything prepared with multiple "layers" —they're all trouble. Instead, order any 2 of the following: crunchy tacos, bean burritos, or anything on the Fresco menu.

Eat This

Fresco Crunchy Tacos
(2) with Pintos 'n Cheese

460 calories
21 g fat
(7 g saturated)
1,440 mg sodium

No question about it, this meal trumps any burger-and-fries pairing in the country. Protein accounts for 20% of the calories, and, thanks in large part to the pinto beans, it contains fully half your day's recommended fiber.

Other Picks

Fresco Ranchero Chicken Soft Tacos (2)
340 calories
8 g fat (3 g saturated)
1,480 mg sodium

Chicken Taquitos
320 calories
11 g fat (4.5 g saturated)
1,000 mg sodium

Steak Gordita Supreme
290 calories
13 g fat (4 g saturated)
550 mg sodium

800 calories

42 g fat
(12 g saturated,
1 g trans)

2,010 mg sodium

Not That!
Volcano Burrito

Want to know the primary ingredient in this burrito's signature "Lava Sauce"? It's soybean oil. Also on the list of offending ingredients: corn syrup, sugar, and phosphoric acid, the same chemical that gives soda its signature bite.

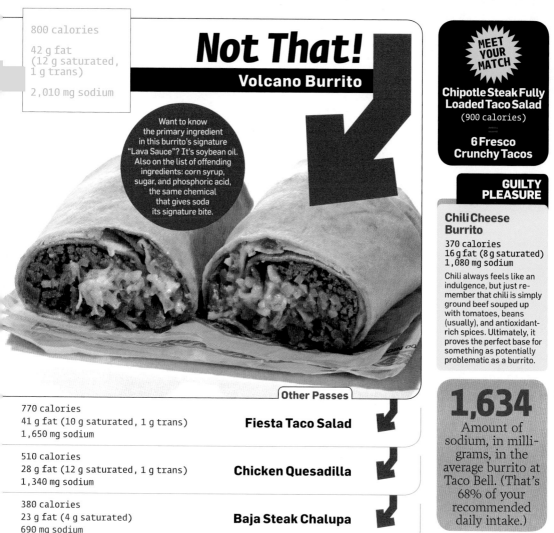

MEET YOUR MATCH

Chipotle Steak Fully Loaded Taco Salad
(900 calories)

6 Fresco Crunchy Tacos

GUILTY PLEASURE

Chili Cheese Burrito

370 calories
16 g fat (8 g saturated)
1,080 mg sodium

Chili always feels like an indulgence, but just remember that chili is simply ground beef souped up with tomatoes, beans (usually), and antioxidant-rich spices. Ultimately, it proves the perfect base for something as potentially problematic as a burrito.

1,634
Amount of sodium, in milligrams, in the average burrito at Taco Bell. (That's 68% of your recommended daily intake.)

Other Passes

770 calories 41 g fat (10 g saturated, 1 g trans) 1,650 mg sodium	**Fiesta Taco Salad**
510 calories 28 g fat (12 g saturated, 1 g trans) 1,340 mg sodium	**Chicken Quesadilla**
380 calories 23 g fat (4 g saturated) 690 mg sodium	**Baja Steak Chalupa**

Tim Horton's

While Tim brings few nutritional superstars to the table, he also manages to avoid the massive calorie land mines that dot nearly every other restaurant menu. In fact, the worst item on the menu is the 470-calorie Frosted Cinnamon Roll. Even though the calorie counts are low, the menu is still littered with refined carbohydrates, from doughnuts to muffins to sugary coffee drinks. Choose wisely.

SURVIVAL STRATEGY

More than ever, it's about the quality of your calories than the quantity. Your best bet at breakfast is the fruit-topped yogurt or brown sugar oatmeal. For lunch, choose either 2 wraps or 1 sandwich and a zero-calorie beverage, and you'll be on solid ground.

Eat This

Apple Fritter Timbits
(4)

200 calories
6 g fat
(4 g saturated)
220 mg sodium

Even when breakfast comes in tiny bites, there are simple, smart ways to slash calories and fat. Here, it means going for the more exciting flavor.

Other Picks

Chicken Salad Wrap
and Minestrone Soup

320 calories
8.5 g fat (1.5 g saturated)
1,280 mg sodium

Chocolate Dip Donut

210 calories
8 g fat (3.5 g saturated)
9 g sugars

Croissant

200 calories
11 g fat (5 g saturated)
2 g sugars

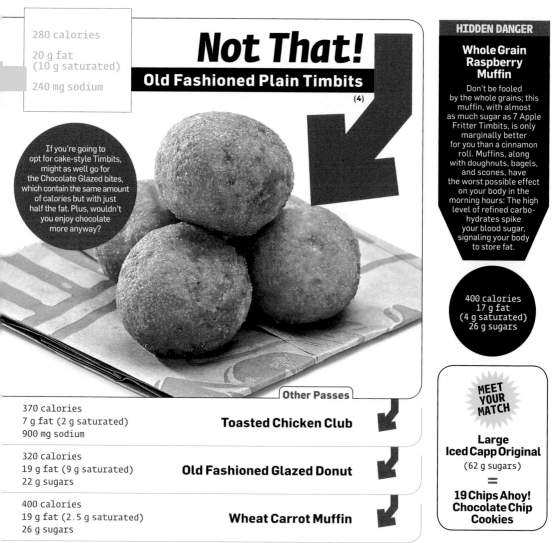

280 calories

20 g fat
(10 g saturated)

240 mg sodium

Not That!

Old Fashioned Plain Timbits

(4)

If you're going to opt for cake-style Timbits, might as well go for the Chocolate Glazed bites, which contain the same amount of calories but with just half the fat. Plus, wouldn't you enjoy chocolate more anyway?

Whole Grain Raspberry Muffin

Don't be fooled by the whole grains; this muffin, with almost as much sugar as 7 Apple Fritter Timbits, is only marginally better for you than a cinnamon roll. Muffins, along with doughnuts, bagels, and scones, have the worst possible effect on your body in the morning hours: The high level of refined carbohydrates spike your blood sugar, signaling your body to store fat.

400 calories
17 g fat
(4 g saturated)
26 g sugars

MEET YOUR MATCH

Large Iced Capp Original
(62 g sugars)

=

19 Chips Ahoy! Chocolate Chip Cookies

Other Passes

370 calories
7 g fat (2 g saturated)
900 mg sodium

Toasted Chicken Club

320 calories
19 g fat (9 g saturated)
22 g sugars

Old Fashioned Glazed Donut

400 calories
19 g fat (2.5 g saturated)
26 g sugars

Wheat Carrot Muffin

Uno Chicago Grill

D+

Uno stikes a curious (if not altogether healthy) balance between oversize sandwiches and burgers, lean grilled steaks and fish entrées, and one of the world's most calorie-dense foods, deep dish pizza, which Uno's invented. It may pride itself on its nutritional transparency, but the only thing that's truly transparent is that there are far too many dishes here that pack 1,000 calories or more.

SURVIVAL STRATEGY

Stick with flatbread instead of deep-dish pizzas—this one move could save you more than 1,000 calories at a sitting. Beyond that, turn to the Smoke, Sizzle & Splash section of the menu for nutritional salvation.

Eat This

Barbecue Chicken Flatbread

(⅓ pizza)

320 calories
11 g fat
(4.5 g saturated)
700 mg sodium

Split this pizza with someone and throw in a house salad. The tab? 560 calories a piece.

Other Picks

Baked Stuffed Chicken

360 calories
18 g fat (6 g saturated)
1,280 mg sodium

Top Sirloin
(8 oz)

400 calories
14 g fat (5 g saturated)
620 mg sodium

Avocado Egg Rolls

480 calories
22 g fat (3 g saturated)
540 mg sodium

680 calories

43 g fat
(12 g saturated)

970 mg sodium

Not That!

Roasted Red Pepper and Chicken Deep Dish

(⅓ pizza)

Considering they list this pizza as an "individual" pie, it's entirely possible to consume all 2,040 calories of it in one sitting.

WEAPON OF MASS DESTRUCTION
Mega-Size Deep Dish Sundae

2,800 calories
136 g fat
(72 g saturated)
272 g sugars

First rule of portion control: Never eat anything that can be described with a word like "mega." Even if you get 3 people to help you wolf this thing down, you'll still be responsible for 700 calories and 68 grams of sugar.

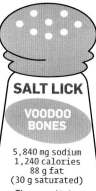

SALT LICK

VOODOO BONES

5,840 mg sodium
1,240 calories
88 g fat
(30 g saturated)

These used to be called ribs, but we think this macabre moniker is more appropriate for a dish with as much salt as 4 pounds of peanuts.

Other Passes

860 calories
58 g fat (10 g saturated)
2,240 mg sodium

Chicken Milanese

580 calories
28 g fat (8 g saturated)
2,060 mg sodium

Sirloin Steak Tips

900 calories
39 g fat (15 g saturated)
2,190 mg sodium

Roasted Vegetable Quesadilla

187

Wendy's

B+

Scoring a decent meal at Wendy's is just about as easy as scoring a bad one, and that's a big compliment to pay a burger joint. Options such as chili and mandarin oranges offer the side-order variety that's missing from less-evolved fast-food chains like Dairy Queen and Carl's Jr. Plus, Wendy's offers a handful of Jr. Burgers that don't stray far above 300 calories. Where Wendy's errs is in the expanded line of desserts and the roster of double- and triple-patty burgers.

SURVIVAL STRATEGY

Choose a grilled chicken sandwich or a wrap—they don't exceed 320 calories. Or opt for a small burger and pair it with chili or a side salad.

Eat This

Jr. Cheeseburger and 5-Piece Crispy Chicken Nuggets

490 calories
26 g fat
(8 g saturated,
0.5 g trans)

1,150 mg sodium

> Pairing two smaller items from Wendy's menu is undoubtedly the best way to go. The Jr. Burgers and Nuggets are fast friends, but try the small chili, side salad, Grilled Chicken Go Wrap, or broccoli and cheese potato, too.

It's impossible to frown while eating a Frosty.™

Other Picks

Mandarin Chicken Salad
with crispy noodles
and oriental sesame dressing

420 calories
14.5 g fat (2 g saturated)
1,180 mg sodium

**Double Stack
and Small Chili**

570 calories
22 g fat (10.5 g saturated, 0.5 g trans)
1,640 mg sodium

Spicy Chicken Go Wrap

320 calories
15 g fat (4 g saturated)
880 mg sodium

630 calories

30 g fat
(10 g saturated)

1,390 mg sodium

Not That!

Chicken Club Sandwich

Chicken clubs rarely deliver on their low-cal reputation, and that's especially true at fast-food joints. Unless it's made with grilled chicken and no mayo, expect it to be on par with the burgers.

BURGER BOMB

¾ lb. Triple with Everything and Cheese

1,030 calories
63 g fat (29 g saturated, 3.5 g trans)
1,860 mg sodium

We're all for big doses of protein, but does one really need a burger made with 12 ounces of meat? In exchange, you give up half a day of calories, a full day of fat, and nearly two days of cholesterol-spiking trans fats.

MENU MAGIC

Your perfect burger is just a few strategic modifications away. Here's an example: A ¼-lb. Single, as served, contains 430 calories. But if you eliminate the mayo, swap out the cheese for a junior cheese serving, and tell them to serve it on a regular-size burger bun—the one typically reserved for Jr. Burgers—you'll cut it down to 320 calories.

Other Passes

790 calories
53.5 g fat (13.5 g saturated)
1,665 mg sodium

Chicken BLT Salad
with homestyle garlic croutons
and honey Dijon dressing

700 calories
40 g fat (17 g saturated, 2 g trans)
1,440 mg sodium

Double Cheeseburger
with everything

550 calories
18 g fat (3.5 g saturated)
2,530 mg sodium

Sweet & Spicy Asian Chicken Boneless Wings

189

Chapter 4

AT THE SUPERMARKET

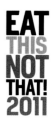

Quantum physics.

Middle East politics. BP's environmental policies.

What do these three things have in common? Each of them is easier to grasp than the average American supermarket.

No matter how meticulously edited our shopping lists are, it's hard not to be overwhelmed the minute we set foot into the electric blue fluorescent glow of the grocery store. More than 50,000 packaged goods line the shelves of the average supermarket, and that's before you take into account the meat, fish, deli, and cheese counters; the produce section, with its exotic greens and 30 different kinds of apples; the precooked quickie dinner area; and the little server with the latex gloves offering a taste of chorizo and bourbon mustard or whatever else they're pushing that day. Go in with a plan to buy 35 items, and you'll come out with 50 of them—and wonder the next day how they ever crept into your kitchen.

And the power of supermarkets (and, um, supermarketers) to have their way with us has never been greater. A February 2009 poll by

MINTEL found that 79 percent of Americans say they're trying to eat at home more, to save money. But are we saving? An April 2009 survey by *Better Homes and Gardens* found that women were spending $34 more every single week at the supermarket. Why? In part because food manufacturers are so sneaky about the ways they trick us into buying their products. That's why it's important for your wallet—and the part of your body that sits on it—to be smart about supermarket strategies.

Nobody wants to have to exercise discipline every time they go on a shopping trip, especially when it comes to the visceral happiness that food can bring us. Yet giving in to temptation or bad judgment at the supermarket can have consequences that last a lifetime. Because we're creatures of habit, we tend to simply grab the same brands every time we hit the store. That's fine, as long as we've chosen wisely. But the wrong choices can cost us thousands, maybe tens of thousands, of calories every year.

Consider this: Let's say that every night you have a modest dessert of two cookies, and your favorite is Oreo Cakesters Chocolate Crème. That means every night you're taking in 250 calories for dessert. Not a terrible nutritional crime by any means—more like a misdemeanor. But if your regular choice was Oreo Fudgees instead of the Cakesters, and you ate the same two cookies every night, by the end of a year you would have saved yourself more than 40,000 calories—the equivalent of a whopping 11½ pounds.

Amazing, right? But every single choice you make in the supermarket comes with the same potential long-term consequences. Think of all the things you and your family consume on a daily or weekly basis—staples like peanut butter, bread, nacho chips, canned fruit, salad dressings, and ice cream. Each choice can add an unnecessary 10, 50, 100 calories or more to your day—and that can very quickly add up. (Imagine those calories were dollars. You'd want to know if you were spending 100 extra dollars every day on something you didn't have to, right?)

So in this chapter, we've surveyed the supermarket shelves and found caloric savings here, there, and everywhere. Some are little savings; some are dramatic, however, and you will be shocked by how quickly and easily they will change your life. Regardless, start rewriting your shopping list—and try these strategies to better stick to it.

STRATEGY #1

STAY AWAY FROM THE SOFT, CREAMY CENTER. That would be the soft, creamy center of the supermarket—aisles 3 through 11 in most grocery stores. While the healthy stuff like dairy, produce, meat, and seafood is usually located around the edges, the interior of the supermarket is almost always packed with highly processed foods made with corn and soy and the 3,000 or more additives manufacturers use to make things that are edible but aren't actually food.

STRATEGY #2

AVERT YOUR EYES! On any grocery shelf, the most highly processed, most caloric, and often most highly priced products are about 5 feet off the ground. Why? Because that's about where your eyes are. That's very valuable real estate, and since supermarkets charge manufacturers for that placement, you can bet that the food marketers are figuring out a way to pass that cost on to you—either by trimming nutrition or amping up cost, or both. Reach up and kneel down, and you'll find both price points and nutrition labels that make a lot more sense.

STRATEGY #3

GET BACK TO THE EARTH. On one hand, we have an apple, a chicken, and a potato. On the other hand, a jar of applesauce, a bag of chicken nuggets, and some chips. Which hand is healthier?

Pretty simple, right? The apple has more nutrients than the sauce, the chicken has fewer carbohydrates than the nuggets, and the potato has less fat than the chips. And the apple/chicken/potato hand is a lot cheaper, too. It's a simple rule: The closer food is to its natural form, the healthier it is for you. So until they start growing apples inside little plastic containers, stick with what Mother Nature gave you.

STRATEGY #4

EAT MORE FOOD, EAT FEWER INGREDIENTS. Another important thing to keep in mind: the fewer ingredients, the better something typically is for you. (Foods with five or fewer deserve a special place in your pantry.) When apples turn into applesauce, they can often double their caloric load because of the addition of high-fructose corn syrup (HFCS). Which would you rather eat: an apple, or a combination of apples, water, and HFCS for twice the calories?

STRATEGY #5

WATCH WHO'S ON FIRST. Reading an ingredients label is like reading a baseball box score: It has plenty of information, but you need to understand what the stats mean. If you know what OBP and ERA mean, you have a good understanding of what's happening in the game. If not, a box score just reads like a bunch of gibberish.

Nutrition labels are the same. There are two things to keep an eye on: The first is the order of ingredients—labels by law must list them in order of volume. So if the number one ingredient is, say, "spinach," that's good. If it's "sugar" or "high-fructose corn syrup" or "canary droppings," that's probably bad. The second thing to look at is the servings per container. You'd be amazed by how a 200-calorie dish really becomes a 400-calorie dish when the little tiny dish supposedly contains two servings—even though you know you're going to eat the whole thing.

STRATEGY #6

ELIMINATE THE DRIVE-BY. A recent study found that shoppers who made "quick trips" to the store end up spending 54 percent more on groceries than they had planned. Instead, be smart about your trips. Bring a list—and a pen to cross off what you've already dropped into your cart. And try doing your shopping on Wednesday evening—that's when supermarkets are the most abandoned. This means a shorter trip and less time in the checkout aisle, eyeing the latest Jen/Brad/Angie brouhaha and those enticing little chocolate-covered crispy crackers that you don't mean to buy, but the kids are complaining and you're hungry and . . .

Log on to
EATTHIS.COM for
more fat-melting,
health-boosting,
money-saving tips.

Cereal
Eat This

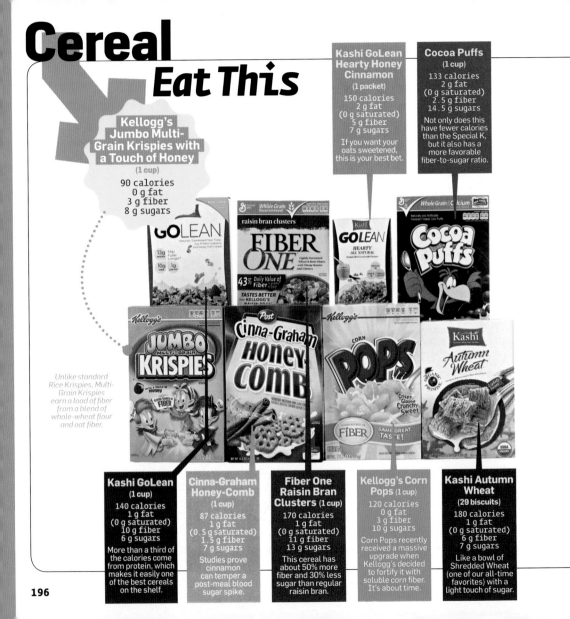

Kashi GoLean Hearty Honey Cinnamon
(1 packet)

150 calories
2 g fat
(0 g saturated)
5 g fiber
7 g sugars

If you want your oats sweetened, this is your best bet.

Cocoa Puffs
(1 cup)

133 calories
2 g fat
(0 g saturated)
2.5 g fiber
14.5 g sugars

Not only does this have fewer calories than the Special K, but it also has a more favorable fiber-to-sugar ratio.

Kellogg's Jumbo Multi-Grain Krispies with a Touch of Honey
(1 cup)

90 calories
0 g fat
3 g fiber
8 g sugars

Unlike standard Rice Krispies, Multi-Grain Krispies earn a load of fiber from a blend of whole-wheat flour and oat fiber.

Kashi GoLean
(1 cup)

140 calories
1 g fat
(0 g saturated)
10 g fiber
6 g sugars

More than a third of the calories come from protein, which makes it easily one of the best cereals on the shelf.

Cinna-Graham Honey-Comb
(1 cup)

87 calories
1 g fat
(0.5 g saturated)
1.5 g fiber
7 g sugars

Studies prove cinnamon can temper a post-meal blood sugar spike.

Fiber One Raisin Bran Clusters (1 cup)

170 calories
1 g fat
(0 g saturated)
11 g fiber
13 g sugars

This cereal has about 50% more fiber and 30% less sugar than regular raisin bran.

Kellogg's Corn Pops (1 cup)

120 calories
0 g fat
(0 g saturated)
3 g fiber
10 g sugars

Corn Pops recently received a massive upgrade when Kellogg's decided to fortify it with soluble corn fiber. It's about time.

Kashi Autumn Wheat
(29 biscuits)

180 calories
1 g fat
(0 g saturated)
6 g fiber
7 g sugars

Like a bowl of Shredded Wheat (one of our all-time favorites) with a light touch of sugar.

Not That!

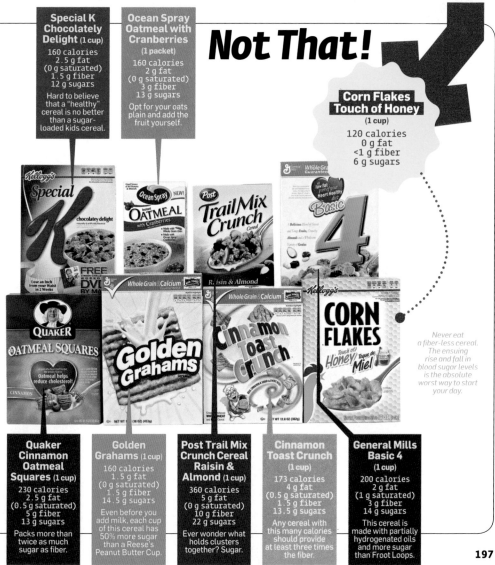

Special K Chocolately Delight (1 cup)

160 calories
2.5 g fat
(0 g saturated)
1.5 g fiber
12 g sugars

Hard to believe that a "healthy" cereal is no better than a sugar-loaded kids cereal.

Ocean Spray Oatmeal with Cranberries (1 packet)

160 calories
2 g fat
(0 g saturated)
3 g fiber
13 g sugars

Opt for your oats plain and add the fruit yourself.

Corn Flakes Touch of Honey (1 cup)

120 calories
0 g fat
<1 g fiber
6 g sugars

Never eat a fiber-less cereal. The ensuing rise and fall in blood sugar levels is the absolute worst way to start your day.

Quaker Cinnamon Oatmeal Squares (1 cup)

230 calories
2.5 g fat
(0.5 g saturated)
5 g fiber
13 g sugars

Packs more than twice as much sugar as fiber.

Golden Grahams (1 cup)

160 calories
1.5 g fat
(0 g saturated)
1.5 g fiber
14.5 g sugars

Even before you add milk, each cup of this cereal has 50% more sugar than a Reese's Peanut Butter Cup.

Post Trail Mix Crunch Cereal Raisin & Almond (1 cup)

360 calories
5 g fat
(0 g saturated)
10 g fiber
22 g sugars

Ever wonder what holds clusters together? Sugar.

Cinnamon Toast Crunch (1 cup)

173 calories
4 g fat
(0.5 g saturated)
1.5 g fiber
13.5 g sugars

Any cereal with this many calories should provide at least three times the fiber.

General Mills Basic 4 (1 cup)

200 calories
2 g fat
(1 g saturated)
3 g fiber
14 g sugars

This cereal is made with partially hydrogenated oils and more sugar than Froot Loops.

Breakfast Breads
Eat This

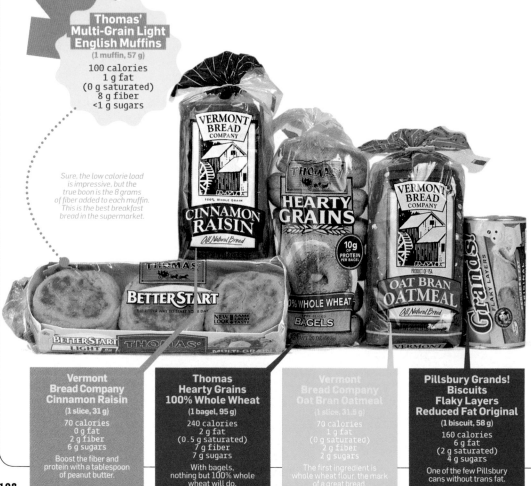

**Thomas'
Multi-Grain Light
English Muffins**

(1 muffin, 57 g)

100 calories
1 g fat
(0 g saturated)
8 g fiber
<1 g sugars

*Sure, the low calorie load
is impressive, but the
true boon is the 8 grams
of fiber added to each muffin.
This is the best breakfast
bread in the supermarket.*

**Vermont
Bread Company
Cinnamon Raisin**

(1 slice, 31 g)

70 calories
0 g fat
2 g fiber
6 g sugars

Boost the fiber and
protein with a tablespoon
of peanut butter.

**Thomas
Hearty Grains
100% Whole Wheat**

(1 bagel, 95 g)

240 calories
2 g fat
(0.5 g saturated)
7 g fiber
7 g sugars

With bagels,
nothing but 100% whole
wheat will do.

**Vermont
Bread Company
Oat Bran Oatmeal**

(1 slice, 31.5 g)

70 calories
1 g fat
(0 g saturated)
2 g fiber
2 g sugars

The first ingredient is
whole wheat flour, the mark
of a great bread.

**Pillsbury Grands!
Biscuits
Flaky Layers
Reduced Fat Original**

(1 biscuit, 58 g)

160 calories
6 g fat
(2 g saturated)
4 g sugars

One of the few Pillsbury
cans without trans fat.

Not That!

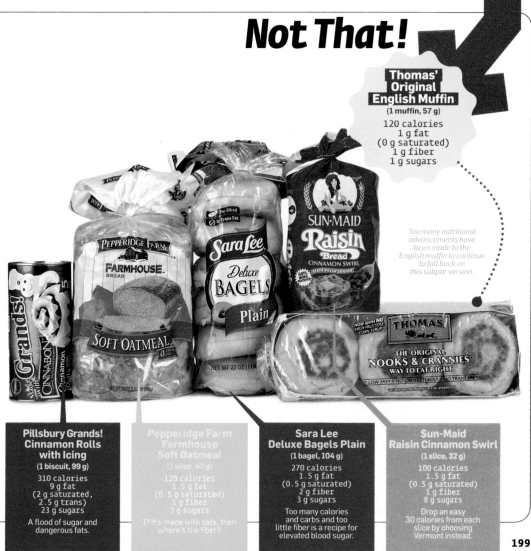

**Thomas'
Original
English Muffin**
(1 muffin, 57 g)

120 calories
1 g fat
(0 g saturated)
1 g fiber
1 g sugars

*Too many nutritional
advancements have
been made to the
English muffin to continue
to fall back on
this subpar version.*

**Pillsbury Grands!
Cinnamon Rolls
with Icing**
(1 biscuit, 99 g)

310 calories
9 g fat
(2 g saturated,
2.5 g trans)
23 g sugars

A flood of sugar and
dangerous fats.

**Pepperidge Farm
Farmhouse
Soft Oatmeal**
(1 slice, 43 g)

120 calories
1.5 g fat
(0.5 g saturated)
1 g fiber
3 g sugars

If it's made with oats, then
where's the fiber?

**Sara Lee
Deluxe Bagels Plain**
(1 bagel, 104 g)

270 calories
1.5 g fat
(0.5 g saturated)
2 g fiber
3 g sugars

Too many calories
and carbs and too
little fiber is a recipe for
elevated blood sugar.

**Sun-Maid
Raisin Cinnamon Swirl**
(1 slice, 32 g)

100 calories
1.5 g fat
(0.5 g saturated)
1 g fiber
8 g sugars

Drop an easy
30 calories from each
slice by choosing
Vermont instead.

199

Yogurt
Eat This

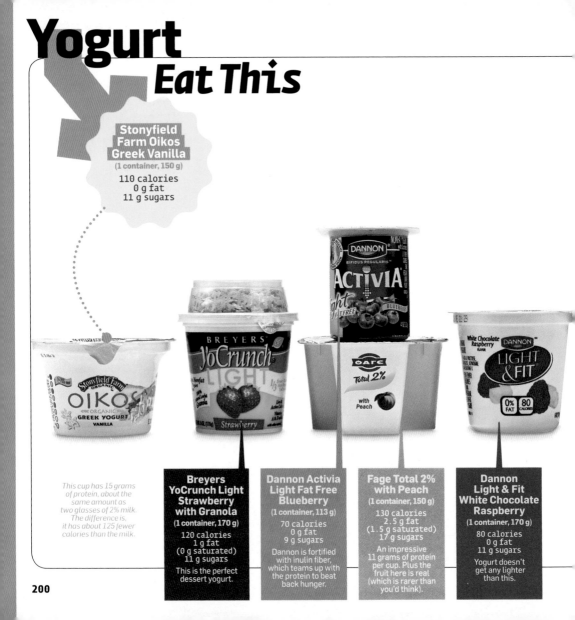

Stonyfield Farm Oikos Greek Vanilla
(1 container, 150 g)

110 calories
0 g fat
11 g sugars

This cup has 15 grams of protein, about the same amount as two glasses of 2% milk. The difference is, it has about 125 fewer calories than the milk.

Breyers YoCrunch Light Strawberry with Granola
(1 container, 170 g)

120 calories
1 g fat
(0 g saturated)
11 g sugars

This is the perfect dessert yogurt.

Dannon Activia Light Fat Free Blueberry
(1 container, 113 g)

70 calories
0 g fat
9 g sugars

Dannon is fortified with inulin fiber, which teams up with the protein to beat back hunger.

Fage Total 2% with Peach
(1 container, 150 g)

130 calories
2.5 g fat
(1.5 g saturated)
17 g sugars

An impressive 11 grams of protein per cup. Plus the fruit here is real (which is rarer than you'd think).

Dannon Light & Fit White Chocolate Raspberry
(1 container, 170 g)

80 calories
0 g fat
11 g sugars

Yogurt doesn't get any lighter than this.

Not That!

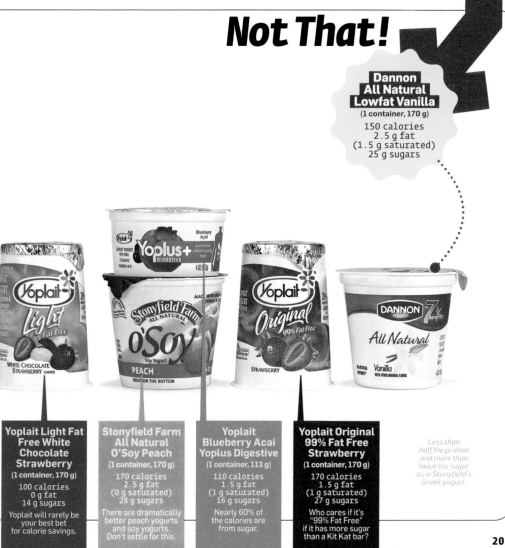

Dannon All Natural Lowfat Vanilla

(1 container, 170 g)

150 calories
2.5 g fat
(1.5 g saturated)
25 g sugars

Yoplait Light Fat Free White Chocolate Strawberry

(1 container, 170 g)

100 calories
0 g fat
14 g sugars

Yoplait will rarely be your best bet for calorie savings.

Stonyfield Farm All Natural O'Soy Peach

(1 container, 170 g)

170 calories
2.5 g fat
(0 g saturated)
28 g sugars

There are dramatically better peach yogurts and soy yogurts. Don't settle for this.

Yoplait Blueberry Acai Yoplus Digestive

(1 container, 113 g)

110 calories
1.5 g fat
(1 g saturated)
16 g sugars

Nearly 60% of the calories are from sugar.

Yoplait Original 99% Fat Free Strawberry

(1 container, 170 g)

170 calories
1.5 g fat
(1 g saturated)
27 g sugars

Who cares if it's "99% Fat Free" if it has more sugar than a Kit Kat bar?

Less than half the protein and more than twice the sugar as in Stonyfield's Greek yogurt.

Cheese
Eat This

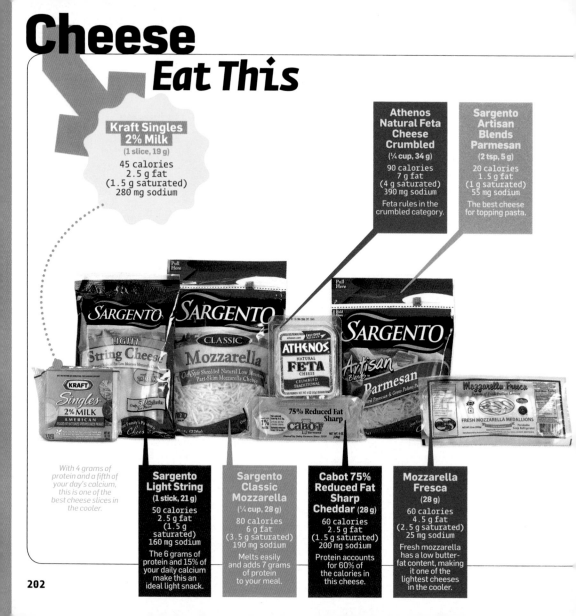

Kraft Singles 2% Milk
(1 slice, 19 g)
45 calories
2.5 g fat
(1.5 g saturated)
280 mg sodium

Athenos Natural Feta Cheese Crumbled
(¼ cup, 34 g)
90 calories
7 g fat
(4 g saturated)
390 mg sodium

Feta rules in the crumbled category.

Sargento Artisan Blends Parmesan
(2 tsp, 5 g)
20 calories
1.5 g fat
(1 g saturated)
55 mg sodium

The best cheese for topping pasta.

With 4 grams of protein and a fifth of your day's calcium, this is one of the best cheese slices in the cooler.

Sargento Light String
(1 stick, 21 g)
50 calories
2.5 g fat
(1.5 g saturated)
160 mg sodium

The 6 grams of protein and 15% of your daily calcium make this an ideal light snack.

Sargento Classic Mozzarella
(¼ cup, 28 g)
80 calories
6 g fat
(3.5 g saturated)
190 mg sodium

Melts easily and adds 7 grams of protein to your meal.

Cabot 75% Reduced Fat Sharp Cheddar (28 g)
60 calories
2.5 g fat
(1.5 g saturated)
200 mg sodium

Protein accounts for 60% of the calories in this cheese.

Mozzarella Fresca
(28 g)
60 calories
4.5 g fat
(2.5 g saturated)
25 mg sodium

Fresh mozzarella has a low butter-fat content, making it one of the lightest cheeses in the cooler.

Not That!

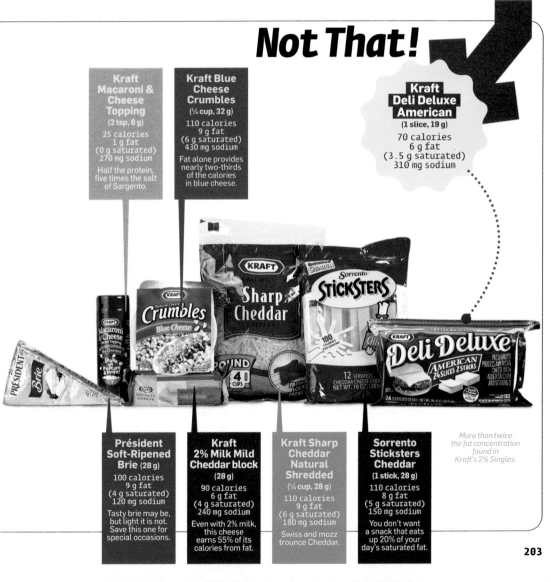

Kraft Macaroni & Cheese Topping (2 tsp, 6 g)

25 calories
1 g fat
(0 g saturated)
270 mg sodium

Half the protein, five times the salt of Sargento.

Kraft Blue Cheese Crumbles (¼ cup, 32 g)

110 calories
9 g fat
(6 g saturated)
430 mg sodium

Fat alone provides nearly two-thirds of the calories in blue cheese.

Kraft Deli Deluxe American (1 slice, 19 g)

70 calories
6 g fat
(3.5 g saturated)
310 mg sodium

Président Soft-Ripened Brie (28 g)

100 calories
9 g fat
(4 g saturated)
120 mg sodium

Tasty brie may be, but light it is not. Save this one for special occasions.

Kraft 2% Milk Mild Cheddar block (28 g)

90 calories
6 g fat
(4 g saturated)
240 mg sodium

Even with 2% milk, this cheese earns 55% of its calories from fat.

Kraft Sharp Cheddar Natural Shredded (¼ cup, 28 g)

110 calories
9 g fat
(6 g saturated)
180 mg sodium

Swiss and mozz trounce Cheddar.

Sorrento Sticksters Cheddar (1 stick, 28 g)

110 calories
8 g fat
(5 g saturated)
150 mg sodium

You don't want a snack that eats up 20% of your day's saturated fat.

More than twice the fat concentration found in Kraft's 2% Singles.

Deli Meats
Eat This

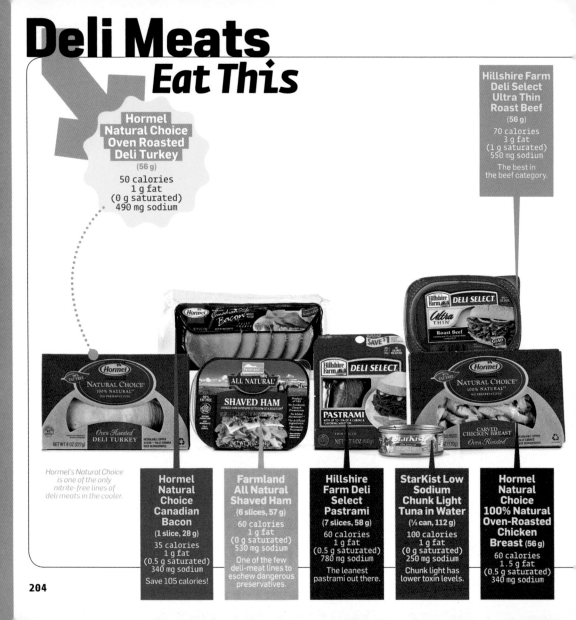

Hormel Natural Choice Oven Roasted Deli Turkey
(56 g)

50 calories
1 g fat
(0 g saturated)
490 mg sodium

Hillshire Farm Deli Select Ultra Thin Roast Beef
(56 g)

70 calories
3 g fat
(1 g saturated)
550 mg sodium

The best in the beef category.

Hormel's Natural Choice is one of the only nitrite-free lines of deli meats in the cooler.

Hormel Natural Choice Canadian Bacon
(1 slice, 28 g)

35 calories
1 g fat
(0.5 g saturated)
340 mg sodium

Save 105 calories!

Farmland All Natural Shaved Ham
(6 slices, 57 g)

60 calories
1 g fat
(0 g saturated)
530 mg sodium

One of the few deli-meat lines to eschew dangerous preservatives.

Hillshire Farm Deli Select Pastrami
(7 slices, 58 g)

60 calories
1 g fat
(0.5 g saturated)
780 mg sodium

The leanest pastrami out there.

StarKist Low Sodium Chunk Light Tuna in Water
(½ can, 112 g)

100 calories
1 g fat
(0 g saturated)
250 mg sodium

Chunk light has lower toxin levels.

Hormel Natural Choice 100% Natural Oven-Roasted Chicken Breast
(56 g)

60 calories
1.5 g fat
(0.5 g saturated)
340 mg sodium

Not That!

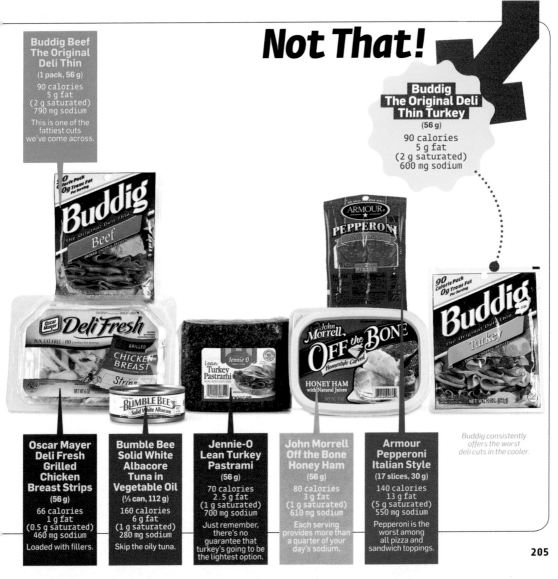

Buddig Beef The Original Deli Thin
(1 pack, 56 g)

90 calories
5 g fat
(2 g saturated)
790 mg sodium

This is one of the fattiest cuts we've come across.

Buddig The Original Deli Thin Turkey
(56 g)

90 calories
5 g fat
(2 g saturated)
600 mg sodium

Oscar Mayer Deli Fresh Grilled Chicken Breast Strips
(56 g)

66 calories
1 g fat
(0.5 g saturated)
460 mg sodium

Loaded with fillers.

Bumble Bee Solid White Albacore Tuna in Vegetable Oil
(⅓ can, 112 g)

160 calories
6 g fat
(1 g saturated)
280 mg sodium

Skip the oily tuna.

Jennie-O Lean Turkey Pastrami
(56 g)

70 calories
2.5 g fat
(1 g saturated)
700 mg sodium

Just remember, there's no guarantee that turkey's going to be the lightest option.

John Morrell Off the Bone Honey Ham
(56 g)

80 calories
3 g fat
(1 g saturated)
610 mg sodium

Each serving provides more than a quarter of your day's sodium.

Armour Pepperoni Italian Style
(17 slices, 30 g)

140 calories
13 g fat
(5 g saturated)
550 mg sodium

Pepperoni is the worst among all pizza and sandwich toppings.

Buddig consistently offers the worst deli cuts in the cooler.

205

Hot Dogs and Sausages

Eat This

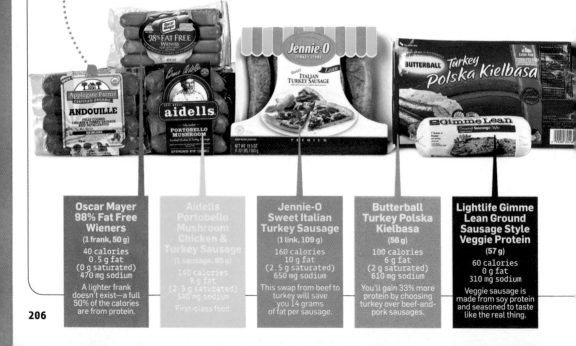

Applegate Farms Andouille Sausage
(1 sausage, 85 g)

120 calories
6 g fat
(2 g saturated)
620 mg sodium

Applegate offers up more protein for less than half the calories and a third of the fat found in the ever-popular Johnsonville brats.

Oscar Mayer 98% Fat Free Wieners
(1 frank, 50 g)

40 calories
0.5 g fat
(0 g saturated)
470 mg sodium

A lighter frank doesn't exist—a full 50% of the calories are from protein.

Aidells Portobello Mushroom Chicken & Turkey Sausage
(1 sausage, 85 g)

140 calories
8 g fat
(2.5 g saturated)
540 mg sodium

First-class food.

Jennie-O Sweet Italian Turkey Sausage
(1 link, 109 g)

160 calories
10 g fat
(2.5 g saturated)
650 mg sodium

This swap from beef to turkey will save you 14 grams of fat per sausage.

Butterball Turkey Polska Kielbasa
(56 g)

100 calories
6 g fat
(2 g saturated)
610 mg sodium

You'll gain 33% more protein by choosing turkey over beef-and-pork sausages.

Lightlife Gimme Lean Ground Sausage Style Veggie Protein
(57 g)

60 calories
0 g fat
310 mg sodium

Veggie sausage is made from soy protein and seasoned to taste like the real thing.

Not That!

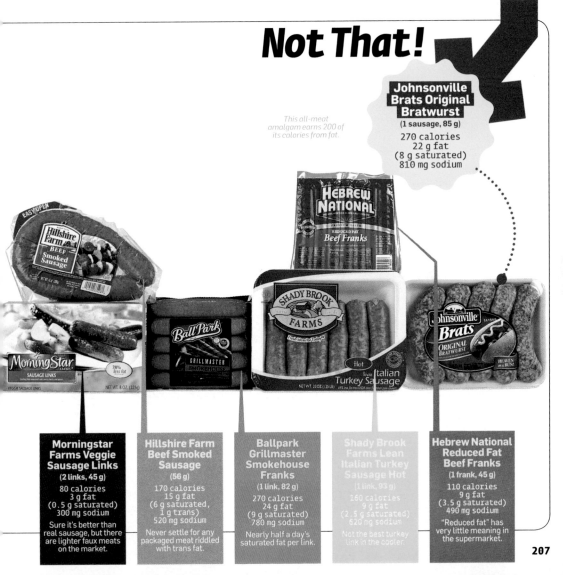

Johnsonville Brats Original Bratwurst
(1 sausage, 85 g)
270 calories
22 g fat
(8 g saturated)
810 mg sodium

This all-meat amalgam earns 200 of its calories from fat.

Morningstar Farms Veggie Sausage Links
(2 links, 45 g)
80 calories
3 g fat
(0.5 g saturated)
300 mg sodium
Sure it's better than real sausage, but there are lighter faux meats on the market.

Hillshire Farm Beef Smoked Sausage
(56 g)
170 calories
15 g fat
(6 g saturated, 1 g trans)
520 mg sodium
Never settle for any packaged meat riddled with trans fat.

Ballpark Grillmaster Smokehouse Franks
(1 link, 82 g)
270 calories
24 g fat
(9 g saturated)
780 mg sodium
Nearly half a day's saturated fat per link.

Shady Brook Farms Lean Italian Turkey Sausage Hot
(1 link, 93 g)
160 calories
9 g fat
(2.5 g saturated)
620 mg sodium
Not the best turkey link in the cooler.

Hebrew National Reduced Fat Beef Franks
(1 frank, 45 g)
110 calories
9 g fat
(3.5 g saturated)
490 mg sodium
"Reduced fat" has very little meaning in the supermarket.

207

Condiments
Eat This

Hellmann's Mayonnaise
with Extra Virgin Olive Oil
(1 Tbsp, 15 g)

50 calories
5 g fat
(0.5 g saturated)
120 mg sodium

By switching over to olive oil-based mayonnaise, not only do you cut the calories nearly in half, but you also increase the amount of heart-healthy monounsaturated fats on your next sandwich.

Annie's Naturals Organic Honey Mustard
(1 Tbsp, 18 g)

30 calories
0 g fat
120 mg sodium

Mustard seeds are rich in omega-3s and the antioxidant selenium.

Hellmann's Dijonnaise
(1 Tbsp, 15 g)

15 calories
0 g fat
210 mg sodium

The Dijonnaise is actually more mustard than mayo, making it far safer than the name implies.

Libby's Crispy Sauerkraut
(2 Tbsp, 30 g)

5 calories
0 g fat
200 mg sodium

Cut calories and sodium in one fell swoop.

Annie's Naturals Organic Ketchup
(1 Tbsp, 17 g)

15 calories
0 g fat
150 mg sodium

Research shows that organic ketchup packs more lycopene.

French's Horseradish Mustard
(2 Tsp, 10 g)

10 calories
0 g fat
160 mg sodium

Get the same kick as horseradish sauce, but without the glut of soybean oil.

Stubb's Mild Bar-B-Q Sauce
(2 Tbsp, 32 g)

30 calories
0 g fat
220 mg sodium

You'd be hard pressed to find a better barbecue sauce in the supermarket.

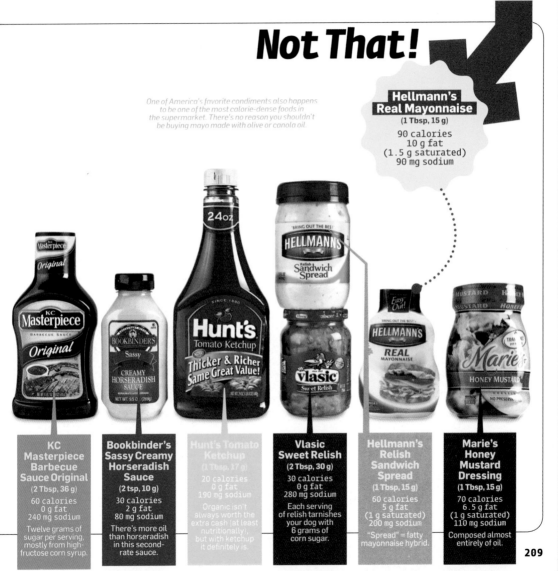

Not That!

One of America's favorite condiments also happens to be one of the most calorie-dense foods in the supermarket. There's no reason you shouldn't be buying mayo made with olive or canola oil.

Hellmann's Real Mayonnaise
(1 Tbsp, 15 g)

90 calories
10 g fat
(1.5 g saturated)
90 mg sodium

KC Masterpiece Barbecue Sauce Original
(2 Tbsp, 36 g)

60 calories
0 g fat
240 mg sodium

Twelve grams of sugar per serving, mostly from high-fructose corn syrup.

Bookbinder's Sassy Creamy Horseradish Sauce
(2 tsp, 10 g)

30 calories
2 g fat
80 mg sodium

There's more oil than horseradish in this second-rate sauce.

Hunt's Tomato Ketchup
(1 Tbsp, 17 g)

20 calories
0 g fat
190 mg sodium

Organic isn't always worth the extra cash (at least nutritionally), but with ketchup it definitely is.

Vlasic Sweet Relish
(2 Tbsp, 30 g)

30 calories
0 g fat
280 mg sodium

Each serving of relish tarnishes your dog with 6 grams of corn sugar.

Hellmann's Relish Sandwich Spread
(1 Tbsp, 15 g)

60 calories
5 g fat
(1 g saturated)
200 mg sodium

"Spread" = fatty mayonnaise hybrid.

Marie's Honey Mustard Dressing
(1 Tbsp, 15 g)

70 calories
6.5 g fat
(1 g saturated)
110 mg sodium

Composed almost entirely of oil.

209

Breads
Eat This

Martin's Whole Wheat Potato
(2 slices, 45 g)

140 calories
2 g fat
(0 g saturated)
8 g fiber

Each slice packs 4 grams of fiber and 6 grams of protein. For our money, this is the best bread in America.

Nature's Own Double Fiber Wheat
(2 slices, 86 g)

200 calories
3 g fat
(0 g saturated)
12 g fiber

Great breads have a favorable fiber-to-calorie ratio. Few can beat this.

Alexia Whole Grain Hearty Rolls
(1 roll, 43 g)

90 calories
1 g fat
(0 g saturated)
2 g fiber

The best roll in the supermarket is actually hiding in the freezer section.

Martin's Long Roll Potato Rolls
(1 bun, 53 g)

130 calories
1.5 g fat
(0 g saturated)
4 g fiber

Martin mines the spud to come up with more fiber than you'll find in whole wheat buns.

Nature's Own Whitewheat
(2 slices, 52 g)

100 calories
2 g fat
(0.5 g saturated)
5 g fiber

There's no longer any excuse to grab a typical, low-fiber white bread.

Mission White Corn
(2 tortillas, 51 g)

110 calories
1.5 g fat
(0 g saturated)
3 g fiber

With more fiber and fewer calories, corn trumps flour every time in the tortilla showdown.

La Tortilla Factory Smart & Delicious Low Carb Whole Wheat
(1 wrap, 62 g)

170 calories
3.5 g fat
(1 g saturated)
5 g fiber

Not That!

You'd have to be a nut to find this bread healthy. It has one of the worst fiber-to-calorie ratios in the bread aisle.

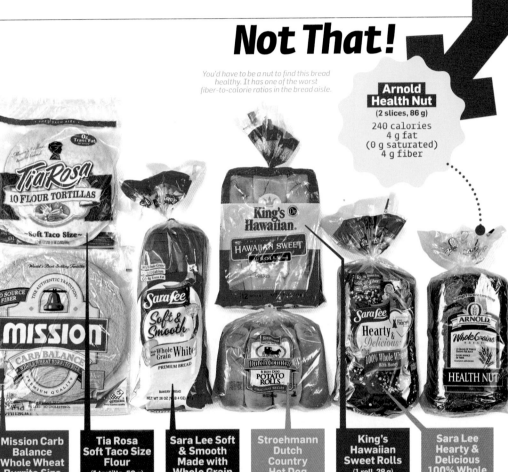

Arnold Health Nut
(2 slices, 86 g)

240 calories
4 g fat
(0 g saturated)
4 g fiber

Mission Carb Balance Whole Wheat Burrito Size
(1 tortilla, 70 g)

200 calories
5 g fat
(2.5 g saturated)
21 g fiber

Fiber-rich, but calorie-dense.

Tia Rosa Soft Taco Size Flour
(1 tortilla, 50 g)

150 calories
4.5 g
(2.5 g saturated)
1 g fiber

Made from oil and refined white flour. Any questions?

Sara Lee Soft & Smooth Made with Whole Grain White
(2 slices, 57 g)

150 calories
2 g fat
(0.5 g saturated)
3 g fiber

Stroehmann Dutch Country Hot Dog Potato Rolls
(1 roll, 53 g)

150 calories
2 g fat
1 g fiber

Don't settle for subpar buns.

King's Hawaiian Sweet Rolls
(1 roll, 28 g)

100 calories
2.5 g fat
(1.5 g saturated)
1 g fiber

Less fiber and five times the sugar as Alexia's Whole Grain Roll.

Sara Lee Hearty & Delicious 100% Whole Wheat with Honey
(2 slices, 86 g)

240 calories
3 g fat
(1 g saturated)
6 g fiber

211

Grains and Noodles
Eat This

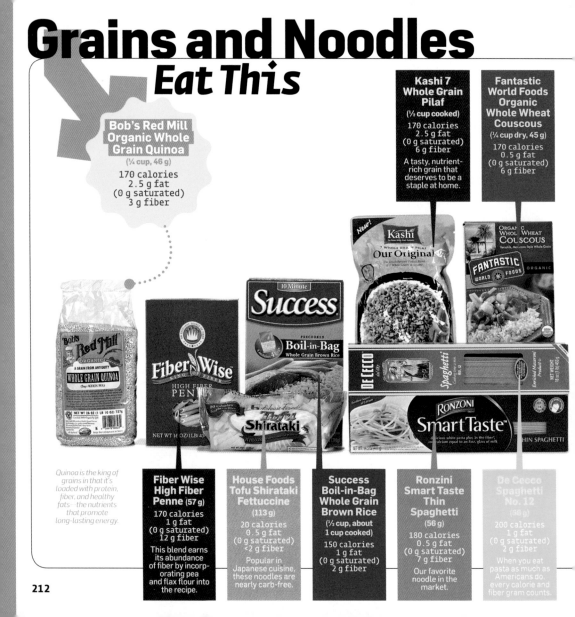

Bob's Red Mill Organic Whole Grain Quinoa
(¼ cup, 46 g)
170 calories
2.5 g fat
(0 g saturated)
3 g fiber

Quinoa is the king of grains in that it's loaded with protein, fiber, and healthy fats—the nutrients that promote long-lasting energy.

Kashi 7 Whole Grain Pilaf
(½ cup cooked)
170 calories
2.5 g fat
(0 g saturated)
6 g fiber
A tasty, nutrient-rich grain that deserves to be a staple at home.

Fantastic World Foods Organic Whole Wheat Couscous
(¼ cup dry, 45 g)
170 calories
0.5 g fat
(0 g saturated)
6 g fiber

Fiber Wise High Fiber Penne (57 g)
170 calories
1 g fat
(0 g saturated)
12 g fiber
This blend earns its abundance of fiber by incorporating pea and flax flour into the recipe.

House Foods Tofu Shirataki Fettuccine
(113 g)
20 calories
0.5 g fat
(0 g saturated)
<2 g fiber
Popular in Japanese cuisine, these noodles are nearly carb-free.

Success Boil-in-Bag Whole Grain Brown Rice
(½ cup, about 1 cup cooked)
150 calories
1 g fat
(0 g saturated)
2 g fiber

Ronzini Smart Taste Thin Spaghetti
(56 g)
180 calories
0.5 g fat
(0 g saturated)
7 g fiber
Our favorite noodle in the market.

De Cecco Spaghetti No. 12
(56 g)
200 calories
1 g fat
(0 g saturated)
2 g fiber
When you eat pasta as much as Americans do, every calorie and fiber gram counts.

Not That!

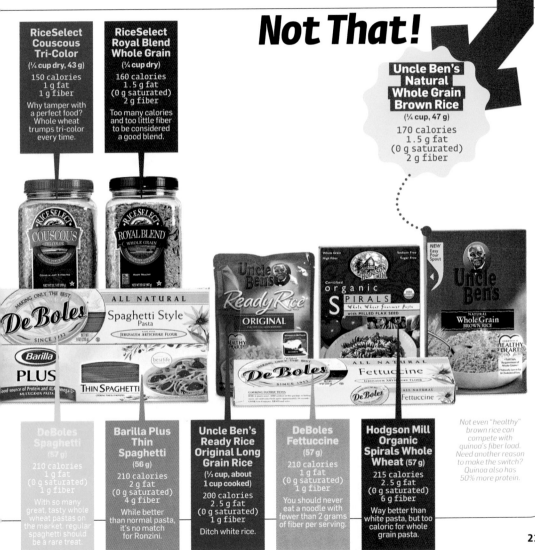

RiceSelect Couscous Tri-Color
(¼ cup dry, 43 g)

150 calories
1 g fat
1 g fiber

Why tamper with a perfect food? Whole wheat trumps tri-color every time.

RiceSelect Royal Blend Whole Grain
(¼ cup dry)

160 calories
1.5 g fat
(0 g saturated)
2 g fiber

Too many calories and too little fiber to be considered a good blend.

Uncle Ben's Natural Whole Grain Brown Rice
(¼ cup, 47 g)

170 calories
1.5 g fat
(0 g saturated)
2 g fiber

DeBoles Spaghetti
(57 g)

210 calories
1 g fat
(0 g saturated)
1 g fiber

With so many great, tasty whole wheat pastas on the market, regular spaghetti should be a rare treat.

Barilla Plus Thin Spaghetti
(56 g)

210 calories
2 g fat
(0 g saturated)
4 g fiber

While better than normal pasta, it's no match for Ronzini.

Uncle Ben's Ready Rice Original Long Grain Rice
(⅓ cup, about 1 cup cooked)

200 calories
2.5 g fat
(0 g saturated)
1 g fiber

Ditch white rice.

DeBoles Fettuccine
(57 g)

210 calories
1 g fat
(0 g saturated)
1 g fiber

You should never eat a noodle with fewer than 2 grams of fiber per serving.

Hodgson Mill Organic Spirals Whole Wheat (57 g)

215 calories
2.5 g fat
(0 g saturated)
6 g fiber

Way better than white pasta, but too caloric for whole grain pasta.

Not even "healthy" brown rice can compete with quinoa's fiber load. Need another reason to make the switch? Quinoa also has 50% more protein.

213

Sauces
Eat This

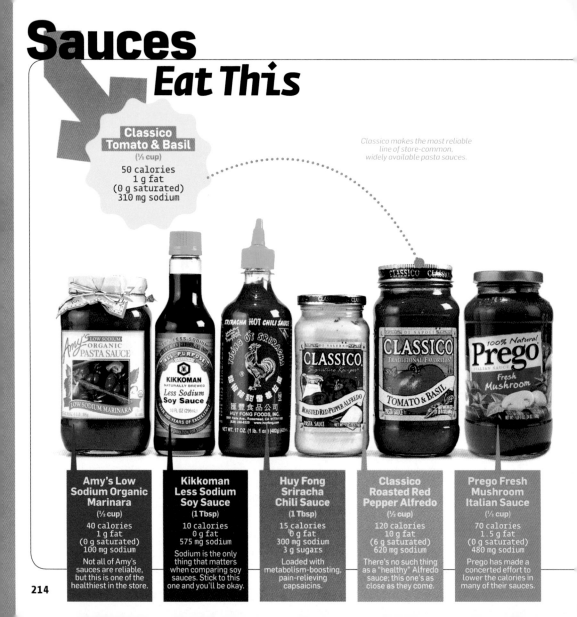

**Classico
Tomato & Basil**
(½ cup)

50 calories
1 g fat
(0 g saturated)
310 mg sodium

*Classico makes the most reliable
line of store-common,
widely available pasta sauces.*

**Amy's Low
Sodium Organic
Marinara**
(½ cup)

40 calories
1 g fat
(0 g saturated)
100 mg sodium

Not all of Amy's
sauces are reliable,
but this is one of the
healthiest in the store.

**Kikkoman
Less Sodium
Soy Sauce**
(1 Tbsp)

10 calories
0 g fat
575 mg sodium

Sodium is the only
thing that matters
when comparing soy
sauces. Stick to this
one and you'll be okay.

**Huy Fong
Sriracha
Chili Sauce**
(1 Tbsp)

15 calories
0 g fat
300 mg sodium
3 g sugars

Loaded with
metabolism-boosting,
pain-relieving
capsaicins.

**Classico
Roasted Red
Pepper Alfredo**
(½ cup)

120 calories
10 g fat
(6 g saturated)
620 mg sodium

There's no such thing
as a "healthy" Alfredo
sauce; this one's as
close as they come.

**Prego Fresh
Mushroom
Italian Sauce**
(½ cup)

70 calories
1.5 g fat
(0 g saturated)
480 mg sodium

Prego has made a
concerted effort to
lower the calories in
many of their sauces.

Not That!

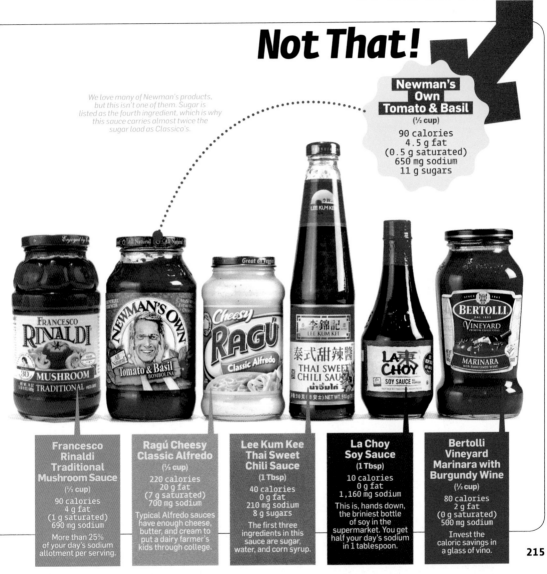

Newman's Own Tomato & Basil
(½ cup)

90 calories
4.5 g fat
(0.5 g saturated)
650 mg sodium
11 g sugars

We love many of Newman's products, but this isn't one of them. Sugar is listed as the fourth ingredient, which is why this sauce carries almost twice the sugar load as Classico's.

Francesco Rinaldi Traditional Mushroom Sauce
(½ cup)

90 calories
4 g fat
(1 g saturated)
690 mg sodium

More than 25% of your day's sodium allotment per serving.

Ragú Cheesy Classic Alfredo
(½ cup)

220 calories
20 g fat
(7 g saturated)
700 mg sodium

Typical Alfredo sauces have enough cheese, butter, and cream to put a dairy farmer's kids through college.

Lee Kum Kee Thai Sweet Chili Sauce
(1 Tbsp)

40 calories
0 g fat
210 mg sodium
8 g sugars

The first three ingredients in this sauce are sugar, water, and corn syrup.

La Choy Soy Sauce
(1 Tbsp)

10 calories
0 g fat
1,160 mg sodium

This is, hands down, the briniest bottle of soy in the supermarket. You get half your day's sodium in 1 tablespoon.

Bertolli Vineyard Marinara with Burgundy Wine
(½ cup)

80 calories
2 g fat
(0 g saturated)
500 mg sodium

Invest the caloric savings in a glass of vino.

215

Soups
Eat This

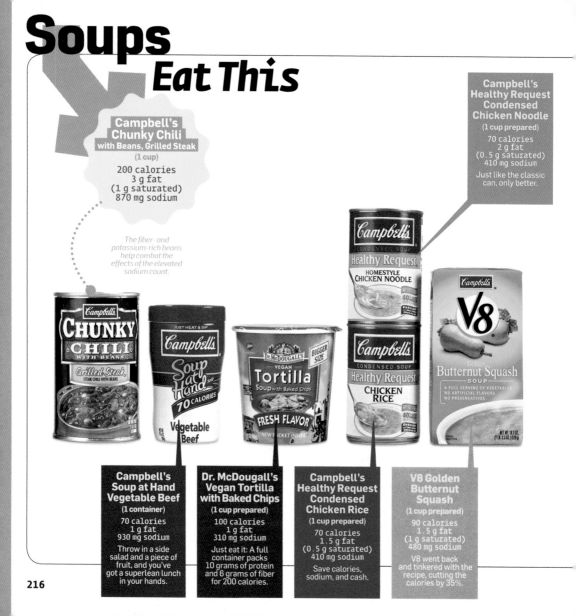

Campbell's Chunky Chili with Beans, Grilled Steak
(1 cup)

200 calories
3 g fat
(1 g saturated)
870 mg sodium

The fiber- and potassium-rich beans help combat the effects of the elevated sodium count.

Campbell's Healthy Request Condensed Chicken Noodle
(1 cup prepared)

70 calories
2 g fat
(0.5 g saturated)
410 mg sodium

Just like the classic can, only better.

Campbell's Soup at Hand Vegetable Beef
(1 container)

70 calories
1 g fat
930 mg sodium

Throw in a side salad and a piece of fruit, and you've got a superlean lunch in your hands.

Dr. McDougall's Vegan Tortilla with Baked Chips
(1 cup prepared)

100 calories
1 g fat
310 mg sodium

Just eat it: A full container packs 10 grams of protein and 6 grams of fiber for 200 calories.

Campbell's Healthy Request Condensed Chicken Rice
(1 cup prepared)

70 calories
1.5 g fat
(0.5 g saturated)
410 mg sodium

Save calories, sodium, and cash.

V8 Golden Butternut Squash
(1 cup prepared)

90 calories
1.5 g fat
(1 g saturated)
480 mg sodium

V8 went back and tinkered with the recipe, cutting the calories by 35%.

Not That!

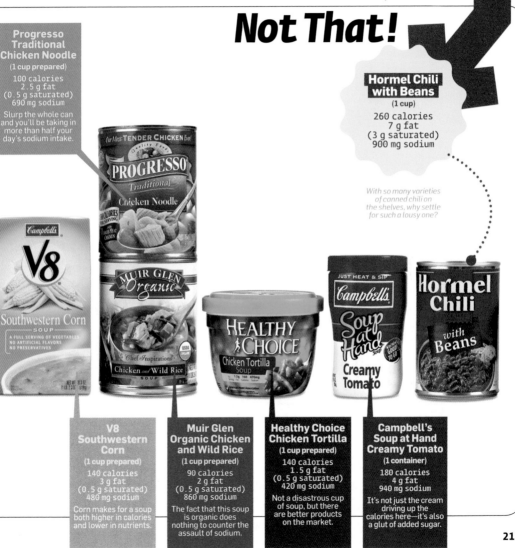

Progresso Traditional Chicken Noodle
(1 cup prepared)
100 calories
2.5 g fat
(0.5 g saturated)
690 mg sodium

Slurp the whole can and you'll be taking in more than half your day's sodium intake.

Hormel Chili with Beans
(1 cup)
260 calories
7 g fat
(3 g saturated)
900 mg sodium

With so many varieties of canned chili on the shelves, why settle for such a lousy one?

V8 Southwestern Corn
(1 cup prepared)
140 calories
3 g fat
(0.5 g saturated)
480 mg sodium

Corn makes for a soup both higher in calories and lower in nutrients.

Muir Glen Organic Chicken and Wild Rice
(1 cup prepared)
90 calories
2 g fat
(0.5 g saturated)
860 mg sodium

The fact that this soup is organic does nothing to counter the assault of sodium.

Healthy Choice Chicken Tortilla
(1 cup prepared)
140 calories
1.5 g fat
(0.5 g saturated)
420 mg sodium

Not a disastrous cup of soup, but there are better products on the market.

Campbell's Soup at Hand Creamy Tomato
(1 container)
180 calories
4 g fat
940 mg sodium

It's not just the cream driving up the calories here—it's also a glut of added sugar.

217

Bars

Eat This

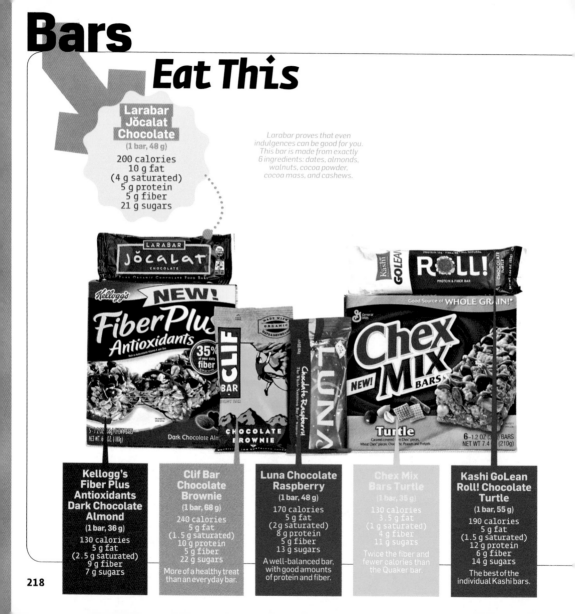

Larabar Jŏcalat Chocolate
(1 bar, 48 g)

200 calories
10 g fat
(4 g saturated)
5 g protein
5 g fiber
21 g sugars

Larabar proves that even indulgences can be good for you. This bar is made from exactly 6 ingredients: dates, almonds, walnuts, cocoa powder, cocoa mass, and cashews.

Kellogg's Fiber Plus Antioxidants Dark Chocolate Almond
(1 bar, 36 g)

130 calories
5 g fat
(2.5 g saturated)
9 g fiber
7 g sugars

Clif Bar Chocolate Brownie
(1 bar, 68 g)

240 calories
5 g fat
(1.5 g saturated)
10 g protein
5 g fiber
22 g sugars

More of a healthy treat than an everyday bar.

Luna Chocolate Raspberry
(1 bar, 48 g)

170 calories
5 g fat
(2 g saturated)
8 g protein
5 g fiber
13 g sugars

A well-balanced bar, with good amounts of protein and fiber.

Chex Mix Bars Turtle
(1 bar, 35 g)

130 calories
3.5 g fat
(1 g saturated)
4 g fiber
11 g sugars

Twice the fiber and fewer calories than the Quaker bar.

Kashi GoLean Roll! Chocolate Turtle
(1 bar, 55 g)

190 calories
5 g fat
(1.5 g saturated)
12 g protein
6 g fiber
14 g sugars

The best of the individual Kashi bars.

Not That!

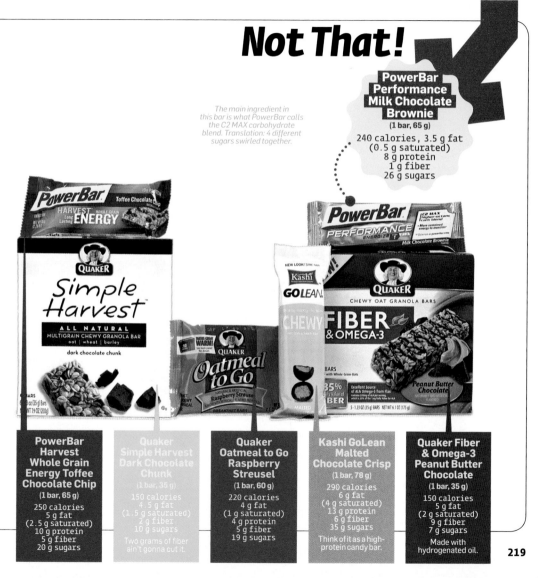

The main ingredient in this bar is what PowerBar calls the C2 MAX carbohydrate blend. Translation: 4 different sugars swirled together.

PowerBar Performance Milk Chocolate Brownie
(1 bar, 65 g)

240 calories, 3.5 g fat
(0.5 g saturated)
8 g protein
1 g fiber
26 g sugars

PowerBar Harvest Whole Grain Energy Toffee Chocolate Chip
(1 bar, 65 g)

250 calories
5 g fat
(2.5 g saturated)
10 g protein
5 g fiber
20 g sugars

Quaker Simple Harvest Dark Chocolate Chunk
(1 bar, 35 g)

150 calories
4.5 g fat
(1.5 g saturated)
2 g fiber
10 g sugars

Two grams of fiber ain't gonna cut it.

Quaker Oatmeal to Go Raspberry Streusel
(1 bar, 60 g)

220 calories
4 g fat
(1 g saturated)
4 g protein
5 g fiber
19 g sugars

Kashi GoLean Malted Chocolate Crisp
(1 bar, 78 g)

290 calories
6 g fat
(4 g saturated)
13 g protein
6 g fiber
35 g sugars

Think of it as a high-protein candy bar.

Quaker Fiber & Omega-3 Peanut Butter Chocolate
(1 bar, 35 g)

150 calories
5 g fat
(2 g saturated)
9 g protein
7 g sugars

Made with hydrogenated oil.

219

Crackers
Eat This

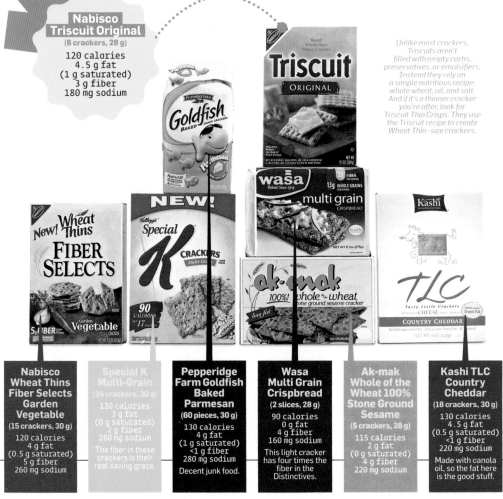

Nabisco Triscuit Original
(6 crackers, 28 g)

120 calories
4.5 g fat
(1 g saturated)
3 g fiber
180 mg sodium

Unlike most crackers, Triscuits aren't filled with empty carbs, preservatives, or emulsifiers. Instead they rely on a simple nutritious recipe: whole wheat, oil, and salt. And if it's a thinner cracker you're after, look for Triscuit Thin Crisps. They use the Triscuit recipe to create Wheat Thin–size crackers.

Nabisco Wheat Thins Fiber Selects Garden Vegetable
(15 crackers, 30 g)

120 calories
4 g fat
(0.5 g saturated)
5 g fiber
260 mg sodium

Special K Multi-Grain
(24 crackers, 30 g)

120 calories
3 g fat
(0 g saturated)
2 g fiber
260 mg sodium

The fiber in these crackers is their real saving grace.

Pepperidge Farm Goldfish Baked Parmesan
(60 pieces, 30 g)

130 calories
4 g fat
(1 g saturated)
<1 g fiber
280 mg sodium

Decent junk food.

Wasa Multi Grain Crispbread
(2 slices, 28 g)

90 calories
0 g fat
4 g fiber
160 mg sodium

This light cracker has four times the fiber in the Distinctives.

Ak-mak Whole of the Wheat 100% Stone Ground Sesame
(5 crackers, 28 g)

115 calories
2 g fat
(0 g saturated)
4 g fiber
220 mg sodium

Kashi TLC Country Cheddar
(18 crackers, 30 g)

130 calories
4.5 g fat
(0.5 g saturated)
<1 g fiber
220 mg sodium

Made with canola oil, so the fat here is the good stuff.

220

Not That!

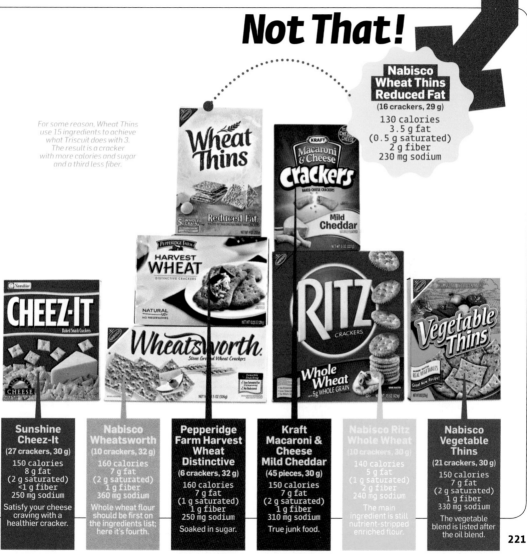

Nabisco Wheat Thins Reduced Fat
(16 crackers, 29 g)

130 calories
3.5 g fat
(0.5 g saturated)
2 g fiber
230 mg sodium

For some reason, Wheat Thins use 15 ingredients to achieve what Triscuit does with 3. The result is a cracker with more calories and sugar and a third less fiber.

Sunshine Cheez-It
(27 crackers, 30 g)

150 calories
8 g fat
(2 g saturated)
<1 g fiber
250 mg sodium

Satisfy your cheese craving with a healthier cracker.

Nabisco Wheatsworth
(10 crackers, 32 g)

160 calories
7 g fat
(2 g saturated)
1 g fiber
360 mg sodium

Whole wheat flour should be first on the ingredients list; here it's fourth.

Pepperidge Farm Harvest Wheat Distinctive
(6 crackers, 32 g)

160 calories
7 g fat
(1 g saturated)
1 g fiber
250 mg sodium

Soaked in sugar.

Kraft Macaroni & Cheese Mild Cheddar
(45 pieces, 30 g)

150 calories
7 g fat
(2 g saturated)
1 g fiber
310 mg sodium

True junk food.

Nabisco Ritz Whole Wheat
(10 crackers, 30 g)

140 calories
5 g fat
(1 g saturated)
2 g fiber
240 mg sodium

The main ingredient is still nutrient-stripped enriched flour.

Nabisco Vegetable Thins
(21 crackers, 30 g)

150 calories
7 g fat
(2 g saturated)
1 g fiber
330 mg sodium

The vegetable blend is listed after the oil blend.

221

Chips

Eat This

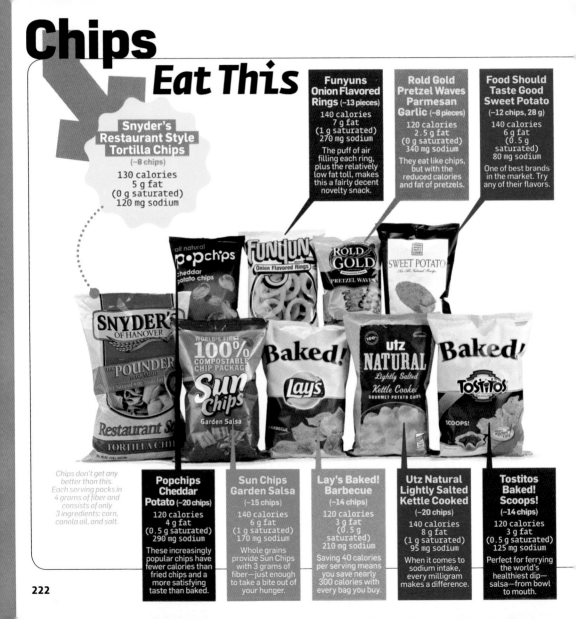

Snyder's Restaurant Style Tortilla Chips (~8 chips)

130 calories
5 g fat
(0 g saturated)
120 mg sodium

Chips don't get any better than this. Each serving packs in 4 grams of fiber and consists of only 3 ingredients: corn, canola oil, and salt.

Funyuns Onion Flavored Rings (~13 pieces)

140 calories
7 g fat
(1 g saturated)
270 mg sodium

The puff of air filling each ring, plus the relatively low fat toll, makes this a fairly decent novelty snack.

Rold Gold Pretzel Waves Parmesan Garlic (~8 pieces)

120 calories
2.5 g fat
(0 g saturated)
340 mg sodium

They eat like chips, but with the reduced calories and fat of pretzels.

Food Should Taste Good Sweet Potato (~12 chips, 28 g)

140 calories
6 g fat
(0.5 g saturated)
80 mg sodium

One of best brands in the market. Try any of their flavors.

Popchips Cheddar Potato (~20 chips)

120 calories
4 g fat
(0.5 g saturated)
290 mg sodium

These increasingly popular chips have fewer calories than fried chips and a more satisfying taste than baked.

Sun Chips Garden Salsa (~15 chips)

140 calories
6 g fat
(1 g saturated)
170 mg sodium

Whole grains provide Sun Chips with 3 grams of fiber—just enough to take a bite out of your hunger.

Lay's Baked! Barbecue (~14 chips)

120 calories
3 g fat
(0.5 g saturated)
210 mg sodium

Saving 40 calories per serving means you save nearly 300 calories with every bag you buy.

Utz Natural Lightly Salted Kettle Cooked (~20 chips)

140 calories
8 g fat
(1 g saturated)
95 mg sodium

When it comes to sodium intake, every milligram makes a difference.

Tostitos Baked! Scoops! (~14 chips)

120 calories
3 g fat
(0.5 g saturated)
125 mg sodium

Perfect for ferrying the world's healthiest dip—salsa—from bowl to mouth.

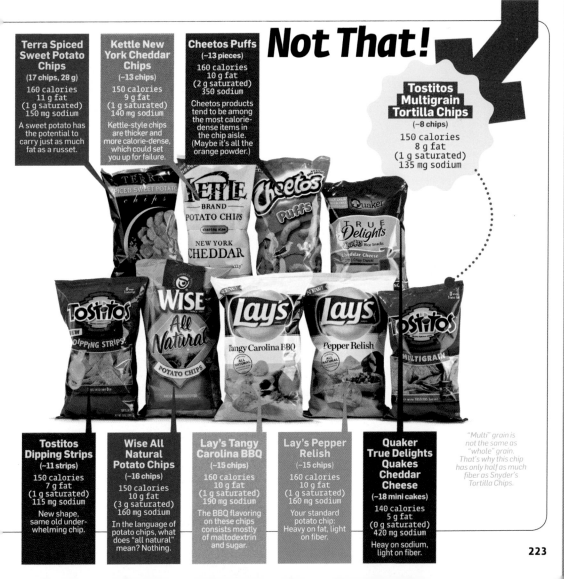

Not That!

Terra Spiced Sweet Potato Chips

(17 chips, 28 g)

160 calories
11 g fat
(1 g saturated)
150 mg sodium

A sweet potato has the potential to carry just as much fat as a russet.

Kettle New York Cheddar Chips

(~13 chips)

150 calories
9 g fat
(1 g saturated)
140 mg sodium

Kettle-style chips are thicker and more calorie-dense, which could set you up for failure.

Cheetos Puffs

(~13 pieces)

160 calories
10 g fat
(2 g saturated)
350 sodium

Cheetos products tend to be among the most calorie-dense items in the chip aisle. (Maybe it's all the orange powder.)

Tostitos Multigrain Tortilla Chips

(~8 chips)

150 calories
8 g fat
(1 g saturated)
135 mg sodium

Tostitos Dipping Strips

(~11 strips)

150 calories
7 g fat
(1 g saturated)
115 mg sodium

New shape, same old underwhelming chip.

Wise All Natural Potato Chips

(~16 chips)

150 calories
10 g fat
(3 g saturated)
160 mg sodium

In the language of potato chips, what does "all natural" mean? Nothing.

Lay's Tangy Carolina BBQ

(~15 chips)

160 calories
10 g fat
(1 g saturated)
190 mg sodium

The BBQ flavoring on these chips consists mostly of maltodextrin and sugar.

Lay's Pepper Relish

(~15 chips)

160 calories
10 g fat
(1 g saturated)
160 mg sodium

Your standard potato chip: Heavy on fat, light on fiber.

Quaker True Delights Quakes Cheddar Cheese

(~18 mini cakes)

140 calories
5 g fat
(0 g saturated)
420 mg sodium

Heavy on sodium, light on fiber.

"Multi" grain is not the same as "whole" grain. That's why this chip has only half as much fiber as Snyder's Tortilla Chips.

Dips and Spreads
Eat This

Ragú Pizza Sauce
(2 Tbsp)
15 calories
0.5 g fat
(0 g saturated)
125 mg sodium

Try dipping vegetables and bread in marinara instead of ranch. You'll cut calories and boost your nutrient intake.

Classico Sun-Dried Tomato Pesto
(¼ cup, 62 g)
90 calories
5 g fat
(1 g saturated)
630 mg sodium

Classico's recipe uses less oil and more tomatoes and basil, so you won't have to sprint to the gym to repent to the nutritional gods.

Calavo Guacamole
(2 Tbsp, 30 g)
66 calories
5 g fat
(1 g saturated)
126 mg sodium

Avocado is teeming with potassium, which helps your body convert sugar into energy.

Tribe Hummus Sweet Roasted Red Pepper
(2 Tbsp, 28 g)
40 calories
2.5 g fat
(0 g saturated)
125 mg sodium

Perfect for dipping and spreading.

Spike's Packing Co. Salsa Con Queso Medium
(2 Tbsp, 31 g)
45 calories
4 g fat
(0.5 g saturated)
200 mg sodium

Fritos Bean Dip
(2 Tbsp, 35 g)
35 calories
1 g fat
(0 g saturated)
190 mg sodium

Whatever you stick into this dip will emerge with a fat-fighting load of fiber and antioxidants.

Heinz Original Cocktail Sauce
(¼ cup, 60 g)
60 calories
0 g fat
690 mg sodium

Heinz's has only 11 grams of sugar per serving, which is half as much as Del Monte's.

Desert Pepper Trading Co. Salsa del Rio
(2 Tbsp, 31 g)
10 calories
0 g fat
230 mg sodium

This tomatillo-based salsa doubles as a sauce for grilled foods.

224

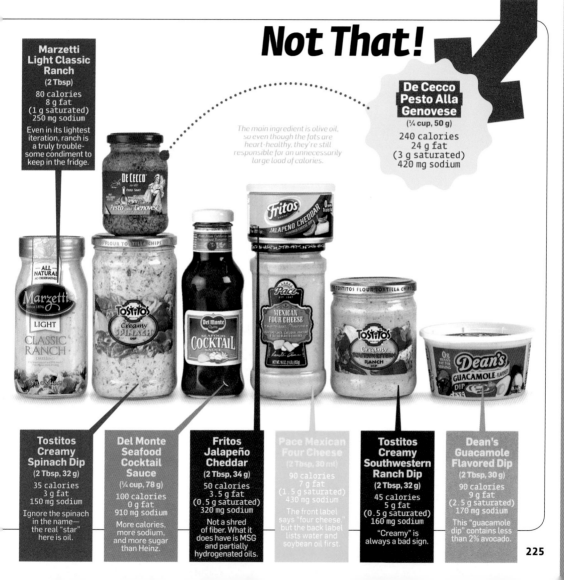

Not That!

Marzetti Light Classic Ranch
(2 Tbsp)

80 calories
8 g fat
(1 g saturated)
250 mg sodium

Even in its lightest iteration, ranch is a truly troublesome condiment to keep in the fridge.

The main ingredient is olive oil, so even though the fats are heart-healthy, they're still responsible for an unnecessarily large load of calories.

De Cecco Pesto Alla Genovese
(¼ cup, 50 g)

240 calories
24 g fat
(3 g saturated)
420 mg sodium

Tostitos Creamy Spinach Dip
(2 Tbsp, 32 g)

35 calories
3 g fat
150 mg sodium

Ignore the spinach in the name—the real "star" here is oil.

Del Monte Seafood Cocktail Sauce
(¼ cup, 78 g)

100 calories
0 g fat
910 mg sodium

More calories, more sodium, and more sugar than Heinz.

Fritos Jalapeño Cheddar
(2 Tbsp, 34 g)

50 calories
3.5 g fat
(0.5 g saturated)
320 mg sodium

Not a shred of fiber. What it does have is MSG and partially hydrogenated oils.

Pace Mexican Four Cheese
(2 Tbsp, 30 ml)

90 calories
7 g fat
(1.5 g saturated)
430 mg sodium

The front label says "four cheese," but the back label lists water and soybean oil first.

Tostitos Creamy Southwestern Ranch Dip
(2 Tbsp, 32 g)

45 calories
5 g fat
(0.5 g saturated)
160 mg sodium

"Creamy" is always a bad sign.

Dean's Guacamole Flavored Dip
(2 Tbsp, 30 g)

90 calories
9 g fat
(2.5 g saturated)
170 mg sodium

This "guacamole dip" contains less than 2% avocado.

225

Salad Dressings
Eat This

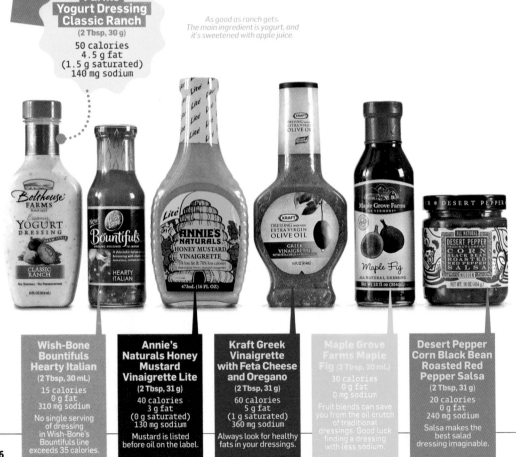

Bolthouse Farms Yogurt Dressing Classic Ranch
(2 Tbsp, 30 g)

50 calories
4.5 g fat
(1.5 g saturated)
140 mg sodium

As good as ranch gets. The main ingredient is yogurt, and it's sweetened with apple juice.

Wish-Bone Bountifuls Hearty Italian
(2 Tbsp, 30 mL)

15 calories
0 g fat
310 mg sodium

No single serving of dressing in Wish-Bone's Bountifuls line exceeds 35 calories.

Annie's Naturals Honey Mustard Vinaigrette Lite
(2 Tbsp, 31 g)

40 calories
3 g fat
(0 g saturated)
130 mg sodium

Mustard is listed before oil on the label.

Kraft Greek Vinaigrette with Feta Cheese and Oregano
(2 Tbsp, 31 g)

60 calories
5 g fat
(1 g saturated)
360 mg sodium

Always look for healthy fats in your dressings.

Maple Grove Farms Maple Fig (2 Tbsp, 30 mL)

30 calories
0 g fat
0 mg sodium

Fruit blends can save you from the oil crutch of traditional dressings. Good luck finding a dressing with less sodium.

Desert Pepper Corn Black Bean Roasted Red Pepper Salsa
(2 Tbsp, 31 g)

20 calories
0 g fat
240 mg sodium

Salsa makes the best salad dressing imaginable.

Not That!

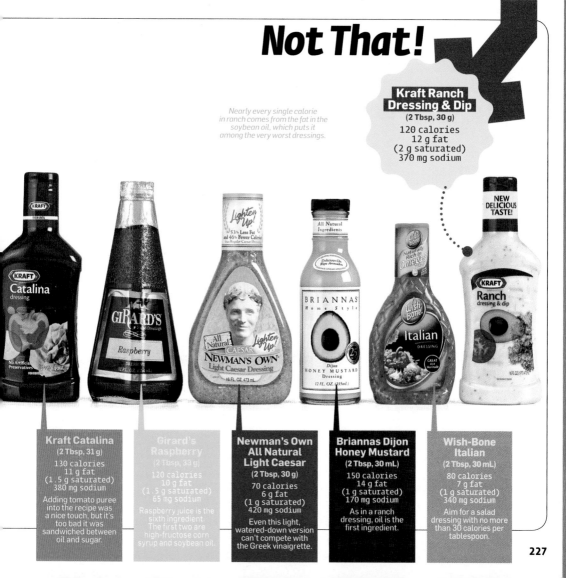

Nearly every single calorie in ranch comes from the fat in the soybean oil, which puts it among the very worst dressings.

Kraft Ranch Dressing & Dip
(2 Tbsp, 30 g)
120 calories
12 g fat
(2 g saturated)
370 mg sodium

NEW DELICIOUS TASTE!

Kraft Catalina
(2 Tbsp, 31 g)
130 calories
11 g fat
(1.5 g saturated)
380 mg sodium

Adding tomato puree into the recipe was a nice touch, but it's too bad it was sandwiched between oil and sugar.

Girard's Raspberry
(2 Tbsp, 33 g)
120 calories
10 g fat
(1.5 g saturated)
65 mg sodium

Raspberry juice is the sixth ingredient. The first two are high-fructose corn syrup and soybean oil.

Newman's Own All Natural Light Caesar
(2 Tbsp, 30 g)
70 calories
6 g fat
(1 g saturated)
420 mg sodium

Even this light, watered-down version can't compete with the Greek vinaigrette.

Briannas Dijon Honey Mustard
(2 Tbsp, 30 mL)
150 calories
14 g fat
(1 g saturated)
170 mg sodium

As in a ranch dressing, oil is the first ingredient.

Wish-Bone Italian
(2 Tbsp, 30 mL)
80 calories
7 g fat
(1 g saturated)
340 mg sodium

Aim for a salad dressing with no more than 30 calories per tablespoon.

227

Cookies
Eat This

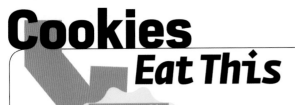

Newman-O's Peanut Butter Crème Filled Chocolate
(2 cookies, 28 g)

120 calories
5 g fat
(1.5 g saturated)
10 g sugars

They're organic, they're made with real peanuts, and instead of the typical generic vegetable oil, Newman's uses omega-3 rich canola oil.

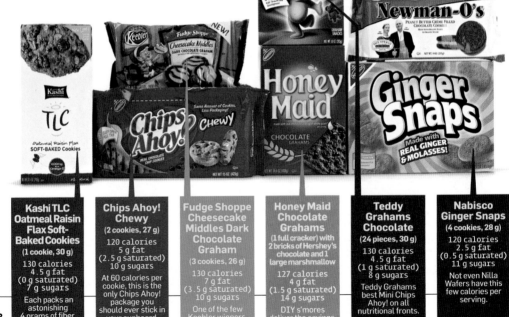

Kashi TLC Oatmeal Raisin Flax Soft-Baked Cookies
(1 cookie, 30 g)

130 calories
4.5 g fat
(0 g saturated)
7 g sugars

Each packs an astonishing 4 grams of fiber.

Chips Ahoy! Chewy
(2 cookies, 27 g)

120 calories
5 g fat
(2.5 g saturated)
10 g sugars

At 60 calories per cookie, this is the only Chips Ahoy! package you should ever stick in your cupboard.

Fudge Shoppe Cheesecake Middles Dark Chocolate Graham
(3 cookies, 26 g)

130 calories
7 g fat
(3.5 g saturated)
10 g sugars

One of the few Keebler winners.

Honey Maid Chocolate Grahams
(1 full cracker) with 2 bricks of Hershey's chocolate and 1 large marshmallow

127 calories
4 g fat
(1.5 g saturated)
14 g sugars

DIY s'mores deliver the savings.

Teddy Grahams Chocolate
(24 pieces, 30 g)

130 calories
4.5 g fat
(1 g saturated)
8 g sugars

Teddy Grahams best Mini Chips Ahoy! on all nutritional fronts.

Nabisco Ginger Snaps
(4 cookies, 28 g)

120 calories
2.5 g fat
(0.5 g saturated)
11 g sugars

Not even Nilla Wafers have this few calories per serving.

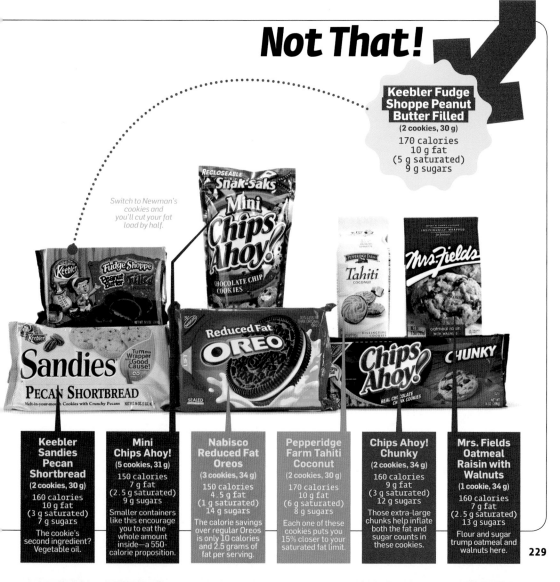

Not That!

Keebler Fudge Shoppe Peanut Butter Filled
(2 cookies, 30 g)
170 calories
10 g fat
(5 g saturated)
9 g sugars

Switch to Newman's cookies and you'll cut your fat load by half.

Keebler Sandies Pecan Shortbread
(2 cookies, 30 g)
160 calories
10 g fat
(3 g saturated)
7 g sugars

The cookie's second ingredient? Vegetable oil.

Mini Chips Ahoy!
(5 cookies, 31 g)
150 calories
7 g fat
(2.5 g saturated)
9 g sugars

Smaller containers like this encourage you to eat the whole amount inside—a 550-calorie proposition.

Nabisco Reduced Fat Oreos
(3 cookies, 34 g)
150 calories
4.5 g fat
(1 g saturated)
14 g sugars

The calorie savings over regular Oreos is only 10 calories and 2.5 grams of fat per serving.

Pepperidge Farm Tahiti Coconut
(2 cookies, 30 g)
170 calories
10 g fat
(6 g saturated)
8 g sugars

Each one of these cookies puts you 15% closer to your saturated fat limit.

Chips Ahoy! Chunky
(2 cookies, 34 g)
160 calories
9 g fat
(3 g saturated)
12 g sugars

Those extra-large chunks help inflate both the fat and sugar counts in these cookies.

Mrs. Fields Oatmeal Raisin with Walnuts
(1 cookie, 34 g)
160 calories
7 g fat
(2.5 g saturated)
13 g sugars

Flour and sugar trump oatmeal and walnuts here.

Candy Bars
Eat This

Reese's Peanut Butter Cups
(1 package, 42 g)

210 calories
13 g fat
(4.5 g saturated)
19 g sugars

Normally chocolate + peanut butter = high calories, but this classic emerges as one of the better candy bars in the grocery store.

Starburst GummiBursts Liquid Filled Gummies
(1 package, 42.5 g)

140 calories
0 g fat
(0 g saturated)
23 g sugars

Surprisingly one of the lowest-calorie candy options you'll find.

Reese's Big Cup
(1 package, 39 g)

200 calories
12 g fat
(4 g saturated)
19 g sugars

There's no cutting corners here: The Big Cup is the size of two regular Reese's Peanut Butter Cups.

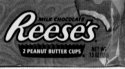

Hershey's Take 5
(1 package, 42 g)

200 calories
11 g fat
(5 g saturated)
18 g sugars

Take 5 cuts big calories by replacing the typical nougat base with chocolatey pretzel.

Hershey's Special Dark
(1 bar, 41 g)

180 calories
12 g fat
(8 g saturated)
21 g sugars

At 45% cocoa, Special Dark is the perfect compromise between the extra-bitter dark chocolate and a regular Hershey's bar.

York Peppermint Pattie
(1 package, 39 g)

140 calories
2.5 g fat
(1.5 g saturated)
25 g sugars

The perfect size for satisfying a serious sweet-tooth hankering.

Kit Kat
(1 package, 43 g)

210 calories
11 g fat
(7 g saturated)
21 g sugars

Your goal: Pawn off one of the four sticks in this package. You'll make a friend and drop your damage down to a very reasonable 160 calories.

Not That!

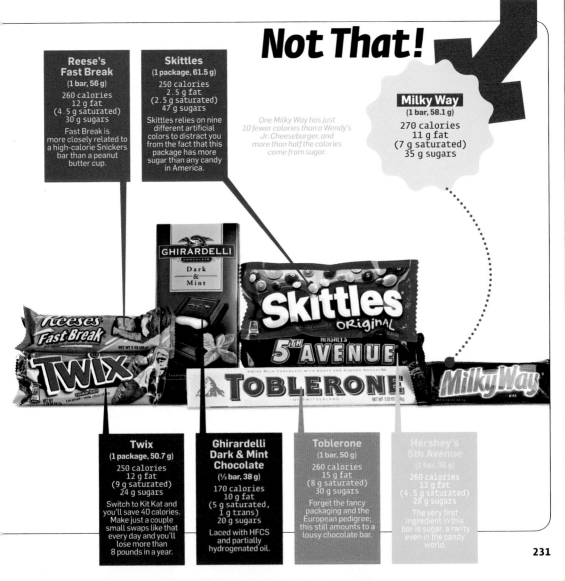

Reese's Fast Break
(1 bar, 56 g)

260 calories
12 g fat
(4.5 g saturated)
30 g sugars

Fast Break is more closely related to a high-calorie Snickers bar than a peanut butter cup.

Skittles
(1 package, 61.5 g)

250 calories
2.5 g fat
(2.5 g saturated)
47 g sugars

Skittles relies on nine different artificial colors to distract you from the fact that this package has more sugar than any candy in America.

One Milky Way has just 10 fewer calories than a Wendy's Jr. Cheeseburger, and more than half the calories come from sugar.

Milky Way
(1 bar, 58.1 g)

270 calories
11 g fat
(7 g saturated)
35 g sugars

Twix
(1 package, 50.7 g)

250 calories
12 g fat
(9 g saturated)
24 g sugars

Switch to Kit Kat and you'll save 40 calories. Make just a couple small swaps like that every day and you'll lose more than 8 pounds in a year.

Ghirardelli Dark & Mint Chocolate
(⅓ bar, 38 g)

170 calories
10 g fat
(5 g saturated, 1 g trans)
20 g sugars

Laced with HFCS and partially hydrogenated oil.

Toblerone
(1 bar, 50 g)

260 calories
15 g fat
(8 g saturated)
30 g sugars

Forget the fancy packaging and the European pedigree; this still amounts to a lousy chocolate bar.

Hershey's 5th Avenue
(1 bar, 56 g)

260 calories
12 g fat
(4.5 g saturated)
28 g sugars

The very first ingredient in this bar is sugar, a rarity even in the candy world.

231

Frozen Breakfast Entrées
Eat This

Eggo Nutri-Grain Filled Strawberry Waffles
(1 waffle, 58 g)

130 calories
3.5 g fat
(1 g saturated)
8 g sugars
300 mg sodium

Amy's Toaster Pops Apple
(1 pastry, 60 g)

160 calories
3.5 g fat
(0 g saturated)
10 g sugars
110 mg sodium

Unlike most toaster pastries, Amy's filling is made with more fruit than sugar.

Golden Blueberry Blintzes
(1 blintz, 61 g)

90 calories
1 g fat
(0 g saturated)
6 g sugars

Most of the sugar comes from the load of blueberries in the filling.

For a gimmicky frozen breakfast, these waffles fare pretty well. The sugar level is moderate, there's real dehydrated fruit inside, and they're loaded with 3 grams of fiber to keep your stomach full until lunch.

Jimmy Dean D-Lights Turkey Sausage Breakfast Bowl
(1 bowl, 198 g)

230 calories
7 g fat
(3 g saturated)
700 mg sodium

A breakfast sandwich, minus the bread.

Jimmy Dean D-Lights Turkey Sausage Muffin
(1 sandwich, 145 g)

260 calories
8 g fat
(3.5 g saturated)
760 mg sodium

Jimmy's D-Lights line is reliable for high-protein, low-calorie meals.

Aunt Jemima Low Fat Waffles
(2 waffles, 71 g)

160 calories
3 g fat
(0.5 g saturated)
3 g sugars
470 mg sodium

"Low fat" usually means high sugar, but this is a top-notch waffle.

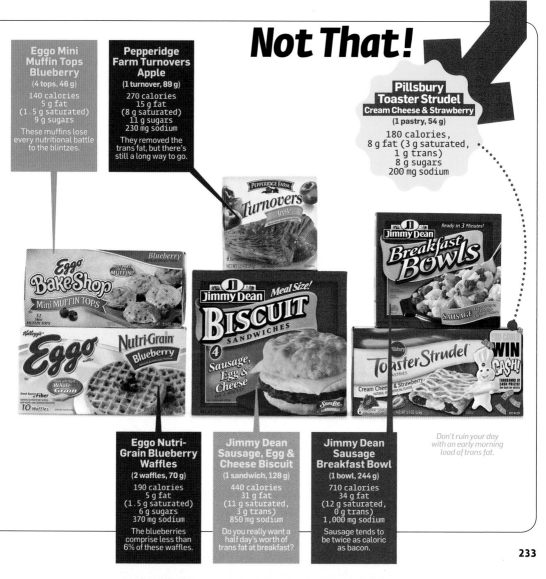

Not That!

Eggo Mini Muffin Tops Blueberry
(4 tops, 46 g)
140 calories
5 g fat
(1.5 g saturated)
9 g sugars

These muffins lose every nutritional battle to the blintzes.

Pepperidge Farm Turnovers Apple
(1 turnover, 89 g)
270 calories
15 g fat
(8 g saturated)
11 g sugars
230 mg sodium

They removed the trans fat, but there's still a long way to go.

Pillsbury Toaster Strudel
Cream Cheese & Strawberry
(1 pastry, 54 g)
180 calories,
8 g fat (3 g saturated,
1 g trans)
8 g sugars
200 mg sodium

Eggo Nutri-Grain Blueberry Waffles
(2 waffles, 70 g)
190 calories
5 g fat
(1.5 g saturated)
6 g sugars
370 mg sodium

The blueberries comprise less than 6% of these waffles.

Jimmy Dean Sausage, Egg & Cheese Biscuit
(1 sandwich, 128 g)
440 calories
31 g fat
(11 g saturated,
3 g trans)
850 mg sodium

Do you really want a half day's worth of trans fat at breakfast?

Jimmy Dean Sausage Breakfast Bowl
(1 bowl, 244 g)
710 calories
34 g fat
(12 g saturated,
0 g trans)
1,000 mg sodium

Sausage tends to be twice as caloric as bacon.

Don't ruin your day with an early morning load of trans fat.

233

Frozen Pizza
Eat This

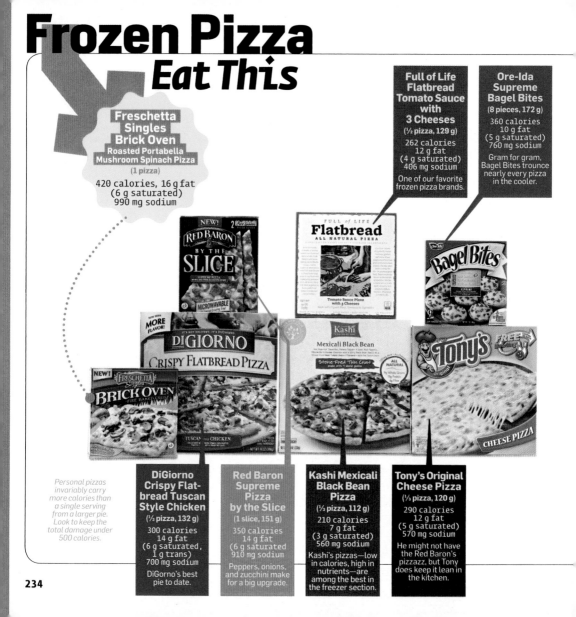

Freschetta Singles Brick Oven
Roasted Portabella Mushroom Spinach Pizza
(1 pizza)

420 calories, 16 g fat
(6 g saturated)
990 mg sodium

Full of Life Flatbread Tomato Sauce with 3 Cheeses
(⅓ pizza, 129 g)

262 calories
12 g fat
(4 g saturated)
406 mg sodium

One of our favorite frozen pizza brands.

Ore-Ida Supreme Bagel Bites
(8 pieces, 172 g)

360 calories
10 g fat
(5 g saturated)
760 mg sodium

Gram for gram, Bagel Bites trounce nearly every pizza in the cooler.

Personal pizzas invariably carry more calories than a single serving from a larger pie. Look to keep the total damage under 500 calories.

DiGiorno Crispy Flatbread Tuscan Style Chicken
(⅓ pizza, 132 g)

300 calories
14 g fat
(6 g saturated, 1 g trans)
700 mg sodium

DiGorno's best pie to date.

Red Baron Supreme Pizza by the Slice
(1 slice, 151 g)

350 calories
14 g fat
(6 g saturated)
910 mg sodium

Peppers, onions, and zucchini make for a big upgrade.

Kashi Mexicali Black Bean Pizza
(⅓ pizza, 112 g)

210 calories
7 g fat
(3 g saturated)
560 mg sodium

Kashi's pizzas—low in calories, high in nutrients—are among the best in the freezer section.

Tony's Original Cheese Pizza
(⅓ pizza, 120 g)

290 calories
12 g fat
(5 g saturated)
570 mg sodium

He might not have the Red Baron's pizzazz, but Tony does keep it lean in the kitchen.

234

Not That!

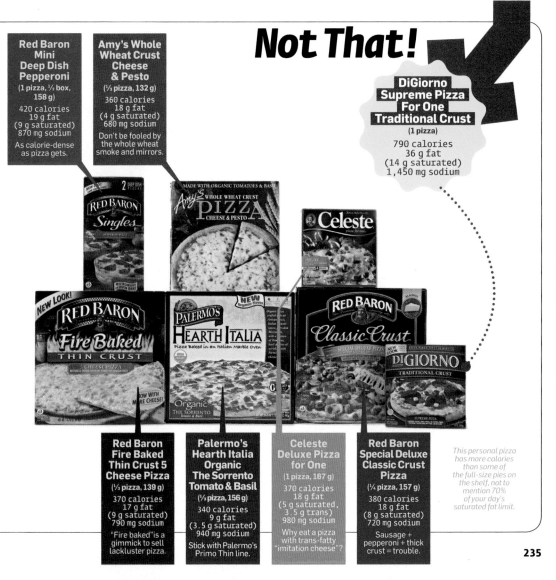

Red Baron Mini Deep Dish Pepperoni
(1 pizza, ½ box, 158 g)

420 calories
19 g fat
(9 g saturated)
870 mg sodium

As calorie-dense as pizza gets.

Amy's Whole Wheat Crust Cheese & Pesto
(⅓ pizza, 132 g)

360 calories
18 g fat
(4 g saturated)
680 mg sodium

Don't be fooled by the whole wheat smoke and mirrors.

DiGiorno Supreme Pizza For One Traditional Crust
(1 pizza)

790 calories
36 g fat
(14 g saturated)
1,450 mg sodium

Red Baron Fire Baked Thin Crust 5 Cheese Pizza
(½ pizza, 139 g)

370 calories
17 g fat
(9 g saturated)
790 mg sodium

"Fire baked" is a gimmick to sell lackluster pizza.

Palermo's Hearth Italia Organic The Sorrento Tomato & Basil
(½ pizza, 156 g)

340 calories
9 g fat
(3.5 g saturated)
940 mg sodium

Stick with Palermo's Primo Thin line.

Celeste Deluxe Pizza for One
(1 pizza, 167 g)

370 calories
18 g fat
(5 g saturated, 3.5 g trans)
980 mg sodium

Why eat a pizza with trans-fatty "imitation cheese"?

Red Baron Special Deluxe Classic Crust Pizza
(¼ pizza, 157 g)

380 calories
18 g fat
(8 g saturated)
720 mg sodium

Sausage + pepperoni + thick crust = trouble.

This personal pizza has more calories than some of the full-size pies on the shelf, not to mention 70% of your day's saturated fat limit.

235

Frozen Pasta Entrées
Eat This

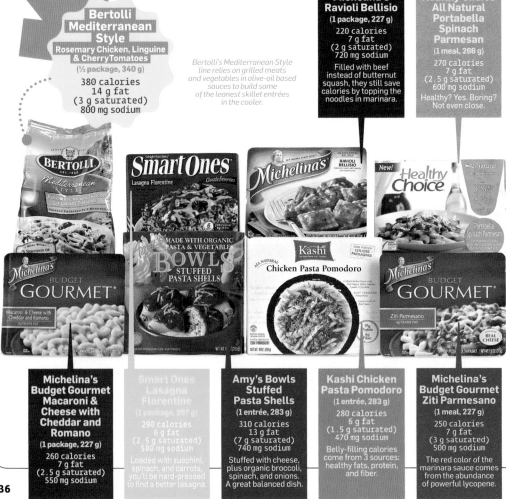

Bertolli Mediterranean Style
Rosemary Chicken, Linguine & CherryTomatoes
(⅓ package, 340 g)

380 calories
14 g fat
(3 g saturated)
800 mg sodium

Bertolli's Mediterranean Style line relies on grilled meats and vegetables in olive-oil based sauces to build some of the leanest skillet entrées in the cooler.

Michelina's Ravioli Bellisio
(1 package, 227 g)

220 calories
7 g fat
(2 g saturated)
720 mg sodium

Filled with beef instead of butternut squash, they still save calories by topping the noodles in marinara.

Healthy Choice All Natural Portabella Spinach Parmesan
(1 meal, 266 g)

270 calories
7 g fat
(2.5 g saturated)
600 mg sodium

Healthy? Yes. Boring? Not even close.

Michelina's Budget Gourmet Macaroni & Cheese with Cheddar and Romano
(1 package, 227 g)

260 calories
7 g fat
(2.5 g saturated)
550 mg sodium

Smart Ones Lasagna Florentine
(1 package, 297 g)

290 calories
6 g fat
(2.5 g saturated)
580 mg sodium

Loaded with zucchini, spinach, and carrots, you'll be hard-pressed to find a better lasagna.

Amy's Bowls Stuffed Pasta Shells
(1 entrée, 283 g)

310 calories
13 g fat
(7 g saturated)
740 mg sodium

Stuffed with cheese, plus organic broccoli, spinach, and onions. A great balanced dish.

Kashi Chicken Pasta Pomodoro
(1 entrée, 283 g)

280 calories
6 g fat
(1.5 g saturated)
470 mg sodium

Belly-filling calories come from 3 sources: healthy fats, protein, and fiber.

Michelina's Budget Gourmet Ziti Parmesano
(1 meal, 227 g)

250 calories
7 g fat
(3 g saturated)
500 mg sodium

The red color of the marinara sauce comes from the abundance of powerful lycopene.

Not That!

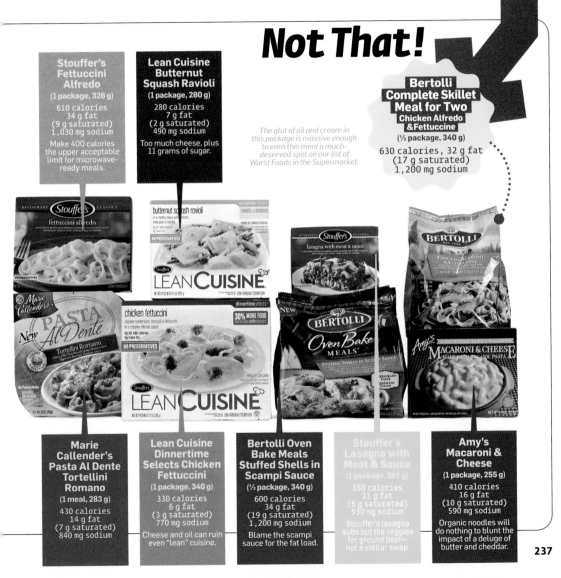

Stouffer's Fettuccini Alfredo
(1 package, 326 g)

610 calories
34 g fat
(9 g saturated)
1,030 mg sodium

Make 400 calories the upper acceptable limit for microwave-ready meals.

Lean Cuisine Butternut Squash Ravioli
(1 package, 280 g)

280 calories
7 g fat
(2 g saturated)
490 mg sodium

Too much cheese, plus 11 grams of sugar.

The glut of oil and cream in this package is massive enough to earn this meal a much-deserved spot on our list of Worst Foods in the Supermarket.

Bertolli Complete Skillet Meal for Two
Chicken Alfredo &Fettuccine
(½ package, 340 g)

630 calories, 32 g fat
(17 g saturated)
1,200 mg sodium

Marie Callender's Pasta Al Dente Tortellini Romano
(1 meal, 283 g)

430 calories
14 g fat
(7 g saturated)
840 mg sodium

Lean Cuisine Dinnertime Selects Chicken Fettuccini
(1 package, 340 g)

330 calories
6 g fat
(3 g saturated)
770 mg sodium

Cheese and oil can ruin even "lean" cuisine.

Bertolli Oven Bake Meals Stuffed Shells in Scampi Sauce
(½ package, 340 g)

600 calories
34 g fat
(19 g saturated)
1,200 mg sodium

Blame the scampi sauce for the fat load.

Stouffer's Lasagna with Meat & Sauce
(1 package, 207 g)

350 calories
11 g fat
(6 g saturated)
930 mg sodium

Stouffer's lasagna subs out the veggies for ground beef—not a stellar swap.

Amy's Macaroni & Cheese
(1 package, 255 g)

410 calories
16 g fat
(10 g saturated)
590 mg sodium

Organic noodles will do nothing to blunt the impact of a deluge of butter and cheddar.

237

Frozen Fish Entrées
Eat This

SeaPak Salmon Burgers
(1 burger, 91 g)

110 calories
3 g fat
(0.5 g saturated)
380 mg sodium

Salmon is one of the world's best sources of omega-3 fats. Try bringing these to your next cookout.

Gorton's Grilled Fillets Garlic Butter
(1 fillet, 108 g)

100 calories
3 g fat
(0.5 g saturated)
290 mg sodium

Most of the fat in this fillet actually comes from olive and canola oils.

Phillips Steamed Spiced Shrimp
(~8 shrimp, 113 g)

120 calories
2 g fat
(0 g saturated)
560 mg sodium

Each individual shrimp has more than 2 grams of protein.

Bantry Bay Mussels in a Garlic Butter Sauce
(½ package, 8 oz)

120 calories
8 g fat
(4 g saturated)
630 mg sodium

Mussels are a great source of lean protein, iron, and zinc, as well as energy-boosting B vitamins.

Contessa Shrimp Stir-Fry
(⅓ package, 215 g)

130 calories
0 g fat
(0 g saturated)
670 mg sodium

Use only half the sauce and you'll cut an extra 50 calories and a bunch of sodium from each serving.

Not That!

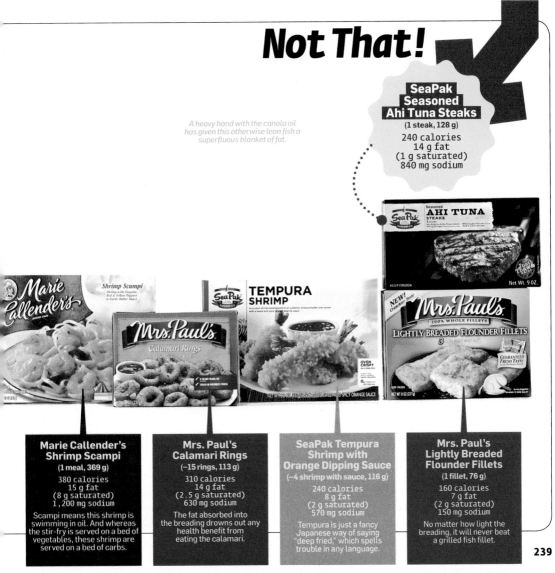

SeaPak Seasoned Ahi Tuna Steaks
(1 steak, 128 g)
240 calories
14 g fat
(1 g saturated)
840 mg sodium

A heavy hand with the canola oil has given this otherwise lean fish a superfluous blanket of fat.

Marie Callender's Shrimp Scampi
(1 meal, 369 g)
380 calories
15 g fat
(8 g saturated)
1,200 mg sodium

Scampi means this shrimp is swimming in oil. And whereas the stir-fry is served on a bed of vegetables, these shrimp are served on a bed of carbs.

Mrs. Paul's Calamari Rings
(~15 rings, 113 g)
310 calories
14 g fat
(2.5 g saturated)
630 mg sodium

The fat absorbed into the breading drowns out any health benefit from eating the calamari.

SeaPak Tempura Shrimp with Orange Dipping Sauce
(~4 shrimp with sauce, 116 g)
240 calories
8 g fat
(2 g saturated)
570 mg sodium

Tempura is just a fancy Japanese way of saying "deep fried," which spells trouble in any language.

Mrs. Paul's Lightly Breaded Flounder Fillets
(1 fillet, 76 g)
160 calories
7 g fat
(2 g saturated)
150 mg sodium

No matter how light the breading, it will never beat a grilled fish fillet.

239

Frozen Chicken Entrées
Eat This

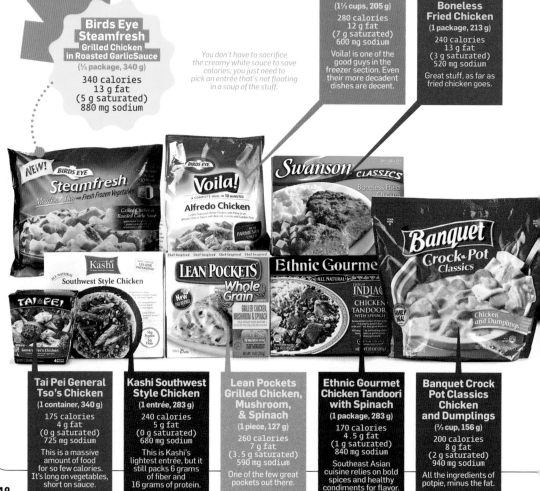

Birds Eye Steamfresh
Grilled Chicken in Roasted Garlic Sauce
(½ package, 340 g)

340 calories
13 g fat
(5 g saturated)
880 mg sodium

You don't have to sacrifice the creamy white sauce to save calories; you just need to pick an entrée that's not floating in a soup of the stuff.

Birds Eye Voila! Alfredo Chicken
(1½ cups, 205 g)

280 calories
12 g fat
(7 g saturated)
600 mg sodium

Voila! is one of the good guys in the freezer section. Even their more decadent dishes are decent.

Swanson Classics Boneless Fried Chicken
(1 package, 213 g)

240 calories
13 g fat
(3 g saturated)
520 mg sodium

Great stuff, as far as fried chicken goes.

Tai Pei General Tso's Chicken
(1 container, 340 g)

175 calories
4 g fat
(0 g saturated)
725 mg sodium

This is a massive amount of food for so few calories. It's long on vegetables, short on sauce.

Kashi Southwest Style Chicken
(1 entrée, 283 g)

240 calories
5 g fat
(0 g saturated)
680 mg sodium

This is Kashi's lightest entrée, but it still packs 6 grams of fiber and 16 grams of protein.

Lean Pockets Grilled Chicken, Mushroom, & Spinach
(1 piece, 127 g)

260 calories
7 g fat
(3.5 g saturated)
590 mg sodium

One of the few great pockets out there.

Ethnic Gourmet Chicken Tandoori with Spinach
(1 package, 283 g)

170 calories
4.5 g fat
(1 g saturated)
840 mg sodium

Southeast Asian cuisine relies on bold spices and healthy condiments for flavor.

Banquet Crock Pot Classics Chicken and Dumplings
(⅔ cup, 156 g)

200 calories
8 g fat
(2 g saturated)
940 mg sodium

All the ingredients of potpie, minus the fat.

Not That!

Banquet Chicken Fried Chicken
(1 package, 228 g)

350 calories
17 g fat
(4 g saturated)
930 mg sodium

Nearly identical dinners, so why would you mess around with one with more calories, fat, and sodium?

TGI Friday's Creamy Chicken Pasta Carbonara Skillet Meals
(1¼ cups, 270 g)

340 calories
9 g fat
(4.5 g saturated)
930 mg sodium

You probably already expect Alfredo sauce to be on the indulgent side, but this is just perilous. It earns more than half your day's fat from heavy doses of whipping cream, cream cheese, soybean oil, half-and-half, and cheese.

Marie Callender's Grilled Chicken Alfredo Bake
(1 meal, 369 g)

500 calories
26 g fat (14 g saturated, 0.5 g trans)
1,230 mg sodium

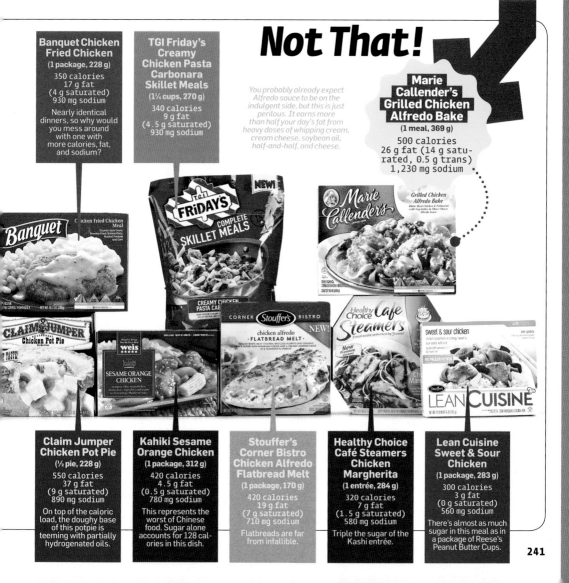

Claim Jumper Chicken Pot Pie
(½ pie, 228 g)

550 calories
37 g fat
(9 g saturated)
890 mg sodium

On top of the caloric load, the doughy base of this potpie is teeming with partially hydrogenated oils.

Kahiki Sesame Orange Chicken
(1 package, 312 g)

420 calories
4.5 g fat
(0.5 g saturated)
780 mg sodium

This represents the worst of Chinese food. Sugar alone accounts for 128 calories in this dish.

Stouffer's Corner Bistro Chicken Alfredo Flatbread Melt
(1 package, 170 g)

420 calories
19 g fat
(7 g saturated)
710 mg sodium

Flatbreads are far from infallible.

Healthy Choice Café Steamers Chicken Margherita
(1 entrée, 284 g)

320 calories
7 g fat
(1.5 g saturated)
580 mg sodium

Triple the sugar of the Kashi entrée.

Lean Cuisine Sweet & Sour Chicken
(1 package, 283 g)

300 calories
3 g fat
(0 g saturated)
560 mg sodium

There's almost as much sugar in this meal as in a package of Reese's Peanut Butter Cups.

Frozen Beef Entrées
Eat This

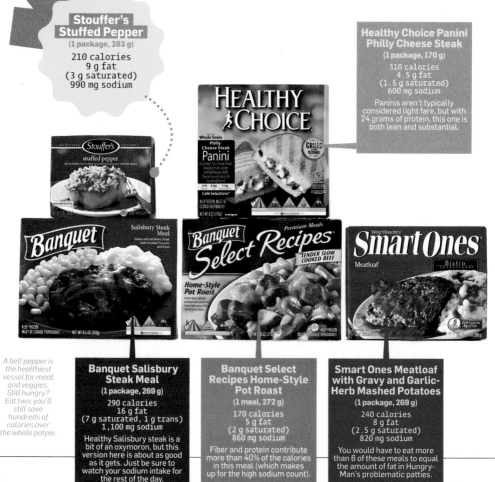

Stouffer's Stuffed Pepper
(1 package, 283 g)

210 calories
9 g fat
(3 g saturated)
990 mg sodium

Healthy Choice Panini Philly Cheese Steak
(1 package, 170 g)

310 calories
4.5 g fat
(1.5 g saturated)
600 mg sodium

Paninis aren't typically considered light fare, but with 24 grams of protein, this one is both lean and substantial.

A bell pepper is the healthiest vessel for meat and veggies. Still hungry? Eat two; you'll still save hundreds of calories over the whole potpie.

Banquet Salisbury Steak Meal
(1 package, 269 g)

290 calories
16 g fat
(7 g saturated, 1 g trans)
1,100 mg sodium

Healthy Salisbury steak is a bit of an oxymoron, but this version here is about as good as it gets. Just be sure to watch your sodium intake for the rest of the day.

Banquet Select Recipes Home-Style Pot Roast
(1 meal, 272 g)

170 calories
5 g fat
(2 g saturated)
860 mg sodium

Fiber and protein contribute more than 40% of the calories in this meal (which makes up for the high sodium count).

Smart Ones Meatloaf with Gravy and Garlic-Herb Mashed Potatoes
(1 package, 269 g)

240 calories
8 g fat
(2.5 g saturated)
820 mg sodium

You would have to eat more than 6 of these meals to equal the amount of fat in Hungry-Man's problematic patties.

Not That!

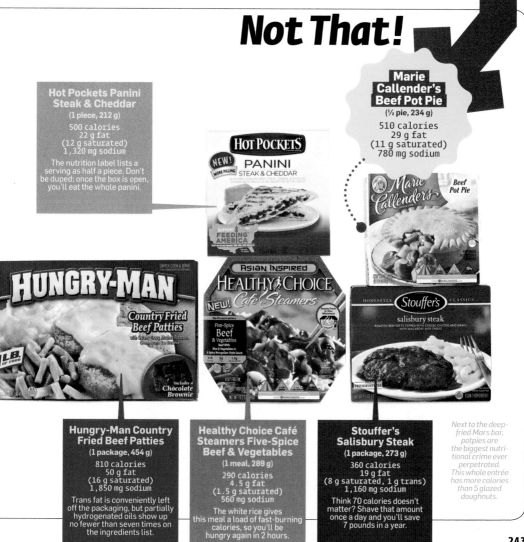

Hot Pockets Panini Steak & Cheddar
(1 piece, 212 g)

500 calories
22 g fat
(12 g saturated)
1,320 mg sodium

The nutrition label lists a serving as half a piece. Don't be duped; once the box is open, you'll eat the whole panini.

Marie Callender's Beef Pot Pie
(½ pie, 234 g)

510 calories
29 g fat
(11 g saturated)
780 mg sodium

Hungry-Man Country Fried Beef Patties
(1 package, 454 g)

810 calories
50 g fat
(16 g saturated)
1,850 mg sodium

Trans fat is conveniently left off the packaging, but partially hydrogenated oils show up no fewer than seven times on the ingredients list.

Healthy Choice Café Steamers Five-Spice Beef & Vegetables
(1 meal, 289 g)

290 calories
4.5 g fat
(1.5 g saturated)
560 mg sodium

The white rice gives this meal a load of fast-burning calories, so you'll be hungry again in 2 hours.

Stouffer's Salisbury Steak
(1 package, 273 g)

360 calories
19 g fat
(8 g saturated, 1 g trans)
1,160 mg sodium

Think 70 calories doesn't matter? Shave that amount once a day and you'll save 7 pounds in a year.

Next to the deep-fried Mars bar, potpies are the biggest nutritional crime ever perpetrated. This whole entrée has more calories than 5 glazed doughnuts.

243

Frozen Sides, Snacks, and

Eat This

Applegate Farms Chicken Nuggets
(7 nuggets, 88 g)

170 calories
9 g fat
(1.5 g saturated)
350 mg sodium

Ore-Ida Steam n' Mash Cut Sweet Potatoes
(1 cup, 123 g)
90 calories
0 g fat
30 mg sodium

This sweet mash brings a ton of vitamin A to the dinner table.

Ore-Ida Potatoes O'Brien with Onions and Peppers
(¾ cup, 85 g)
60 calories
0 g fat
40 mg sodium

The best of the bagged potatoes.

The light breading on these nuggets makes up less than 2% of the total weight, making them the lightest nuggets we've ever come across.

Morningstar Farms Veggie Bites Broccoli Cheddar
(3 pieces, 85 g)
180 calories
10 g fat
(2.5 g saturated)
550 mg sodium

Less fat, more fiber and protein.

Alexia Mushroom Bites
(~5 pieces, 60 g)
110 calories
4 g fat
(0.5 g saturated)
280 mg sodium

Mushrooms are packed with energy-boosting vitamins.

Foster Farms Mini Corn Dogs, Honey Crunchy
(4 dogs, 76 g)
220 calories
13 g fat
(3.5 g saturated)
510 mg sodium

A meager 55 calories per dog.

El Monterey Grilled Quesadillas Chicken & Cheese
(1 quesadilla, 85 g)
190 calories
7 g fat
(3 g saturated)
460 mg sodium

Cascadian Farm Straight Cut French Fries (85 g)
100 calories
4 g fat
(1 g saturated)
10 mg sodium

Just potatoes, a dash of oil, and apple juice to help them brown.

244

Appetizers

Not That!

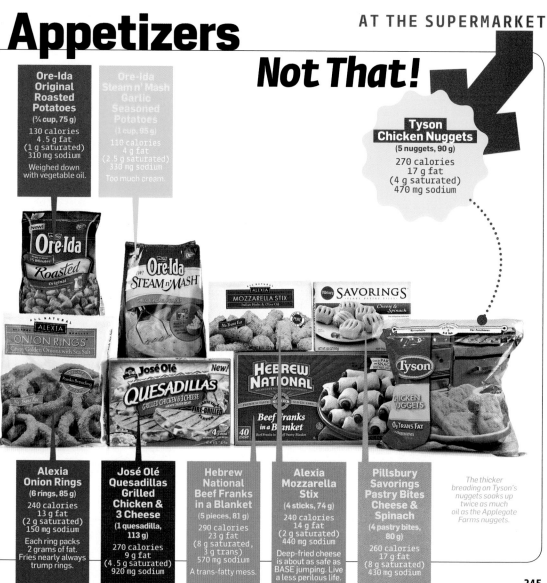

Ore-Ida Original Roasted Potatoes
(¾ cup, 75 g)

130 calories
4.5 g fat
(1 g saturated)
310 mg sodium

Weighed down with vegetable oil.

Ore-Ida Steam n' Mash Garlic Seasoned Potatoes
(1 cup, 95 g)

110 calories
4 g fat
(2.5 g saturated)
330 mg sodium

Too much cream.

Tyson Chicken Nuggets
(5 nuggets, 90 g)

270 calories
17 g fat
(4 g saturated)
470 mg sodium

Alexia Onion Rings
(6 rings, 85 g)

240 calories
13 g fat
(2 g saturated)
150 mg sodium

Each ring packs 2 grams of fat. Fries nearly always trump rings.

José Olé Quesadillas Grilled Chicken & 3 Cheese
(1 quesadilla, 113 g)

270 calories
9 g fat
(4.5 g saturated)
920 mg sodium

Hebrew National Beef Franks in a Blanket
(5 pieces, 81 g)

290 calories
23 g fat
(8 g saturated, 3 g trans)
570 mg sodium

A trans-fatty mess.

Alexia Mozzarella Stix
(4 sticks, 74 g)

240 calories
14 g fat
(2 g saturated)
440 mg sodium

Deep-fried cheese is about as safe as BASE jumping. Live a less perilous life.

Pillsbury Savorings Pastry Bites Cheese & Spinach
(4 pastry bites, 80 g)

260 calories
17 g fat
(8 g saturated)
430 mg sodium

The thicker breading on Tyson's nuggets soaks up twice as much oil as the Applegate Farms nuggets.

245

Ice Cream
Eat This

Breyers Reese's Peanut Butter Cups Ice Cream
(½ cup)

160 calories
6 g fat
(2.5 g saturated)
18 g sugars

To compensate for the extra load of fat from the peanuts, Breyers uses regular milk, rather than cream, as the base for this ice cream.

Stonyfield Frozen Yogurt Minty Chocolate Chip
(½ cup, 85 g)

140 calories
2.5 g fat
(1.5 g saturated)
21 g sugars

Made from hormone-free milk.

Blue Bunny Premium Vanilla
(½ cup, 68 g)

140 calories
8 g fat
(5 g saturated)
15 g sugars

Everyone needs a reliable vanilla in the freezer. Look no further.

Häagen-Dazs Low Fat Chocolate Sorbet
(½ cup, 105 g)

130 calories
0.5 g fat
(0 g saturated)
21 g sugars

Sorbets are the one frozen dessert that Häagen-Dazs does well.

Turkey Hill Stuff'd Chocolate Pretzel
(½ cup, 65 g)

130 calories
3.5 g fat
(2.5 g saturated)
15 g sugars

Even Turkey Hill's most indulgent flavors have fewer than 150 calories.

Edy's Fun Flavors Espresso Chip
(½ cup, 60 g)

120 calories
5 g fat
(3.5 g saturated)
14 g sugars

Contains real coffee, but with half the calories and a third of the fat.

Edy's Slow Churned Chocolate Fudge Chunk
(½ cup, 82 g)

120 calories
4.5 g fat
(3 g saturated)
15 g sugars

One of the most reliable ice cream lines in the cooler.

Breyers Smooth & Dreamy Dark Chocolate Velvet
(½ cup, 66 g)

140 calories
7 g fat
(4.5 g saturated)
16 g sugars

One more reason to love Breyers.

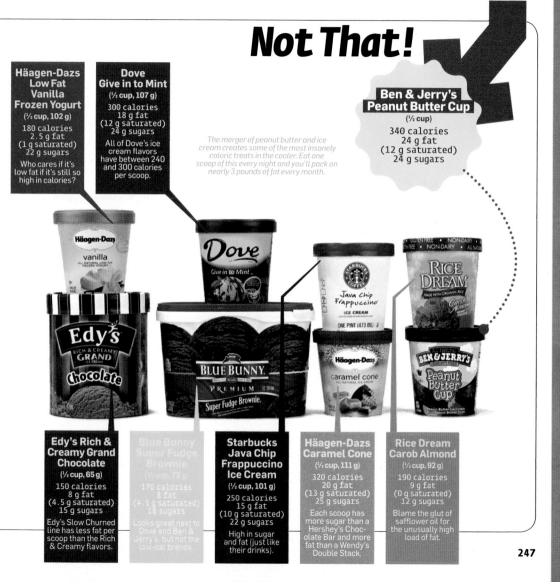

Not That!

Häagen-Dazs Low Fat Vanilla Frozen Yogurt
(½ cup, 102 g)

180 calories
2.5 g fat
(1 g saturated)
22 g sugars

Who cares if it's low fat if it's still so high in calories?

Dove Give in to Mint
(½ cup, 107 g)

300 calories
18 g fat
(12 g saturated)
24 g sugars

All of Dove's ice cream flavors have between 240 and 300 calories per scoop.

The merger of peanut butter and ice cream creates some of the most insanely caloric treats in the cooler. Eat one scoop of this every night and you'll pack on nearly 3 pounds of fat every month.

Ben & Jerry's Peanut Butter Cup
(½ cup)

340 calories
24 g fat
(12 g saturated)
24 g sugars

Edy's Rich & Creamy Grand Chocolate
(½ cup, 65 g)

150 calories
8 g fat
(4.5 g saturated)
15 g sugars

Edy's Slow Churned line has less fat per scoop than the Rich & Creamy flavors.

Blue Bunny Super Fudge Brownie
(½ cup, 72 g)

170 calories
8 fat
(4.5 g saturated)
18 sugars

Looks great next to Dove and Ben & Jerry's, but not the low-cal brands.

Starbucks Java Chip Frappuccino Ice Cream
(½ cup, 101 g)

250 calories
15 g fat
(10 g saturated)
22 g sugars

High in sugar and fat (just like their drinks).

Häagen-Dazs Caramel Cone
(½ cup, 111 g)

320 calories
20 g fat
(13 g saturated)
25 g sugars

Each scoop has more sugar than a Hershey's Chocolate Bar and more fat than a Wendy's Double Stack.

Rice Dream Carob Almond
(½ cup, 92 g)

190 calories
9 g fat
(0 g saturated)
12 g sugars

Blame the glut of safflower oil for the unusually high load of fat.

Frozen Treats
Eat This

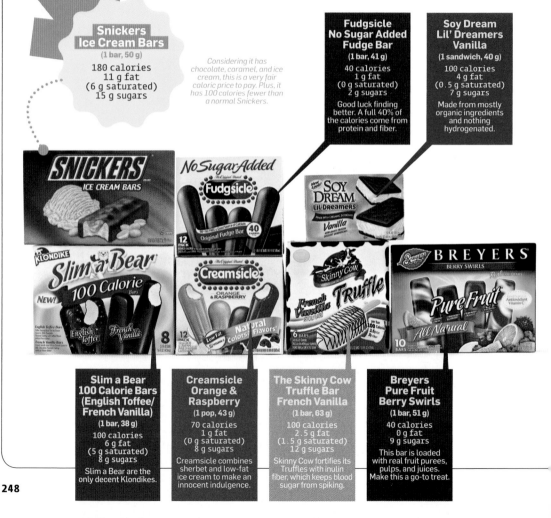

Snickers Ice Cream Bars
(1 bar, 50 g)
180 calories
11 g fat
(6 g saturated)
15 g sugars

Considering it has chocolate, caramel, and ice cream, this is a very fair caloric price to pay. Plus, it has 100 calories fewer than a normal Snickers.

Fudgsicle No Sugar Added Fudge Bar
(1 bar, 41 g)
40 calories
1 g fat
(0 g saturated)
2 g sugars
Good luck finding better. A full 40% of the calories come from protein and fiber.

Soy Dream Lil' Dreamers Vanilla
(1 sandwich, 40 g)
100 calories
4 g fat
(0.5 g saturated)
7 g sugars
Made from mostly organic ingredients and nothing hydrogenated.

Slim a Bear 100 Calorie Bars (English Toffee/ French Vanilla)
(1 bar, 38 g)
100 calories
6 g fat
(5 g saturated)
8 g sugars
Slim a Bear are the only decent Klondikes.

Creamsicle Orange & Raspberry
(1 pop, 43 g)
70 calories
1 g fat
(0 g saturated)
8 g sugars
Creamsicle combines sherbet and low-fat ice cream to make an innocent indulgence.

The Skinny Cow Truffle Bar French Vanilla
(1 bar, 63 g)
100 calories
2.5 g fat
(1.5 g saturated)
12 g sugars
Skinny Cow fortifies its Truffles with inulin fiber, which keeps blood sugar from spiking.

Breyers Pure Fruit Berry Swirls
(1 bar, 51 g)
40 calories
0 g fat
9 g sugars
This bar is loaded with real fruit purees, pulps, and juices. Make this a go-to treat.

Not That!

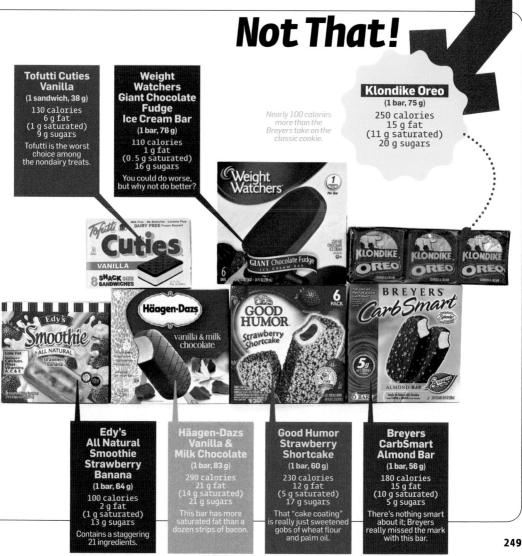

Tofutti Cuties Vanilla
(1 sandwich, 38 g)

130 calories
6 g fat
(1 g saturated)
9 g sugars

Tofutti is the worst choice among the nondairy treats.

Weight Watchers Giant Chocolate Fudge Ice Cream Bar
(1 bar, 76 g)

110 calories
1 g fat
(0.5 g saturated)
16 g sugars

You could do worse, but why not do better?

Nearly 100 calories more than the Breyers take on the classic cookie.

Klondike Oreo
(1 bar, 75 g)

250 calories
15 g fat
(11 g saturated)
20 g sugars

Edy's All Natural Smoothie Strawberry Banana
(1 bar, 64 g)

100 calories
2 g fat
(1 g saturated)
13 g sugars

Contains a staggering 21 ingredients.

Häagen-Dazs Vanilla & Milk Chocolate
(1 bar, 83 g)

290 calories
21 g fat
(14 g saturated)
21 g sugars

This bar has more saturated fat than a dozen strips of bacon.

Good Humor Strawberry Shortcake
(1 bar, 60 g)

230 calories
12 g fat
(5 g saturated)
17 g sugars

That "cake coating" is really just sweetened gobs of wheat flour and palm oil.

Breyers CarbSmart Almond Bar
(1 bar, 56 g)

180 calories
15 g fat
(10 g saturated)
5 g sugars

There's nothing smart about it; Breyers really missed the mark with this bar.

249

Juice
Drink This

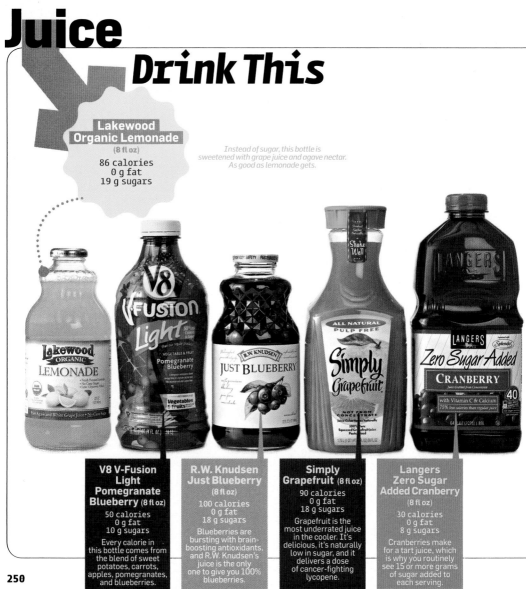

Lakewood Organic Lemonade
(8 fl oz)

86 calories
0 g fat
19 g sugars

Instead of sugar, this bottle is sweetened with grape juice and agave nectar. As good as lemonade gets.

V8 V-Fusion Light Pomegranate Blueberry (8 fl oz)

50 calories
0 g fat
10 g sugars

Every calorie in this bottle comes from the blend of sweet potatoes, carrots, apples, pomegranates, and blueberries.

R.W. Knudsen Just Blueberry
(8 fl oz)

100 calories
0 g fat
18 g sugars

Blueberries are bursting with brain-boosting antioxidants, and R.W. Knudsen's juice is the only one to give you 100% blueberries.

Simply Grapefruit (8 fl oz)

90 calories
0 g fat
18 g sugars

Grapefruit is the most underrated juice in the cooler. It's delicious, it's naturally low in sugar, and it delivers a dose of cancer-fighting lycopene.

Langers Zero Sugar Added Cranberry
(8 fl oz)

30 calories
0 g fat
8 g sugars

Cranberries make for a tart juice, which is why you routinely see 15 or more grams of sugar added to each serving.

Not That!

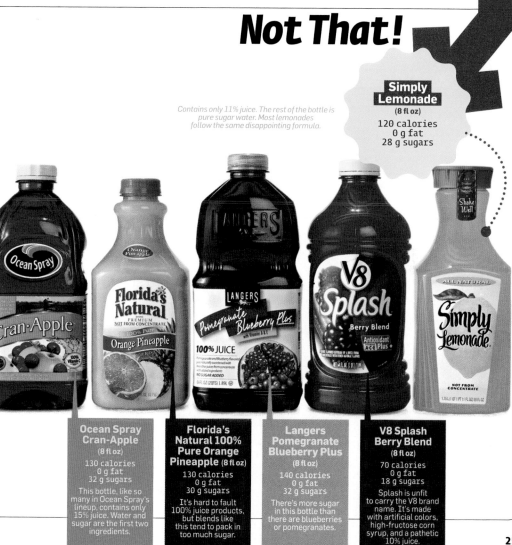

Contains only 11% juice. The rest of the bottle is pure sugar water. Most lemonades follow the same disappointing formula.

Ocean Spray Cran-Apple
(8 fl oz)

130 calories
0 g fat
32 g sugars

This bottle, like so many in Ocean Spray's lineup, contains only 15% juice. Water and sugar are the first two ingredients.

Florida's Natural 100% Pure Orange Pineapple (8 fl oz)

130 calories
0 g fat
30 g sugars

It's hard to fault 100% juice products, but blends like this tend to pack in too much sugar.

Langers Pomegranate Blueberry Plus
(8 fl oz)

140 calories
0 g fat
32 g sugars

There's more sugar in this bottle than there are blueberries or pomegranates.

V8 Splash Berry Blend
(8 fl oz)

70 calories
0 g fat
18 g sugars

Splash is unfit to carry the V8 brand name. It's made with artificial colors, high-fructose corn syrup, and a pathetic 10% juice.

251

Coffee and Energy Drinks
Drink This

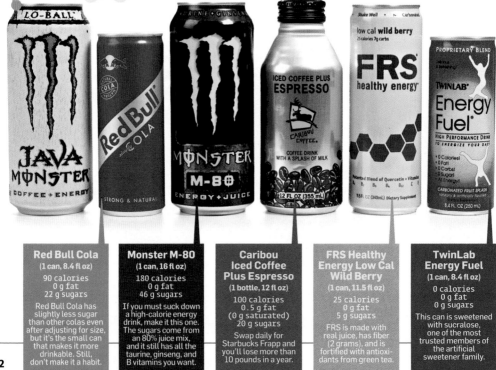

Java Monster Lo-Ball
(1 can, 15 fl oz)

100 calories
3 g fat
(2 g saturated)
8 g sugars

A lighter dose of sugar makes this can much more manageable than most of the alternatives.

Red Bull Cola
(1 can, 8.4 fl oz)

90 calories
0 g fat
22 g sugars

Red Bull Cola has slightly less sugar than other colas even after adjusting for size, but it's the small can that makes it more drinkable. Still, don't make it a habit.

Monster M-80
(1 can, 16 fl oz)

180 calories
0 g fat
46 g sugars

If you must suck down a high-calorie energy drink, make it this one. The sugars come from an 80% juice mix, and it still has all the taurine, ginseng, and B vitamins you want.

Caribou Iced Coffee Plus Espresso
(1 bottle, 12 fl oz)

100 calories
0.5 g fat
(0 g saturated)
20 g sugars

Swap daily for Starbucks Frapp and you'll lose more than 10 pounds in a year.

FRS Healthy Energy Low Cal Wild Berry
(1 can, 11.5 fl oz)

25 calories
0 g fat
5 g sugars

FRS is made with real juice, has fiber (2 grams), and is fortified with antioxidants from green tea.

TwinLab Energy Fuel
(1 can, 8.4 fl oz)

0 calories
0 g fat
0 g sugars

This can is sweetened with sucralose, one of the most trusted members of the artificial sweetener family.

Not That!

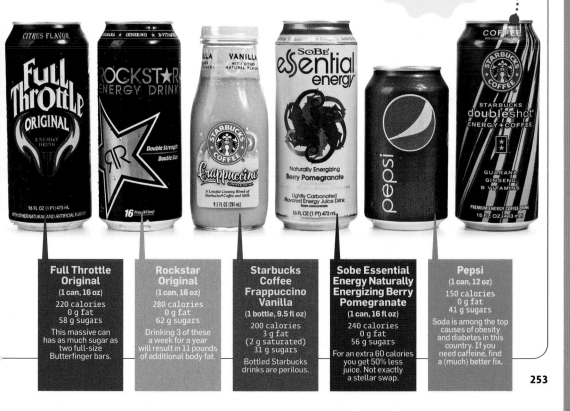

Starbucks Doubleshot
(1 can, 16 fl oz)
220 calories
3 g fat
(2 g saturated)
28 g sugars

If the goal was to bring something new to the sugar-saturated energy-drink market, consider this a failure. It's right up there with the worst offenders.

Full Throttle Original
(1 can, 16 oz)
220 calories
0 g fat
58 g sugars

This massive can has as much sugar as two full-size Butterfinger bars.

Rockstar Original
(1 can, 16 oz)
280 calories
0 g fat
62 g sugars

Drinking 3 of these a week for a year will result in 11 pounds of additional body fat.

Starbucks Coffee Frappuccino Vanilla
(1 bottle, 9.5 fl oz)
200 calories
3 g fat
(2 g saturated)
31 g sugars

Bottled Starbucks drinks are perilous.

Sobe Essential Energy Naturally Energizing Berry Pomegranate
(1 can, 16 fl oz)
240 calories
0 g fat
56 g sugars

For an extra 60 calories you get 50% less juice. Not exactly a stellar swap.

Pepsi
(1 can, 12 oz)
150 calories
0 g fat
41 g sugars

Soda is among the top causes of obesity and diabetes in this country. If you need caffeine, find a (much) better fix.

253

Tea

Drink This

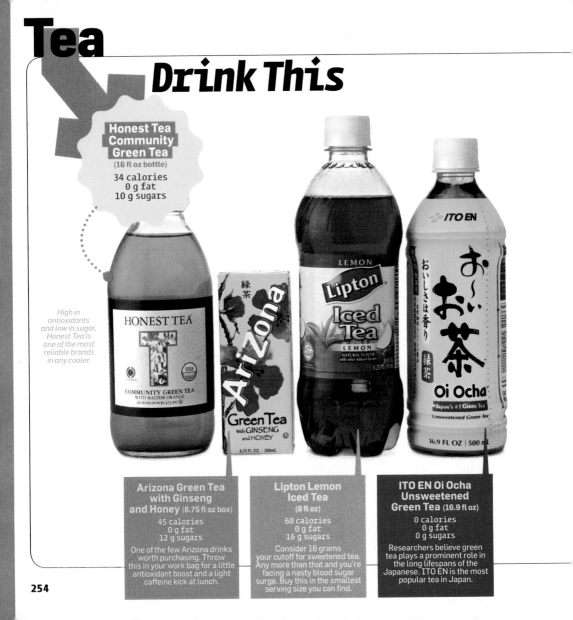

Honest Tea Community Green Tea
(16 fl oz bottle)

34 calories
0 g fat
10 g sugars

High in antioxidants and low in sugar, Honest Tea is one of the most reliable brands in any cooler.

Arizona Green Tea with Ginseng and Honey (6.75 fl oz box)

45 calories
0 g fat
12 g sugars

One of the few Arizona drinks worth purchasing. Throw this in your work bag for a little antioxidant boost and a light caffeine kick at lunch.

Lipton Lemon Iced Tea
(8 fl oz)

60 calories
0 g fat
16 g sugars

Consider 16 grams your cutoff for sweetened tea. Any more than that and you're facing a nasty blood sugar surge. Buy this in the smallest serving size you can find.

ITO EN Oi Ocha Unsweetened Green Tea (16.9 fl oz)

0 calories
0 g fat
0 g sugars

Researchers believe green tea plays a prominent role in the long lifespans of the Japanese. ITO EN is the most popular tea in Japan.

Not That!

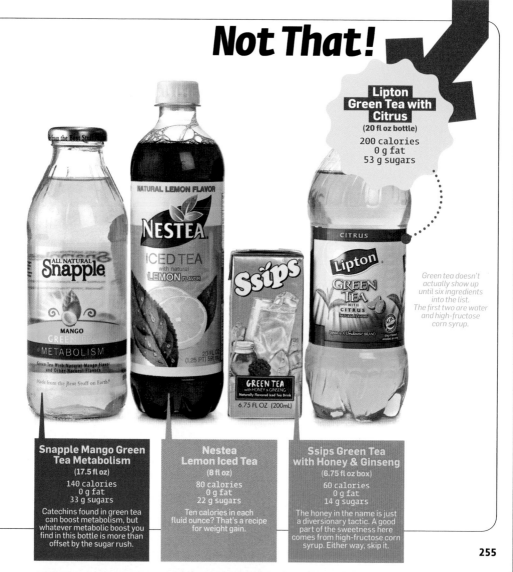

Lipton Green Tea with Citrus
(20 fl oz bottle)
200 calories
0 g fat
53 g sugars

Green tea doesn't actually show up until six ingredients into the list. The first two are water and high-fructose corn syrup.

Snapple Mango Green Tea Metabolism
(17.5 fl oz)
140 calories
0 g fat
33 g sugars

Catechins found in green tea can boost metabolism, but whatever metabolic boost you find in this bottle is more than offset by the sugar rush.

Nestea Lemon Iced Tea
(8 fl oz)
80 calories
0 g fat
22 g sugars

Ten calories in each fluid ounce? That's a recipe for weight gain.

Ssips Green Tea with Honey & Ginseng
(6.75 fl oz box)
60 calories
0 g fat
14 g sugars

The honey in the name is just a diversionary tactic. A good part of the sweetness here comes from high-fructose corn syrup. Either way, skip it.

255

Mixers

Drink This

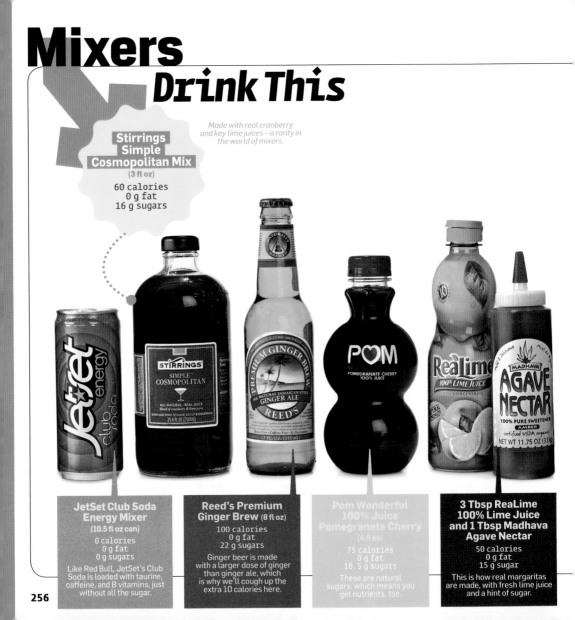

Made with real cranberry and key lime juices—a rarity in the world of mixers.

Stirrings Simple Cosmopolitan Mix
(3 fl oz)

60 calories
0 g fat
16 g sugars

JetSet Club Soda Energy Mixer
(10.5 fl oz can)

0 calories
0 g fat
0 g sugars

Like Red Bull, JetSet's Club Soda is loaded with taurine, caffeine, and B vitamins, just without all the sugar.

Reed's Premium Ginger Brew (8 fl oz)

100 calories
0 g fat
22 g sugars

Ginger beer is made with a larger dose of ginger than ginger ale, which is why we'll cough up the extra 10 calories here.

Pom Wonderful 100% Juice Pomegranate Cherry
(4 fl oz)

75 calories
0 g fat
16.5 g sugars

These are natural sugars, which means you get nutrients, too.

3 Tbsp ReaLime 100% Lime Juice and 1 Tbsp Madhava Agave Nectar

50 calories
0 g fat
15 g sugar

This is how real margaritas are made, with fresh lime juice and a hint of sugar.

Not That!

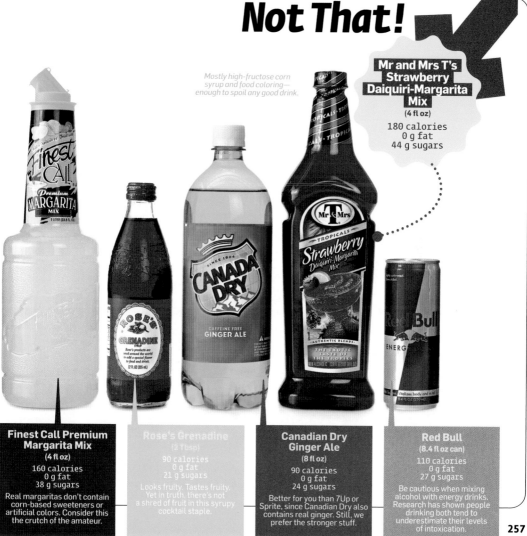

Mostly high-fructose corn syrup and food coloring—enough to spoil any good drink.

Mr and Mrs T's Strawberry Daiquiri-Margarita Mix
(4 fl oz)

180 calories
0 g fat
44 g sugars

Finest Call Premium Margarita Mix
(4 fl oz)

160 calories
0 g fat
38 g sugars

Real margaritas don't contain corn-based sweeteners or artificial colors. Consider this the crutch of the amateur.

Rose's Grenadine
(2 Tbsp)

90 calories
0 g fat
21 g sugars

Looks fruity. Tastes fruity. Yet in truth, there's not a shred of fruit in this syrupy cocktail staple.

Canadian Dry Ginger Ale
(8 fl oz)

90 calories
0 g fat
24 g sugars

Better for you than 7Up or Sprite, since Canadian Dry also contains real ginger. Still, we prefer the stronger stuff.

Red Bull
(8.4 fl oz can)

110 calories
0 g fat
27 g sugars

Be cautious when mixing alcohol with energy drinks. Research has shown people drinking both tend to underestimate their levels of intoxication.

257

Beer

Drink This

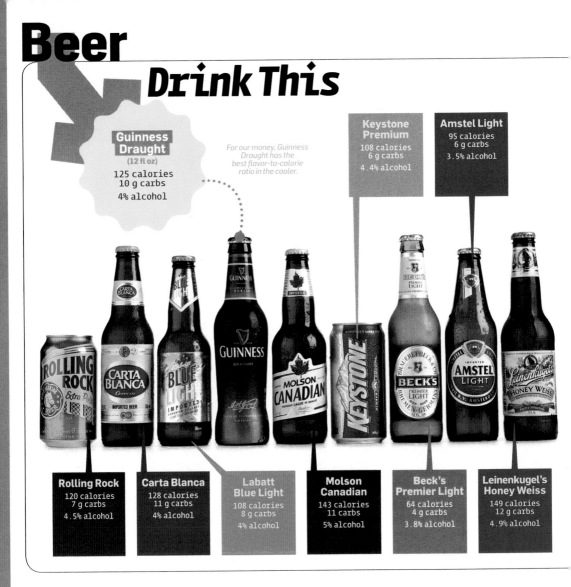

Guinness Draught
(12 fl oz)
125 calories
10 g carbs
4% alcohol

For our money, Guinness Draught has the best flavor-to-calorie ratio in the cooler.

Keystone Premium
108 calories
6 g carbs
4.4% alcohol

Amstel Light
95 calories
6 g carbs
3.5% alcohol

Rolling Rock
120 calories
7 g carbs
4.5% alcohol

Carta Blanca
128 calories
11 g carbs
4% alcohol

Labatt Blue Light
108 calories
8 g carbs
4% alcohol

Molson Canadian
143 calories
11 carbs
5% alcohol

Beck's Premier Light
64 calories
4 g carbs
3.8% alcohol

Leinenkugel's Honey Weiss
149 calories
12 g carbs
4.9% alcohol

Not That!

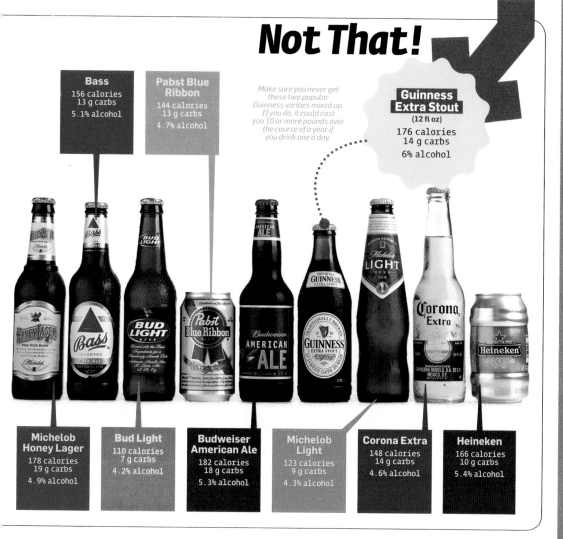

Bass
156 calories
13 g carbs
5.1% alcohol

Pabst Blue Ribbon
144 calories
13 g carbs
4.7% alcohol

Make sure you never get these two popular Guinness varieties mixed up. If you do, it could cost you 10 or more pounds over the course of a year if you drink one a day.

Guinness Extra Stout
(12 fl oz)
176 calories
14 g carbs
6% alcohol

Michelob Honey Lager
178 calories
19 g carbs
4.9% alcohol

Bud Light
110 calories
7 g carbs
4.2% alcohol

Budweiser American Ale
182 calories
18 g carbs
5.3% alcohol

Michelob Light
123 calories
9 g carbs
4.3% alcohol

Corona Extra
148 calories
14 g carbs
4.6% alcohol

Heineken
166 calories
10 g carbs
5.4% alcohol

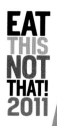

Chapter

5

HOLIDAYS &
SPECIAL OCCASIONS

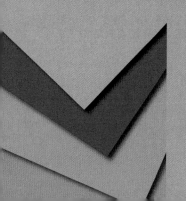

There's an old joke that says...

every Jewish holiday celebrates the same idea: "They tried to kill us, we won, let's eat." Sadly, too many holiday traditions in too many cultures today focus only on those last two words: "Let's eat." Whether you're cooking up a ham for Christmas, turkey for Thanksgiving, jerked chicken for Kwanzaa, or flanken for Passover, every holiday on the American calendar seems to carry an egregious caloric load. And that's before the Thanksgiving wine, the Christmas egg nog, the Easter brunch mimosas, and the brewskis on the Fourth of July.

Consider that most astronomically caloric, gastronomically uneconomic of holidays, Thanksgiving. According to the Calorie Control Council, the average American will consume 4,500 calories and 229 grams of fat on

Thanksgiving day, a feat worthy of competitive eating accolades on any other day. But that doesn't mean you can't stuff your face without testing the fortitude of your new designer jeans. We imagine you'll want turkey. Cranberry sauce. Potatoes, sure. Gravy. Maybe some veggies on the side. Oh, and pie? Yeah, go for it! But just by making a couple of smart at-the-table swaps (like choosing pumpkin over pecan pie, or white meat over the drumstick), you could eat to your heart's content and still take in 700 fewer calories than you did last year.

Now imagine if you could do that at every holiday: whack off 700 calories from Christmas, New Year's, Fourth of July, and Halloween, and you've just shaved an entire pound off your body. And the sacrifice? Well, there is none. You can still raid the kids' stockings and trick-or-treat bags, feast on grilled goodies and all the fixings at the summer barbecue, and drink Champagne toasts aplenty to welcome in the new year.

You'll just look leaner and fitter while you do it.

Thanksgiving
Eat This

Turkey is the least of your concerns on Turkey Day. Pick smart sides and a reasonable dessert and you can save 500 calories or more.

White Meat Turkey Dinner

900 calories
37 g fat
(11.5 g saturated)
1,115 mg sodium

Pumpkin pie with low-fat whipped cream
(1 medium slice; ¼ pie)

335 calories
15 g fat
(6.5 g saturated)
38 g sugars

In the pantheon of pies, pumpkin ranks among one of the lower-calorie slices.

Green bean casserole
(½ cup)

100 calories
6 g fat
(1 g saturated)
300 mg sodium

Can the cream of mushroom and fried onions and make it with fresh green beans and sautéed onions.

Mashed potatoes (½ cup) with turkey gravy (¼ cup)

140 calories
7 g fat
(2 g saturated)
340 mg sodium

Don't nix the mash—just go easy with the butter and use low-fat milk to prepare them.

Turkey breast (4 oz) with homemade cranberry sauce (2 Tbsp)

195 calories
4 g fat
265 mg sodium

White meat turkey is as lean as meat gets. Homemade cranberry sauce cuts the sugar.

Dinner roll with butter

130 calories
5 g fat
(2 g saturated)
210 mg sodium

A small pat of butter helps lower the glycemic index of the roll, meaning the carbs will have less of an effect on blood sugar.

Not That!

Stuffing, sweet potatoes, and cornbread are among the worst of the Thanksgiving staples. Combined, they bring 615 calories to this plate.

Dark Meat Turkey Dinner

1,475 calories
62 g fat
(23 g saturated)
1,370 mg sodium

Cornbread with butter

190 calories
9 g fat
(4 g saturated)
360 mg sodium

Sweeter, saltier, and fattier than a regular roll.

Dark turkey meat
(4 oz)
with jellied cranberry sauce
(¼-inch slice)

410 calories
10 g fat
(4 g saturated)
320 mg sodium

Dark meat is about twice as fatty as white meat.

Candied sweet potatoes with marshmallow topping (½ cup)

250 calories
8 g fat
(5 g saturated)
270 mg sodium

Sweet potatoes lose their nutrutitional edge once they're covered in marshmallows.

Stuffing
(½ cup)

175 calories
14 g fat
(6 g saturated)
420 mg sodium

Stuffing is nothing more than a pile of croutons moistened with fat and loaded with sodium. Double this number if it was cooked inside the bird.

Pecan pie
(1 medium slice; ⅛ pie)

450 calories
21 g fat
(4 g saturated)
70 g sugars

The healthy fat from the pecans is not enough to justify the extra load of corn syrup calories.

265

Christmas
Eat This

Beef Tenderloin Dinner

815 calories
30 g fat
(11 g saturated)
665 mg sodium

Medium-rare beef, crispy potatoes, red wine, and chocolate: What more could you ask for from a Christmas feast?

Chocolate fondue (1 oz) with fruit (½ cup)

200 calories
8 g fat
(4 g saturated)
18 g sugars

Go with dark instead of milk chocolate and you'll get a deeper-flavored fondue with more antioxidants and less added sugar.

Beef tenderloin (6 oz)

300 calories
15 g fat
(6 g saturated)
400 mg sodium

Save cash by purchasing a whole tenderloin. Rub the lean hunk of beef with olive oil, garlic and rosemary, and roast at 450°F.

Roasted red potatoes (½ cup)

100 calories
5 g fat
(1 g saturated)
170 mg sodium

Any roasted vegetable will be a welcome addition to a holiday feast.

Peas and pearl onions (½ cup)

90 calories
2 g fat
95 mg sodium

Fend off the food coma: The fiber in the peas and the chromium in the onions both help to regulate blood sugar levels.

Glass of red wine (5 oz)

125 calories
5.3 g carbohydrates

Research shows that pinot noir has the highest concentration of the flavonoids in wine that may protect your cardio-vascular system.

Not That!

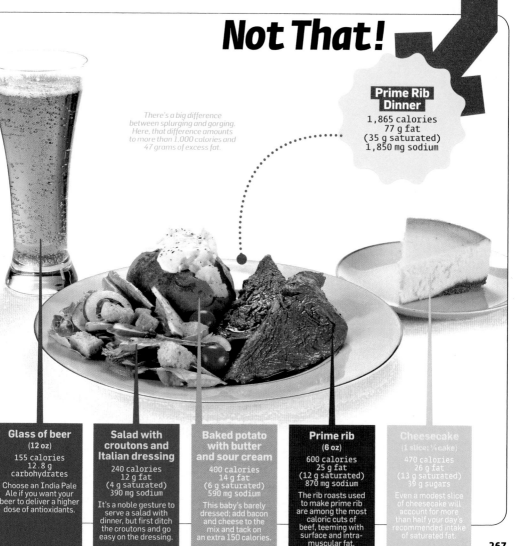

There's a big difference between splurging and gorging. Here, that difference amounts to more than 1,000 calories and 47 grams of excess fat.

Prime Rib Dinner
1,865 calories
77 g fat
(35 g saturated)
1,850 mg sodium

Glass of beer
(12 oz)
155 calories
12.8 g carbohydrates

Choose an India Pale Ale if you want your beer to deliver a higher dose of antioxidants.

Salad with croutons and Italian dressing
240 calories
12 g fat
(4 g saturated)
390 mg sodium

It's a noble gesture to serve a salad with dinner, but first ditch the croutons and go easy on the dressing.

Baked potato with butter and sour cream
400 calories
14 g fat
(6 g saturated)
590 mg sodium

This baby's barely dressed; add bacon and cheese to the mix and tack on an extra 150 calories.

Prime rib
(6 oz)
600 calories
25 g fat
(12 g saturated)
870 mg sodium

The rib roasts used to make prime rib are among the most caloric cuts of beef, teeming with surface and intramuscular fat.

Cheesecake
(1 slice; ⅛ cake)
470 calories
26 g fat
(13 g saturated)
39 g sugars

Even a modest slice of cheesecake will account for more than half your day's recommended intake of saturated fat.

267

Cocktail Party
Eat This

Jumbo shrimp
(6) with cocktail sauce (2 Tbsp)

60 calories
<1 g fat
470 mg sodium

Shrimp are essentially fat free and protein packed, which makes them one of the few foods you can gorge on without paying the price. But limit yourself on the cocktail sauce—it's mostly tomatoes, but it's heavy on sodium.

Meatballs
(3)

240 calories
12 g fat
(4.5 g saturated)
650 mg sodium

Start off with protein-based bites and you'll fill your belly quickly, saving you from senseless snacking the rest of the night.

Glass of Champagne
(6 oz)

130 calories
6 g carbohydrates

Turns out the perfect New Year's drink can also help reduce heart-threatening inflammation. Cheers to that!

Tomato bruschetta
(2 pieces)

200 calories
4 g fat
(1 g saturated)
230 mg sodium

Other than the bread, it's a bunch of A-list players: tomatoes, garlic, basil, and extra-virgin olive oil.

Mojito
(8 oz)

180 calories
15 g carbohydrates

Made with a bevy of healthy components, including lime juice, fresh mint, and sugar-free club soda.

Vodka soda
(8 oz)

120 calories
0 g carbohydrates

All clear spirits pack around the same amount of calories and carbs, so the only variable with cocktails is mixers. Here, soda trumps tonic for one reason: It's calorie free.

Not That!

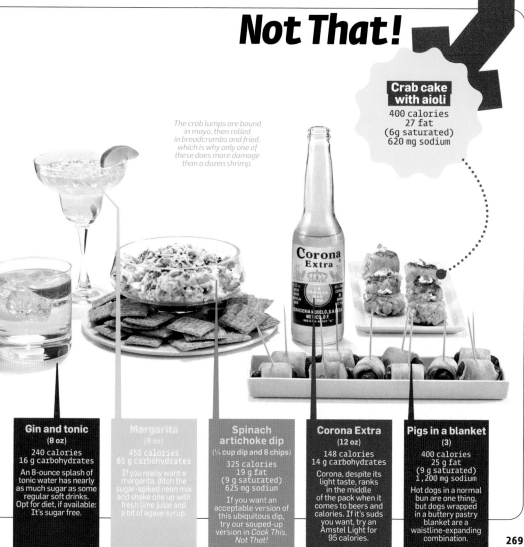

Crab cake with aioli
400 calories
27 fat
(6g saturated)
620 mg sodium

The crab lumps are bound in mayo, then rolled in breadcrumbs and fried, which is why only one of these does more damage than a dozen shrimp.

Gin and tonic
(8 oz)

240 calories
16 g carbohydrates

An 8-ounce splash of tonic water has nearly as much sugar as some regular soft drinks. Opt for diet, if available: It's sugar free.

Margarita
(8 oz)

450 calories
65 g carbohydrates

If you really want a margarita, ditch the sugar-spiked neon mix and shake one up with fresh lime juice and a bit of agave syrup.

Spinach artichoke dip
(¼ cup dip and 8 chips)

325 calories
19 g fat
(9 g saturated)
625 mg sodium

If you want an acceptable version of this ubiquitous dip, try our souped-up version in *Cook This, Not That!*

Corona Extra
(12 oz)

148 calories
14 g carbohydrates

Corona, despite its light taste, ranks in the middle of the pack when it comes to beers and calories. If it's suds you want, try an Amstel Light for 95 calories.

Pigs in a blanket
(3)

400 calories
25 g fat
(9 g saturated)
1,200 mg sodium

Hot dogs in a normal bun are one thing, but dogs wrapped in a buttery pastry blanket are a waistline-expanding combination.

269

At the Ballpark
Eat This

Hot dog with relish, ketchup, and mustard
320 calories
18 g fat
(8 g saturated)
960 mg sodium

Not only will a hot dog save you calories over a plate of nachos, but it will also give a bellyful of protein to help ward off late-game munchies.

Cotton candy
(1 serving)
220 calories
0 g fat
56 g sugars

We're not going to pretend this is healthy; it is, after all, pure sugar. But in terms of weight, it's ultralight, helping to minimize the overall calorie count.

Neapolitan ice cream sandwich
190 calories
7 g fat
(3.5 g saturated)
15 g sugars

Ice cream sandwiches all come in the same small portion, so you know you're getting less than 200 calories, regardless of brand.

Cracker Jacks
420 calories
7 g fat
(0 g saturated)
245 mg sodium

See that regular fat to saturated fat ratio? That's because the fat in this classic box is the healthy monounsaturated variety found in peanuts.

Beef kabob
220 calories
9 g fat
(4.5 g saturated)
120 mg sodium

Most kabobs are made with lean sirloin. Find one with vegetables on the skewer and you've located the best meal in the ballpark.

Light beer
(20 oz)
174 calories
0 g fat
9.6 g carbohydrates

When it comes to stadium-size cups, you'd be wise to stick to light beer.

Not That!

This is a nutritionist's nightmare. It's loaded with sodium, has close to a day's worth of saturated fat, and offers nothing by way of redeeming nutrients.

Nachos
(40 chips and 4 oz cheese)

1,101 calories
59 g fat
(18.5 g saturated)
1,580 mg sodium

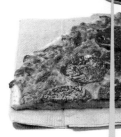

Cola
(20 oz)

243 calories
0 g fat
67.5 g
carbohydrates

Once again soda proves to be the nutritional loser. It's just a cupful of carbonated water and high-fructose corn syrup.

Pepperoni pizza
(1 slice)

425 calories
19 g fat
(7 g saturated)
820 mg sodium

In order to charge $5 or $6 a pop, vendors tend to sell slices that are larger than your typical delivery pie.

French fries

600 calories
32 g fat
(10 g saturated)
890 mg sodium

Make this your regular ballpark snack and you'll need to turn the seventh inning stretch into a full-game workout to keep the pounds off.

French vanilla soft-serve ice cream
(1 cup)

380 calories
22 g fat
(13 g saturated)
36 g sugars

Malts and soft serve come in huge portion sizes, making them a dangerous choice.

Chocolate ice cream in a helmet (1½ cups)

429 calories
21 g fat
(12 g saturated)

Mini helmets house about a cup and a half of cream, i.e., three times too much for you. Only order this if you're prepared to share.

271

At the Mall
Eat This

Ask for your pretzel with no butter and you'll save 90 calories of pure fat.

Subway 6-inch Oven Roasted Chicken Breast

320 calories
4.5 g fat
(1 g saturated)
750 mg sodium

Who says you can't eat light at the mall? If you're fortunate enough to find a Subway in the food court, make a beeline for it.

Panda Express Mushroom Chicken with Mixed Vegetables

255 calories
13 g fat
(3 g saturated)
1,040 mg sodium

As long as you skip the orange chicken (and the rice and noodles), Panda Express can be a solid spot to squash a growing hunger.

McDonald's Vanilla Ice Cream Cone

150 calories
3.5 g fat
(2 g saturated)
18 g sugars

Slice the saturated fat from the chocolate chip treat in half with Mickey D's well-portioned cone.

Orange Julius
(20 oz)

160 calories
0.5 g fat
38 g sugars

Short of unsweetened iced tea, H₂O, and black coffee, this is the best beverage you'll find in the food court.

272

Not That!

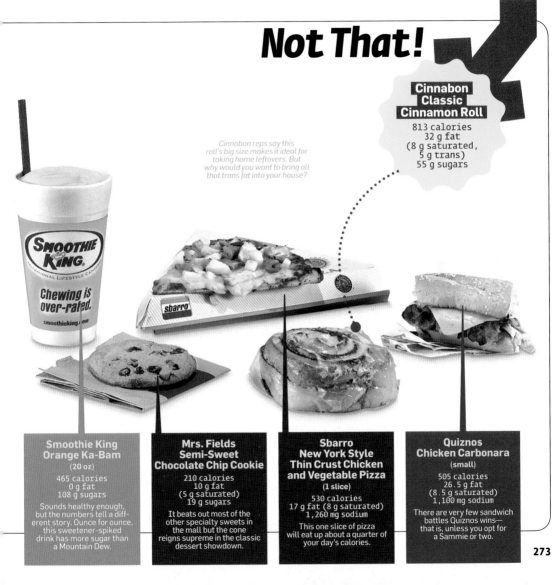

Cinnabon Classic Cinnamon Roll

813 calories
32 g fat
(8 g saturated,
5 g trans)
55 g sugars

Cinnabon reps say this roll's big size makes it ideal for taking home leftovers. But why would you want to bring all that trans fat into your house?

Smoothie King Orange Ka-Bam

(20 oz)

465 calories
0 g fat
108 g sugars

Sounds healthy enough, but the numbers tell a different story. Ounce for ounce, this sweetener-spiked drink has more sugar than a Mountain Dew.

Mrs. Fields Semi-Sweet Chocolate Chip Cookie

210 calories
10 g fat
(5 g saturated)
19 g sugars

It beats out most of the other specialty sweets in the mall but the cone reigns supreme in the classic dessert showdown.

Sbarro New York Style Thin Crust Chicken and Vegetable Pizza

(1 slice)

530 calories
17 g fat (8 g saturated)
1,260 mg sodium

This one slice of pizza will eat up about a quarter of your day's calories.

Quiznos Chicken Carbonara

(small)

505 calories
26.5 g fat
(8.5 g saturated)
1,100 mg sodium

There are very few sandwich battles Quiznos wins—that is, unless you opt for a Sammie or two.

273

At the Movie Theater
Eat This

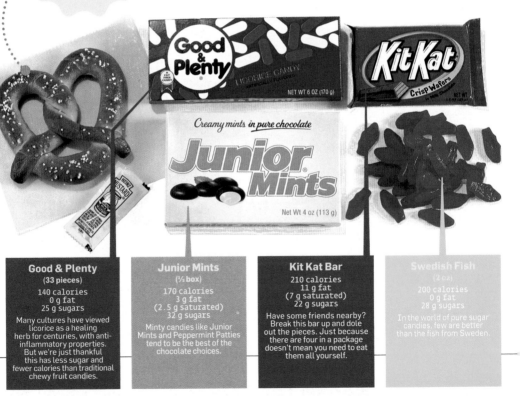

As long as you're not dipping it into molten cheese, a large soft pretzel makes a reasonable movie theater or street corner snack. Be really good and ask them to skip the salt—mustard packs plenty of sodium as it is.

Good & Plenty
LICORICE CANDY
ARTIFICIAL FLAVORS
NET WT 6 OZ (170 g)

Kit Kat
Crisp Wafers
NET WT

Creamy mints *in pure chocolate*
Junior Mints
Net Wt 4 oz (113 g)

Good & Plenty
(33 pieces)

140 calories
0 g fat
25 g sugars

Many cultures have viewed licorice as a healing herb for centuries, with anti-inflammatory properties. But we're just thankful this has less sugar and fewer calories than traditional chewy fruit candies.

Junior Mints
(½ box)

170 calories
3 g fat
(2.5 g saturated)
32 g sugars

Minty candies like Junior Mints and Peppermint Patties tend to be the best of the chocolate choices.

Kit Kat Bar

210 calories
11 g fat
(7 g saturated)
22 g sugars

Have some friends nearby? Break this bar up and dole out the pieces. Just because there are four in a package doesn't mean you need to eat them all yourself.

Swedish Fish
(2 oz)

200 calories
0 g fat
28 g sugars

In the world of pure sugar candies, few are better than the fish from Sweden.

Not That!

Popcorn can be a great, fiber-rich snack, as long as you stay away from the dreaded butter pump. Besides tripling the calories of a bag of popcorn, many movie theater "butters" are teeming with trans fat. Instead, seek flavor from the spice mixes many theaters carry now.

Buttered popcorn
(medium; 10 to 12 cups)

600 calories
39 g fat
(12 g saturated)
1,120 mg sodium

HERSHEY'S Milk Chocolate
NET WT. 1.55 OZ. (43 g)

Twizzlers
MAKES MOUTHS HAPPY!®
NET WT. 2.5 OZ. (70 g)
STRAWBERRY ARTIFICIALLY FLAVORED *TWISTS*

Milk Chocolate **m&m's**®
CHOCOLATE CANDIES
NET WT. 1.69 OZ. (47.9 g)

Dots
(22 pieces)

260 calories
0 g fat
42 g sugars

They stick to your teeth just like they stick to your waistline. You're better off going for nearly any other gummy product besides these.

Hershey's Milk Chocolate Bar

210 calories
13 g fat
(8 g saturated)
24 g sugars

If you're going to eat pure chocolate, you're better off picking up a bar with at least 65% cacao. That way, you lower your sugar intake while maximizing antioxidants.

M&M's
(1 bag)

240 calories
10 g fat
(6 g saturated)
31 g sugars

They may seem harmless and fun in their tiny candy-coated vessels, but a few generous handfuls of M&M's can wipe out a meal's worth of calories before you know it.

Twizzlers
(⅓ 6-oz package)

320 calories
1 g fat
38 g sugars

Ignore the "low fat" claims on the side of the package—these are nothing more than ropes of corn syrup.

Vending Machine
Eat This

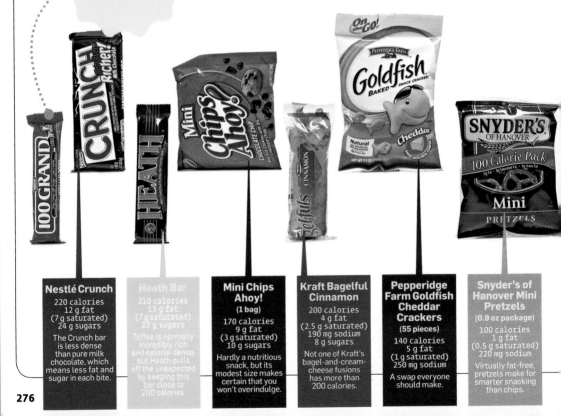

100 Grand
190 calories
8 g fat
(5 g saturated)
23 g sugars

The "best" (we use that term loosely) candy bar in America. This is the only full-size chocolate bar we've ever seen under 200 calories.

Nestlé Crunch
220 calories
12 g fat
(7 g saturated)
24 g sugars

The Crunch bar is less dense than pure milk chocolate, which means less fat and sugar in each bite.

Heath Bar
210 calories
13 g fat
(7 g saturated)
23 g sugars

Toffee is normally incredibly rich and calorie-dense, but Heath pulls off the unexpected by keeping this bar close to 200 calories.

Mini Chips Ahoy!
(1 bag)
170 calories
9 g fat
(3 g saturated)
10 g sugars

Hardly a nutritious snack, but its modest size makes certain that you won't overindulge.

Kraft Bagelful Cinnamon
200 calories
4 g fat
(2.5 g saturated)
190 mg sodium
8 g sugars

Not one of Kraft's bagel-and-cream-cheese fusions has more than 200 calories.

Pepperidge Farm Goldfish Cheddar Crackers
(55 pieces)
140 calories
5 g fat
(1 g saturated)
250 mg sodium

A swap everyone should make.

Snyder's of Hanover Mini Pretzels
(0.9 oz package)
100 calories
1 g fat
(0.5 g saturated)
220 mg sodium

Virtually fat-free, pretzels make for smarter snacking than chips.

Not That!

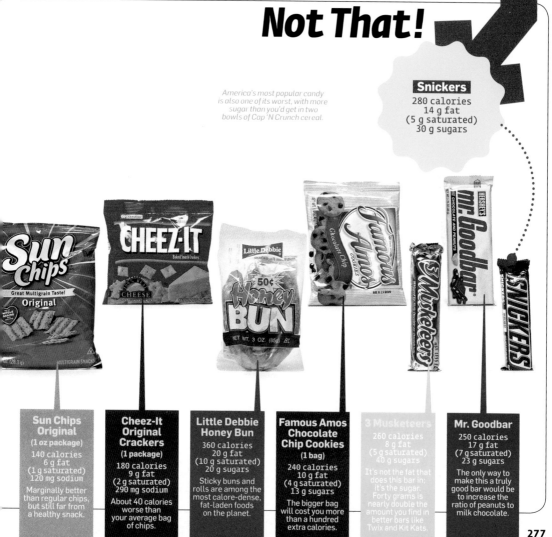

America's most popular candy is also one of its worst, with more sugar than you'd get in two bowls of Cap 'N Crunch cereal.

Snickers
280 calories
14 g fat
(5 g saturated)
30 g sugars

Sun Chips Original
(1 oz package)

140 calories
6 g fat
(1 g saturated)
120 mg sodium

Marginally better than regular chips, but still far from a healthy snack.

Cheez-It Original Crackers
(1 package)

180 calories
9 g fat
(2 g saturated)
290 mg sodium

About 40 calories worse than your average bag of chips.

Little Debbie Honey Bun

360 calories
20 g fat
(10 g saturated)
20 g sugars

Sticky buns and rolls are among the most calorie-dense, fat-laden foods on the planet.

Famous Amos Chocolate Chip Cookies
(1 bag)

240 calories
10 g fat
(4 g saturated)
13 g sugars

The bigger bag will cost you more than a hundred extra calories.

3 Musketeers

260 calories
8 g fat
(5 g saturated)
40 g sugars

It's not the fat that does this bar in; it's the sugar. Forty grams is nearly double the amount you find in better bars like Twix and Kit Kats.

Mr. Goodbar

250 calories
17 g fat
(7 g saturated)
23 g sugars

The only way to make this a truly good bar would be to increase the ratio of peanuts to milk chocolate.

277

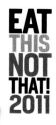

Chapter
6

FOR KIDS

Being a great parent

has always been a challenge. Think of Adam and Eve, figuring out the whole parenting thing without a guidebook. (Eve: "Should we be concerned about Cain picking on his brother?" Adam: "Nah, they're fine. Hand me an apple.") Or how about Oedipus, who killed his dad, married his mom, and brought disaster to their kingdom? (And you thought your kids feeding Fido their green beans was a big deal.)

But while headaches, backaches, and wallet aches have always been part of the penalty we pay for having children we love, it seems as though parenting has gotten even more complicated in recent years. Technology deserves a lot of the blame: Facebook, texting, and a dozen other wizardly wonders have given our progeny plenty of ways to get around the rules. But the technology that's complicating our lives as parents is a different kind of science entirely.

FOOD SCIENCE.

See, the foods our kids are eating today are very different from the foods we ate as children. The foods in today's supermarkets and on restaurant kids' menus come not from the great green earth, but from the minds of marketers. They're assembled not in warm, welcoming kitchens, but in cold, bright science labs, and their nutritional labels read like the contents of a chemistry set.

Consider, if you will, the humble Cheerio. A little round O of goodness, the Cheerio that you and I grew up with contains only ground oats, a little sugar, some starch, some salt, and two preservatives—one of which is good old vitamin E. Pretty simple.

Until it got complicated. Because now we have not only Cheerios, but also Berry Burst Cheerios, MultiGrain Cheerios, Apple Cinnamon Cheerios, Honey Nut Cheerios, and something called Yogurt Burst Cheerios. Which of these variations are good for your kids? Which are not?

It's hard to tell. Is the "fractionated palm kernel oil" in the Yogurt Burst Cheerios something you should feed your kids? What about the dextrose, the maltodextrin, the corn syrup, the brown sugar syrup, and oh yes the actual sugar (which is listed twice!)? In fact, this breakfast concoction is a great example of how today's food marketers are taking healthy foods and making them unhealthy by messing around with a complicated combination of confusing chemicals.

The result of all this fiddling about with our food supply is easy to see all around us: Kids are getting fatter. And with that fat comes more than just pleated pants and jokes about

What Our Kids Need Each Day

	1–3 YEARS	4–8 YEARS	9–13 YEARS	14–18 YEARS
CALORIES	1,000–1,400	1,400–1,600	1,800–2,200 (B)	2,200–2,400 (B)
			1,600–2,200 (G)	2,000 (G)
FAT (g)	33–54	39–62	62–85	61–95 (B) 55–78 (G)
SATURATED FAT (g)	<12–16	<16–18	<20–24 (B) <18–22 (G)	<24–27 (B) <22 (G)
SODIUM (mg)	1,000–1,500	1,200–1,900	1,500–2,200	1,500–2,300
CARBS (g)	130	130	130	130
FIBER (g)	19	25	31 (B) 26 (G)	38 (B) 26 (G)
PROTEIN (g)	13	19	31 (B) 26 (G)	52 (B) 46 (G)

being junk-food junkies. Being over-weight as a child is a serious health problem. Consider this:

Ten years ago, type 2 diabetes was known as "adult-onset diabetes" because it took several decades of overeating to get your body to the point where it was at risk. But we have so hyperinflated the calories in our foods that even children—children as young as 4!—are now develop-ing this disease. And it's not a pretty disease: Among its complications are blindness, heart attack, stroke, and sexual dysfunction. And the Centers for Disease Control and Prevention (CDC) recently predicted that one in three children born in the year 2000 will develop diabetes at some point in his or her lifetime.

Yet much of the food on offer as "for kids" in America's restaurants and super-markets is a practical invitation to diabetes and other health complications—from heart disease to cancer to high blood pressure to asthma—later in life.

That's why we've included this chapter. We've analyzed the offerings of all the major restaurant chains and uncovered the real truth about what America is feeding its children. And the great news is this: You can have a major impact on your children's health and future, simply by making a few smart choices.

The power is in your hands.

Eat This Pyramid, Not That One

The USDA has its pyramid, of course, but the iconic image young students learn so well in school leaves a lot to be desired in terms of specifics. According to the vagaries of the image, a serving of white rice and quinoa both count the same toward the recommended six daily servings, despite the fact that one is packed with fiber, healthy fat, and essential amino acids (quinoa) and the other is a nutritional black hole (rice).

It's time for parental discretion. One-quarter of all vegetables consumed by kids are French fries, and according to a government study of 4,000 kids between the ages of 2 and 19, the overwhelming bulk of their nutrients comes from fruit juice and sugary cereals. While those might have a place in the USDA's pyramid, they have no place in ours. It's still important for your kids to go about constructing their pyramids each day—you just need to be sure they have the right building blocks.

FATS AND OILS (USE SPARINGLY)

Eat This
Healthy fats: olive oil; canola oil; monounsaturated fats from nuts, avocado, and salmon

Not That!
Unhealthy fats: stick margarine, lard, palm oil, anything with partially hydrogenated oil

DAIRY (2 OR 3 1-CUP SERVINGS)

Eat This
2 percent milk, string cheese, cottage cheese, plain yogurt sweetened with fresh fruit

Not That!
Chocolate milk, ice cream, hot cheese dip, yogurt with fruit on the bottom

MEAT, POULTRY, FISH, EGGS, AND BEANS (2 OR 3 2-OUNCE SERVINGS)

Eat This
Grilled chicken breast; roast pork tenderloin; sirloin steak; scrambled, boiled, or poached eggs; stewed black beans; almonds; unsweetened peanut butter

Not That!
Chicken fingers, crispy chicken sandwiches, cheeseburgers, strip or ribeye steak, peanut butter with added sugars

VEGETABLES (5½ 1-CUP SERVINGS)

Eat This
Sautéed spinach, steamed broccoli, romaine or mixed green salads, roasted mushrooms, grilled pepper and onion skewers, baby carrots, tomato sauce, salsa, homemade guacamole

Not That!
French fries, potato chips, onion rings, vegetables dipped in ranch dressing

FRUIT (3½ 1-CUP SERVINGS)

Eat This
Sliced apples or pears; berries; grapes; stone fruit like peaches, plums, and apricots; 100 percent fruit smoothies

Not That!
More than one 8-ounce glass of juice a day; more than a few tablespoons of dried fruit a day; smoothies made with sherbet, frozen yogurt, or added sugar

(6 1-OUNCE SERVINGS)

Eat This
Brown rice, whole grain bread, quinoa, whole grain pasta, oatmeal

Not That!
White rice, white bread, pasta, muffins, tortillas, pancakes, waffles, heavily sweetened cereal

6 Rules of Good Nutrition

GREAT FOR YOUR KIDS, AND GREAT FOR YOU

Rule #1
NEVER SKIP BREAKFAST. EVER.

Yes, mornings are crazy. But they're also our best hope at regaining our nutritional sanity. A 2005 study synthesized the results of 47 other studies that examined the impact of starting the day with a healthy breakfast. Here's what they found.

Children skipped breakfast more than any other meal. Skipping is more prevalent in girls, older children, and adolescents.

People who skip breakfast are more likely to take up smoking or drinking, less likely to exercise, and more likely to follow fad diets or express concerns about body weight. Common reasons cited for skipping were lack of time, lack of hunger, or dieting.

▶ The day that one national breakfast survey was administered, 8 percent of 1- to 7-year-olds skipped, 12 percent of 8- to 10-year-olds skipped, 20 percent of 11- to 14-year-olds skipped, and 30 percent of 15- to 18-year-olds skipped.

Bad news. Sure, it would seem to make sense that skipping breakfast means eating fewer calories, which means weighing less. But it doesn't work that way. Consider:

People who eat breakfast tend to have higher total calorie intakes throughout the day, but they also get significantly more fiber, calcium, and other micronutrients than skippers do. Breakfast eaters also tended to consume less soda and French fries and more fruits, vegetables, and milk.

Breakfast eaters were approximately 30 percent less likely to be overweight or obese. (Think about that—kids who eat breakfast eat more food, but weigh less!)

Rule #2
SNACK WITH PURPOSE.

There's a big difference between mindless munching and strategic snacking. Snacking with purpose means reinforcing good habits, keeping your metabolic rate high, and filling the gaps between meals with the nutrients your child's body craves.

▶ In the 20 years leading up to the 21st century (1977 to 1996), salty snack portions increased by 93 calories, and soft drink portions increased by 49 calories. So when you give your kid an individual bag of chips and a soda—the same snack you might have enjoyed when you were 10—he's ingesting 142 more calories than you did. Feeding him that just twice a week means he'll weigh 4 more pounds within a year.

Combat portion distortion by sending your kid off to school with healthy snacks that you'll both feel good about: Triscuits and peanut butter; string cheese; a sandwich bag filled with homemade popcorn; or that classic of kid's snacktime nourishment, ants on a log.

Rule #3
BEWARE OF PORTION DISTORTION.
Snack portions aren't the only things that have increased wildly in size. Since 1977, hamburgers have increased by 97 calories, French fries by 68 calories, and Mexican foods by 133 calories, according to an analysis of the Nationwide Food Consumption Survey.

▶ A study published in the *American Journal of Preventive Medicine* looked at 63,380 individuals' drinking habits over a span of 19 years. The results show that for children ages 2 to 18, portions of sweetened beverages increased from 13.1 ounces in 1977 to 18.9 ounces in 1996.

One easy way to short-circuit this growing trend? *Buy smaller bowls and cups.* A recent study at the Children's Nutrition Research Center in Houston, Texas, shows that 5- and 6-year-old children will consume a third more calories when presented with a larger portion. The findings are based on a sample of 53 children who were served either 1- or 2-cup portions of macaroni and cheese.

Rule #4
DRINK RESPONSIBLY.
Too many of us keep in mind the adage "watch what you eat," and we forget another serious threat to our health: We don't watch what we drink. In fact, according to research from the University of North Carolina, Americans now slurp

up nearly 25 percent of their calories in liquid form—nearly double the rate we used to drink just 20 years ago. One study found that sweetened beverages constituted more than half (51 percent) of all beverages consumed by fourth- through sixth-grade students. The students who consumed the most sweetened beverages took in approximately 330 extra calories per day, and on average they ate less than half the amount of real fruit than did their peers who drank unsweetened or lightly sweetened beverages.

One important strategy is to keep cold, filtered water in a pitcher in the fridge. You might even want to keep some cut-up limes, oranges, or lemons nearby for kids to flavor their own water with. A UK study showed that in classrooms with limited access to water, only 29 percent of students met their daily needs; free access to water led to higher intake.

Be extra careful about the juice you purchase. Too many "juices" are little more than sugar water masquerading as the real thing. Ocean Spray Cran-Raspberry, for instance, has just 15 percent real fruit juice. The other 85 percent?

High-fructose corn syrup and water. Make sure the juice you buy says "100 percent Fruit Juice" on the label, and try to choose one made from a single fruit, not a mix of high-sugar fruits like white grapes, which are commonly used in fruit juice blends. And after you find the perfect juice, limit kids to one 8-ounce glass a day. If they want more, hand them a glass of water and a piece of fruit.

Rule #5
EAT MORE WHOLE FOODS AND FEWER SCIENCE EXPERIMENTS.

Here's a rule of healthy eating that will serve you well when picking out foods for your family: The shorter the ingredients list, the healthier the food. (One of the worst foods we ever found, the Baskin-Robbins Heath Shake, had 73 ingredients—and, by the way, a whopping 2,310 calories and more than 3 days' worth of saturated fat! What happened to the idea that a milk shake was, um, milk and ice cream? Let's be grateful that Baskin-Robbins finally pulled this monstrosity from its menus.) The FDA maintains a list of more than 3,000 ingredients that are considered safe to eat, but we've found reasons for concern for a number of the additives on that long list, and any one of them could wind up in your next box of mac 'n' cheese.

▶ According to USDA reports, most of the sodium in the American diet comes from packaged and processed foods. Naturally occurring salt accounts for only 12 percent of total intake, while 77 percent is added by food manufacturers.

Rule #6
SET THE TABLE.

Children in families with more structured mealtimes exhibit healthier eating habits. Among middle- and high-school girls, those whose families ate together only once or twice per week were more than twice as likely to exhibit weight control issues, compared with those who ate together three or four times per week.

Of course, the notion of a 6 P.M. dinnertime and then everyone into their pj's is a quaint one, but it's hardly realistic in a society where our kids have such highly scheduled social lives that the delineation between "parent" and "chauffeur" is sometimes difficult to parse. While we can't always bring the family together like Ozzie Nelson's (or, heck, even like Ozzy Osbourne's), we can make some positive steps in that direction. One busy family I know keeps Sunday night dinner sacred—no social plans, no school projects, no extra work brought home from the office. Even keeping the family ritual just once a week gives parents the opportunity to point out what is and isn't healthy at the dinner table.

Another smart move: Get your kids involved in cooking. Make a game of trying to pack the most healthful ingredients into your meals. A Texas study showed that children can be encouraged to eat more fruits and vegetables by giving them goals and allowing them to help with preparation. So buy the kids their own aprons and cutting boards and let them peel carrots and stir sauces, and if at the end of the day they've done their duties as dilligent sous chefs, reward them with that priceless kitchen treasure: a few licks of the cake batter off the back of the beaters.

Eat the Rainbow!

Let's not pretend that getting a child to eat what's good for him isn't sometimes a struggle. "A lot of parents tell me, 'My kids don't like healthy foods,'" says David Katz, MD, an associate clinical professor of epidemiology and public health at Yale Medical School. "'Finicky' is not an excuse. You never hear a parent say, 'My child doesn't like to look both ways before he crosses the street.' They tell him to do it. More kids today will die of complications from bad foods they eat than will die from tobacco, drugs, and alcohol."

So how do you teach the basics of nutrition to a 7-year-old? Even we grown-ups have trouble understanding how many calories we're supposed to take in each day, which vitamins and minerals we need more of, and which of the complicated chemical ingredients flooding our food system we need to avoid.

Well, here's a simple trick: Just teach your kids to eat as many different colors as they can. And no, we're not talking about red, green, and purple Skittles. We're talking about eating as much of a mix of fruits and vegetables as possible. That's because the colors represented in foods are indicators of nutritional value—and different colors mean different vitamins and minerals.

Not everything on this list is going to appeal to your child. But there's enough variation here that he or she can squeeze one food from each category into a day's eating. For a fun project, make a multicolor checklist and have your kid check off each color as he or she eats it throughout the day.

Or do what our parents did and sell them on the kid-friendly benefits trapped inside of spinach, carrots, and the like. Each group of produce offers seriously cool "superpowers" that appeal to kids' deepest desires to dominate math quizzes and monkey bars alike. Feel free to sell these as hard as you want. Hey, even if it didn't end up making you as strong as Popeye, you still ate your spinach, right?

Red

Rosy-hued fruits and vegetables offer a payload of an important antioxidant called lycopene. Lycopene is a carotenoid that is associated with a cache of health benefits, including protecting the skin from sun damage and decreasing the risk of heart disease and certain forms of cancer. Lycopene is most strongly concentrated in the most red of all red fruits: the tomato. What is surprising, though, is that cooked and processed tomatoes have higher concentrations of lycopene, so don't shy away from the salsa or marinara sauce.
SUPERPOWER: Red food makes you dash like the Flash! There's a reason he wore red: Lycopene-rich foods have been shown to decrease symptoms of wheezing, asthma, and shortness of breath in people when they exercise.

TOMATO
This queen of lycopene is also packed with antioxidant-rich vitamins A and C, as well as vitamin K, which is important for maintaining healthy bones. Canned and cooked tomatoes have been shown to contain more lycopene than fresh, so go crazy with the salsa and marinara sauce. When possible, buy organic: USDA researchers found that organic ketchup has three times the lycopene as normal ketchup.

RED BELL PEPPER
The red ones pack twice the vitamin C and nine times the vitamin A as their green relatives. They've been shown to aid in the fight against everything from asthma to cancer to cataracts. Slice them up raw and serve with hummus for an after-school snack, or buy jarred roasted peppers and puree them into a soup. (It tastes just like tomato soup.)

GUAVA
Like most lycopene vessels, guava is packed with vitamins A and C. It also contains heart-healthy omega-3 fatty acids and belly-filling fiber. Get your hands on these in the produce aisles of larger supermarkets or Latin grocers, or simply keep a bottle of guava nectar in the fridge.

WATERMELON
This summertime favorite is also a big provider of vitamins A and C, which help to neutralize cancer-causing free radicals. Spike a fruit salad with big hunks of watermelon; blend it with yogurt, ice, and OJ for a refreshing smoothie; or just hand over a big hunk to the little ones the next time you fire up the grill.

PINK GRAPEFRUIT
This contains one of the highest concentrations of antioxidants in the produce aisle. Mix segments into yogurt and granola in the morning for breakfast, slip them into salads, or just swap out the OJ for the occasional glass of ruby red grapefruit juice.

Orange

Beta-carotene is the nutrient responsible for fruits and vegetables' dramatic orange color, and although the carotenoid is present in a host of other vegetables (spinach, kale, and broccoli, for instance), the orange ones have the highest concentrations. But the conspicuous hue of this carotenoid does more than just attract your attention; once inside your body, it is converted into vitamin A, a powerful antioxidant that contributes to immune health, improves communication between cells, and helps fight off cell-damaging free radicals. **SUPERPOWER:** Orange foods give you night vision! That's because vitamin A is vital for creating the pigment in the retina responsible for vision in low-light situations. Just think of the benefits: It'll help them beat their friends at hide-and-seek, spy on their brothers or sisters, and spot bogeymen before they can hide under their beds.

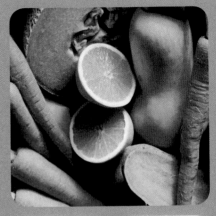

SWEET POTATO

The best thing about sweet potatoes, outside of the beta-carotene, is that they're loaded with fiber. That means they have a gentler effect on your kid's blood sugar levels than regular potatoes do. Substitute baked sweet potatoes for baked potatoes, mash them up like you would an Idaho, or make fries out of them by tossing spears with olive oil and roasting in a 400°F oven for 30 minutes.

ORANGE

This vaunted vitamin C monster has a cadre of critical phytonutrients known to lower blood pressure and contain strong anti-inflammatory properties. Juice is fine, but the real fruit is even better. The secret, though, is that the orange's most powerful healing properties are found in the peel; use a zester to grate the peel over bowls of yogurt, salads, or directly into smoothies.

WINTER SQUASH

A true grab bag of nutrients, winter squash is a great source of a dozen different vitamins, including a host of B vitamins, folate, manganese, and fiber. What does that all mean? It means feed it to your kid! And lots of it! The best way is to cut the squash into 1-inch wedges and bake them at 375°F for 40 minutes, until they're soft and caramelized.

CANTALOUPE

The surge of vitamin A is important not just for your eyes, but also for healthy lungs, and the megadose of vitamin C helps white blood cells ward off infection. Sliced cantaloupe and yogurt make a killer breakfast, or combine the two in a food processor with a touch of honey and lemon, and puree into a soup. It makes a great low-cal dessert.

CARROT

The snack of choice for Bugs Bunny happens to be the richest carotene source of all. Raw baby carrots are perfect for dipping or snacking on, of course, but also try shredding carrots into a salad or marinara for a hint of natural sweetness, or roasting them slowly in the oven with olive oil and salt.

Yellow

Yellow foods are close relatives to orange foods, and they are similarly rich in carotenoids. The more common yellow carotenoid is beta-cryptoxanthin, which supplies about half the vitamin A as beta-carotene. Studies show it decreases the likelihood of such diseases as lung cancer and arthritis, but since youngsters have more important things to worry about, you're better off selling yellow foods on the superpowers they bestow. **SUPERPOWER:** Yellow foods make you jump higher and play harder! Research shows that foods rich in beta-cryptoxanthin help decrease inflammation in the joints, ensuring a springy step in kids for years to come. Studies also show that this potent carotenoid may improve the functioning of the respiratory system, making beating their classmates in dodgeball and relay races that much easier.

BANANA

Bananas are loaded with potassium, which will help your kids grow strong, durable bones. They also contain a compound called a prebiotic, which makes it easier for eaters to absorb nutrients of all kinds. Shopping tip: Not all ananas are equally rich in carotenoids. Search for those with a deeper gold to their peels.

YELLOW BELL PEPPER

Yellow bells are vitamin C treasure troves, providing 2½ times the amount you'd get from an orange. Their sweet, mellow flavor is perfect for kids, making them a good addition to stir-fries and sandwiches, and they're great cooked on the grill and served as a side to chicken.

PINEAPPLE

This fruit might be high on the list of carotenoid-containing fruits, but it has other benefits, as well—notably an abundance of bromelain, which has strong digestive benefits. Skewer chunks and cook them on a hot grill for a killer dessert.

CORN

This king of the summer barbecue is loaded with thiamin, which plays a central role in energy production and cognitive function. Boost their brains and their energy levels by carefully removing the kernels from the cob with a kitchen knife and sautéing with a bit of olive oil. Eat as is, or sprinkle the toasty corn niblets on top of soups and salads.

YELLOW SQUASH

With huge doses of fiber, manganese, magnesium, and folate, summer squash proves to be a serious nutritional player. Drizzle grilled slices with a bit of pesto.

Green

Not just potent vitamin vessels capable of strengthening bones, muscles, and brains, green foods are also among the most abundant sources of lutein and zeaxanthin, an antioxidant tag team that, among other things, promotes healthy vision. **SUPERPOWER:** Green foods give you sharp vision and superhuman healing abilities! Beyond the peeper protection kids get from lutein and zeaxanthin, green fruits and vegetables get their color from chlorophyll, which studies show plays an important role in stimulating the growth of new tissue and hindering the growth of bacteria. As a topical treatment, it can speed healing time by 25 percent.

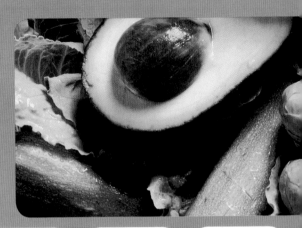

AVOCADO

This creamy fruit is bursting with monounsaturated fats, the kind that are proven to be great for your heart. Tossing avocado slices into sandwiches and soups is one way to add some healthy fat, but your best bet for slipping them into your kid's diet is to mash 'em up with garlic, onion, and lemon juice for a tasty homemade guacamole.

ASPARAGUS

These potent spears contain a special kind of carbohydrate called inulin, which promotes the growth of healthy bacteria in our large intestines, forcing out the more mischievous kind. Wrap spears in thin slices of ham and bake in a 400°F oven until the ham is crispy.

ROMAINE LETTUCE

Whereas the ubiquitous iceberg has nary a nutrient to its name, romaine is bursting at the leaves with everything from bone-strengthening vitamin K to folic acid, which is essential to cardiovascular health. Other good, nutrient-dense lettuces for salads and sandwiches include Bibb, red leaf, and arugula.

BRUSSELS SPROUTS

One of the strongest natural cancer-fighters on the planet, brussels sprouts too often get a bad rap for being boring. Combat the boredom by roasting in a 450°F oven until crispy and caramelized, then tossing them with sliced almonds and golden raisins.

SPINACH

This is one of your best sources of folate, which keeps your body in good supply of oxygen-carrying red blood cells. If your kid isn't ready to eat it from the can like Popeye, try sauteeing it in olive oil until fully wilted, then scrambling it into eggs or mixing it into pasta.

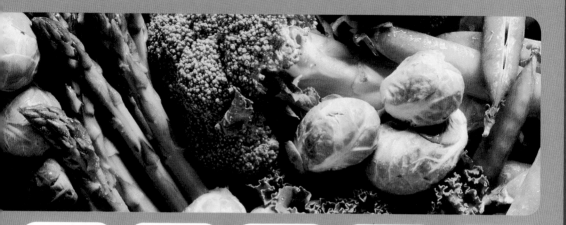

KALE
Aside from containing nearly 2 weeks' worth of bone-strengthening vitamin K, each serving of these deep green leaves has fewer than 40 calories and nearly 10% of your RDA of calcium. Sauté in olive oil until wilted, then add raisins and toasted pine nuts.

BROCCOLI
These little trees have 2 days' worth of vitamins C and K in each serving. Top a baked potato with a few steamed florets and a bit of shredded cheese, or serve chopped-up pieces alongside a tub of hummus and see if the dip doesn't get the kids interested.

KIWI
Not only do kiwis pack more vitamin C than oranges, they also lay claim to a bulky portfolio of polyphoneols and carotenoids, some of which may have protective effects on our respiratory health. An Italian study found that children who consumed more kiwis had fewer problems with shortness of breath, wheezing, and coughing. Try layering the slices of kiwi with yogurt and granola for a kid-friendly parfait.

ZUCCHINI
A dense and diverse source of nutrients, this summer squash comes with everything from omega-3s to copper. Toss sautéed zucchini with a drizzle of balsamic vinegar, or add grated zucchini to your favorite bread or muffin recipe.

GREEN PEAS
Beyond the abundance of vitamins and minerals, a cup of peas contains more than a third of your kid's daily fiber intake—more than most whole-wheat breads. Add frozen peas to a pasta sauce at the last second, or puree them with garlic and olive oil as a simple, sweet dip.

Blue
and Purple

Blue and purple foods get their colors from the presence of a unique set of flavonoids called anthocyanins. Flavonoids in general are known to improve cardiovascular health and prevent short-term memory loss, but the deeply pigmented anthocyanins go even further. Researchers at Tufts University have found that blueberries may make brain cells respond better to incoming messages and might even spur the growth of new nerve cells, giving new meaning to "smart eating." **SUPERPOWER:** Blue foods make you the smartest kid in the class!

EGGPLANT

A pigment called nasunin is concentrated in the peel of the eggplant, and studies have shown that it has powerful disease-fighting properties. Simplify eggplant parmesan by layering ½-inch-thick slices with marinara and mozzarella cheese and baking in a 375˚F oven for 25 minutes.

RADISH

Nutritional benefits vary among the many varieties of radishes, but they all share an abundance of vitamin C and a tendency to facilitate the digestive process. Try thinly sliced radishes on a bagel with low-fat cream cheese and black pepper.

PURPLE GRAPE

Some researchers believe that, despite their high-fat diets, the French are protected from heart disease by their mass consumption of grapes and wine. Look for a deeper shade of purple—that indicates a high flavonoid concentration. Try freezing grapes in the dead of summer for a cool, healthy treat—or use the frozen orbs as sweet little ice cubes.

BEET

This candy-sweet vegetable gets most of its color from a cancer-fighting pigment called betacyanin. The edible root is replete with fiber, potassium, and manganese. Toss roasted beet chunks with toasted walnuts and orange segments, or grate raw beets into salads.

BLACKBERRY

One cup of berries contains 5% of your child's daily folate and half the day's vitamin C. Try pureeing blackberries, then combining them with olive oil and balsamic vinegar for a superhealthy salad dressing.

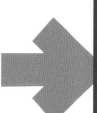

Kids' Restaurant Report Card

Just as your kids are tested every day on state capitals and basic arithmetic, restaurants need to be closely examined based on the fare they serve to our future doctors, lawyers, and Twitteratti. After all, the difference between one restaurant's chicken finger meal and another's can be 500 calories or more. That's why we've put 21 major chain restaurants under the microscope, picking apart the details of their kiddie concessions, in order to help you make better decisions about where and what your family should eat next time you venture out. Do your kids' favorite restaurants make the grade?

APPLEBEE'S

C+ Applebee's finally gave up the nutritional goods and the results are mixed. High-impact items like the burgers, grilled cheese, and the 790-calorie Oreo shake are balanced out by a handful of sound entrees, plus plenty of healthy sides and juice options.

SURVIVAL STRATEGY
Two Mini Cheeseburgers, fries, and a soft drink add up to a shocking 1,200 calories, making it one of the worst kids' meals in America. The better bet is to pair a hot dog or a grilled chicken sandwich with applesauce or celery sticks and milk, juice, or water.

BLUEBERRY
The most abundant source of anthocyanins has more antioxidant punch than red wine, and it helps vitamin C do its job better. Sprinkle blueberries into oatmeal, cereal, or yogurt, or mix with almonds and a few chocolate chips for an easy trail mix.

PLUM
Another rich source of antioxidants, plums have also been shown to help the body better absorb iron. Roast plum halves in the oven and serve warm over a small scoop of vanilla ice cream.

BASKIN-ROBBINS

D+ It's hard to serve just ice cream and still make the grade, but Baskin-Robbins does nothing to help its case. It serves up some of the fattiest scoops in the industry, plus 900-calorie soft serve concoctions, smoothies with more sugar than fruit, and a handful of the worst shakes and sundaes on the planet.

SURVIVAL STRATEGY

Baskin does deserve credit for offering plenty of lighter options, such as sherbets, sorbets, and low-sugar ice creams; each of these lines offers ample opportunity to feel indulgent without really being so.

BURGER KING

B- The standard kids' fare—hamburger, cheeseburger, French fries— is no better or worse here than it is at most fast-food joints, but BK does offer a lower-calorie chicken tender than most. It also finally cut most of the trans fats from the menu, which is why its grade moves up a few notches this year.

SURVIVAL STRATEGY

Burger King deserves credit for one of the finest inventions of the 21st century: apple fries, the ultimate healthy decoy for deep-fried potatoes. Pair

them with a 4-piece Chicken Tenders and water or milk for an impressive kids' meal.

CHILI'S

C- Chili's Pepper Pals program gets the award for the longest, most diverse kids' menu we've seen, and many of the items on it represent reasonable nutritional options. Typical burgers and mac and cheese are available, but so is a solid corn dog option and an excellent grilled chicken platter.

SURVIVAL STRATEGY

Skip over any item with the word "cheese" in the title (they all have more than 400 calories) and make sure the kids pick a healthy side like black beans, mandarin oranges, or seasonal veggies. (Note: Cinnamon apples do not count as a healthy side.)

DOMINO'S PIZZA

C+ Domino's suffers the same pitfalls as any other pizza purveyor: too much cheese, bread, and greasy toppings. If you don't know the pitfalls, you might bag your child a pizza with more than 350 calories per slice. To its credit, Domino's does keep the trans fat off the

pizza, and it also offers the lowest-calorie thin crust option out there.

SURVIVAL STRATEGY

Stick with the Crunchy Thin Crust pizzas sans sausage and pepperoni. Whenever possible, try to sneak a vegetable or two onto each pie.

DUNKIN' DONUTS

C+ Dunkin' has shown encouraging signs of health-consciousness with their new lines of flatbread sandwiches and DD Smart options, but those appeal more to Mom and Dad than they do Suzy and Tommy. Kids are most likely at Dunkin' for one reason: the namesake breakfast treat, which means mitagating the damage should be the main goal here.

SURVIVAL STRATEGY

If doughnuts are unavoidable, limit them to one, and make it a raised doughnut instead of a cake doughnut. Otherwise, opt for sandwiches made on English muffins for breakfast, and flatbread sandwiches (preferably the ham and swiss) at all other times.

IHOP

F IHOP refuses to serve up nutritional information, but thanks to the New York City Board of Health, it was forced to publish calorie counts on its menus in April 2008. The big reveal shocked New York diners: 1,700-calorie cheeseburgers and salads with more than 1,000 calories. For the kids, the only real trouble comes with the 850-calorie Cheese Omelette.

SURVIVAL STRATEGY

Write letters, make phone calls, beg, scream, and plead for IHOP to provide nutritional information on all of its products. While those complaints are being processed, know that the best breakfast option for kids is the Silver Five pancakes at 390 calories and the best option the rest of the day is the Crispy Chicken Strips at 360 calories, or the 380-calorie Grilled Cheese Sandwich—both (thankfully) served with fresh fruit.

KFC

B- For a place with the word "fried" in its acronymic title, KFC manages to downplay the damage of its namesake goods by offering low-calorie Snacker sandwiches and a variety of relatively healthy vegetable sides. The new line of grilled chicken is a good sign that the Colonel is willing to step away from the fryer.

SURVIVAL STRATEGY

Skip over the fried chicken—unless your family likes it skinless, in which case, have at it—and look instead to the Snackers, the Crispy Strips, and the grilled chicken. Don't miss the opportunity to sneak a serving or two of vegetables into your kid's diet, assuming those veggies don't come out of the fryer.

MCDONALD'S

B Though not blessed with an abundance of healthy options for kids, Mickey D's isn't burdened with any major calorie bombs, either. Kid standards like McNuggets and cheeseburgers both come in right around the 300-calorie mark.

SURVIVAL STRATEGY

Apple Dippers and 2 percent milk with a small entrée make for a pretty decent meal. McDonald's quintessential Happy Meal makes this possible—just beware the usual French fries and soda pitfalls.

OLIVE GARDEN

C We're happy to see Olive Garden finally offer up full nutritional info on its menu items. We're not so happy to see, however, that the pasta purveyor is serving up 800-calorie portions of fettuccine Alfredo to young eaters.

SURVIVAL STRATEGY

The kids' menu is short and straightforward, which makes finding the high points and avoiding the caloric potholes that much easier. Skip the Alfredo, the cheese pizza, and anything with a 400-calorie serving of fries. The 250-calorie plate of spaghetti and the grilled chicken and pasta both make fine meals.

OUTBACK STEAKHOUSE

D Outback's new interactive nutritional tool reveals some scary numbers for the adult fare, but the kids' dishes don't score much better. Both the chicken fingers and the ribs top 1,000 calories when paired with fries, and the cheeseburger and mac and cheese aren't far off.

SURVIVAL STRATEGY

The 240-calorie Joey Sirloin, the 390-calorie Grilled Cheese-A-Roo, and the 209-calorie Grilled Chicken on the Barbie all make great meals, as long as you pair them with smart sides (i.e., the baked potato or the veggies).

PAPA JOHN'S

C Pizza joints suffer the curse of bad report cards because of their thick crusts, fat-speckled meats, and blankets of cheese. That said, Papa John's does have a few advantages over the competition: the absence of trans fat, the assortment of nonsoda beverage options, and the first whole-wheat crust offered by a big US pizza chain.

SURVIVAL STRATEGY

Order chicken strips with pizza sauce to blunt the family's collective hunger. Follow with a slice of thin or wheat crust cheese or spinach Alfredo pizza. Whatever you do, be sure to avoid Papa's pan crust like it's the plague.

PIZZA HUT

D+ Expect no surprises from this quintessential pizza parlor. The chain offers no kid-friendly beverage or side options, and with nothing else to choose from, a couple of breadsticks and a soda tack hundreds of calories onto a pizza dinner. A thin-crust delivery can be a lifesaver in a pinch, but as for truly nourishing options, you won't find many here.

SURVIVAL STRATEGY

First off, nix the pepperoni. If the kids want meat, stick to ham

and chicken, but try to add veggies whenever possible. The best possible scenario? Fit 'N Delicious Pizzas. Any of them.

QUIZNOS

C+ Toasty or not, Quiznos offers some of America's worst sandwiches, including the 1,760-calorie large tuna melt. Cookies and fatty salads don't make matters any better. What does improve matters is the line of kid-size Sammies—the rare bright spot on an otherwise dark menu.

SURVIVAL STRATEGY

With a handful of Sammies at 200 calories each, they make perfect meals for younger kids. You can double up for the older eaters—even two of the healthier Sammies will be better than many small sandwiches.

RED LOBSTER

B+ Red Lobster boasts one of America's healthiest adult menus, and some of that magic rubs off on its kids' offerings: broiled fish, crab legs, and even popcorn shrimp all make good picks, as do a few of the eight side options. Still, the ever-appealing chicken fingers and fries together pack 740 calories and more

than 2,000 milligrams of sodium—some choppy seas in an otherwise smooth sail.

SURVIVAL STRATEGY

The biggest battle here is fought on the sides front. Broccoli, salad, and a baked potato are all strong options; the fries, Caesar, and Cheddar Bay Biscuit, not so much. Match one of the former options with grilled chicken or any of the seafood choices for a great meal.

RUBY TUESDAY

C- To its credit, Ruby Tuesday's has made some real improvements to the kids' menu in the past year. Previously limited to a single dish with fewer than 400 calories, now the chicken breast, fried shrimp, chicken tenders and chop steak all bear that distinction. But beyond that safe zone lies a dangerous milieu of high-cal pastas, fat-strewn fried fare, and "mini" burgers with more calories than Wendy's infamous Baconator.

SURVIVAL STRATEGY

Pair one of the four dishes mentioned above with a fresh vegetable side and there is hope for a happy, healthy dinner. If not, your kid could very well end up consuming half her day's calories in one sitting.

STARBUCKS

C- As any caffeine-addicted parent knows, there are few options for kids at a coffee shop. Starbucks is no exception. Whether due to an excess of sugar or a surge of caffeine (or both), nearly every drink here will have your kid treating your furniture like a trampoline. The food isn't much better, though Starbucks has started to show real signs of improvement in the edibles department.

SURVIVAL STRATEGY

Try giving your kid one of the fiber-rich, fruit-based Vivanno smoothies—he'll think he's getting a reward for good behavior. As for food, skip the baked goods in favor of Perfect Oatmeal or a hot breakfast wrap.

SUBWAY

A- A menu based on lean protein and vegetables is always going to score well in our book. With four kid-friendly sandwiches at less than 300 calories, plus a slew of soups and healthy sides to boot, Subway can satisfy even the pickiest eater without breaking the caloric bank. But despite what Jared may want you to believe, Subway is not nutritionally infallible: Most of those rosy calorie counts posted on the menu boards include neither cheese nor mayo (add 170 calories per 6-inch sub), and some of the toasted subs, like the meatball marinara, contain hefty doses of calories, saturated fat, and sodium.

SURVIVAL STRATEGY

Cornell researchers have discovered a "health halo" at Subway—this refers to the tendency to reward yourself or your kid with chips, cookies, and large soft drinks because your entrée is healthy. Avoid the halo, and all will be well.

TGI FRIDAY'S

F We applaud Friday's efforts to offer smaller portion sizes for high-calorie dishes, but we don't approve of its reluctance to provide hard nutritional data on any of its dishes. Between the array of deep-fried starters and mammoth sandwiches, it's clear it has something to hide.

SURVIVAL STRATEGY

Calls to Friday's revealed that the chicken fingers and pasta have 700 calories, the ribs 600 calories, and the burger and mac and cheese have 500. Your child would be better off ordering the 480-calorie Dragonfire Chicken or the 400-calorie Shrimp Key West from the adult menu.

TACO BELL

C Diners live and die by the mix-and-match opportunities Taco Bell presents, where any two items can either be a reasonable 400-calorie meal or a 900-calorie saturated fat and sodium fest.

SURVIVAL STRATEGY

Cut out the big-ticket items like Mexican pizzas and nachos, and direct your kid's attention to the crunchy tacos, bean burritos, and anything on the Fresco menu.

WENDY'S

A- Wendy's official kids' menu may be a tiny concession to little eaters, but it is free of the belly-busters that hamper most menus. Plus, the rest of the menu offers ample options for a growing kid; a cup of chili and a baked potato, chicken salad, or even a burger with a cup of mandarin oranges all qualify as nutritionally commendable meals.

SURVIVAL STRATEGY

The Super Value Menu is full of solid choices, as long as you avoid the 320-calorie add-on of fries and a regular soft drink.

Burger King

Eat This

Chicken Tender

(5-piece) with barbecue dipping sauce and Apple Fries with caramel sauce

At just 46 calories a piece, these rank among the best nuggets/tenders/fingers in the fast-food world. Add to that the genius product that is Apple Fries and you have a pretty sound kid's meal.

330 calories

13.5 g fat
(2.5 g saturated)

820 mg sodium

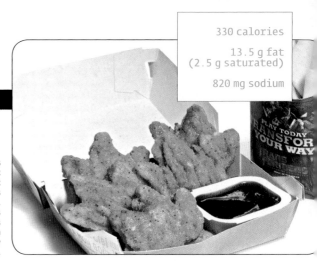

Dunkin' Donuts

Eat This

Glazed Chocolate Cake Munchkins
(4)

No, this is not a typo. A pile of chocolate doughnut holes is better for you than a bagel with light cream cheese in almost every major nutritional category. Still, don't let your kids make a habit of it, since they are really just a glorified dessert.

240 calories

12 g fat
(6 g saturated)

32 g carbohydrates

650 calories

32 g fat
(10.5 g saturated,
0.5 g trans)

1,270 mg sodium

Not That!

Cheeseburger
with French fries (small)

The cheeseburger, with 310 calories and 7 grams of saturated fat, gets trounced by the tenders, while the small French fries double the meal's caloric load without adding any real nutrition to the equation.

420 calories

10.5 g fat
(5.5 g saturated)

68 g carbohydrates

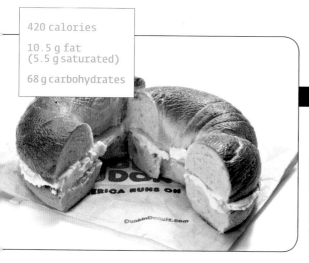

Not That!

Plain Bagel
with reduced fat cream cheese

The reduced fat cream cheese will save you 50 calories over the regular stuff, but it won't cut any of the refined carbs—and those are to blame for the high calorie count and the denigrated reputation of the bagel in this book series.

KFC

Eat This

KFC Snacker Honey BBQ

with macaroni and cheese

Outside the recent
addition of grilled
chicken, the series
of Snackers is
the best thing to ever
happen to the KFC
menu. They're the
perfect size for a kid,
and the Honey BBQ
(the best of them all)
has just 210 calories.

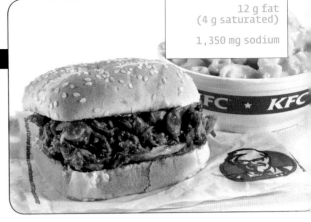

390 calories

12 g fat
(4 g saturated)

1,350 mg sodium

McDonald's

Eat This

Happy Meal

**(Chicken McNuggets (4 piece),
Apple Dippers with caramel sauce,
and 1% Low-Fat White Milk Jug)**

This is one of the most
well-rounded meals a
parent could hope to
find in a drive-thru.
Kids will get protein
from the chicken, more
protein (plus calcium)
from the milk, and
a much-needed full
serving of fruit with
the beloved dippers.

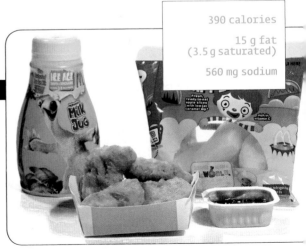

390 calories

15 g fat
(3.5 g saturated)

560 mg sodium

550 calories

32 g fat
(6 g saturated)

1,590 mg sodium

KFC

Caution: Hot

Not That!

Kids Popcorn Chicken

with potato wedges

If your kid really wants fried chicken at KFC, let her order the Crispy Strips. Two substantial fingers run 230 calories. As for potato products, swap in the mashed taters with gravy for the wedges and save 140 calories.

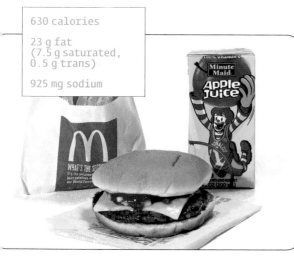

630 calories

23 g fat
(7.5 g saturated,
0.5 g trans)

925 mg sodium

Not That!

Happy Meal

(Cheeseburger with small French fries and apple juice box)

Even a juice box can't save this unhappy meal from itself. Combined, it packs in nearly half a day's caloric allotment for an 8-year-old. At the very least, insist that the kids get Apple Dippers instead of fries—it will cut out 125 empty calories.

Subway

Eat This

**Turkey Breast
and Swiss Cheese**

(6-inch, with lettuce, tomatoes, and onions)

Turkey and swiss:
a classic combination
that proves to be
the blueprint for a great
kids' meal at Subway.
It has everything
your kid needs: lean
protein, fresh produce,
calcium, and a
bit of cheesy incentive.

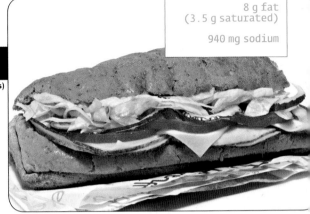

330 calories

8 g fat
(3.5 g saturated)

940 mg sodium

Taco Bell

Eat This

Crunchy Fresco Tacos

(2)

Kids love crunchy
stuff and parents love
fresh produce, and
these tacos satisfy both
affections. If you
can get your kids to
take the Fresco
treatment, then Taco
Bell ranks among the
best eateries for the
younger set.

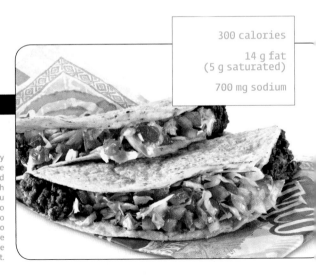

300 calories

14 g fat
(5 g saturated)

700 mg sodium

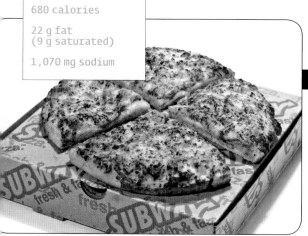

680 calories

22 g fat
(9 g saturated)

1,070 mg sodium

Not That!

Individual Cheese Pizza

(8-inch)

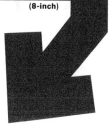

Let's hope this new addition to the Subway menu becomes discontinued soon. In the meantime, don't let your kids fall for the allure of pizza in a sub shop. This pie packs more calories and fat than most footlong sandwiches.

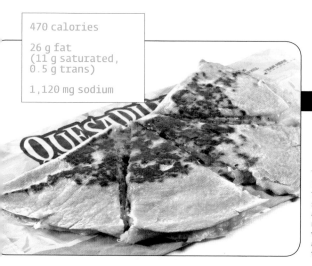

470 calories

26 g fat
(11 g saturated,
0.5 g trans)

1,120 mg sodium

Not That!

Cheese Quesadilla

The quesadilla is Mexico's answer to the grilled cheese sandwich, and this one at the Bell delivers more than half a day's worth of saturated fat and sodium between the toasty tortillas.

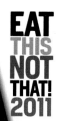

Chapter

7

ON A BUDGET

307

Waiting for some good news

that finally scratches off the tarry black outlook of the economy and reveals a shiny silver lining beneath? We've got it for you. The past 3 years have been a challenge—both in the United States and around the world—thanks to what appears to be a small group of balding men in suits and ties with private jets and mysterious jobs and the magic power to make everyone else's money instantly disappear.

How do they do that?

Well, we're still working on an answer to that one. We're not quite sure what happened to the other half of our 401(k), except that it had something to do with things called credit-default swaps, subprime loans, and the Glass-Steagall Act, which only the very smart guys who lost all the money in the first place supposedly comprehend. (And we thought understanding "high-fructose corn syrup" was a challenge.) But we do know that when the economy gets tough, the tough do one smart thing: They cook at home.

And there's the silver lining.

You see, the power to control your weight and your health comes down to the power to control the foods you feed into your body.

Once you hop into the car and head to your local eatery—whether it's the eggs-and-bacon diner you've been going to for 20 years or the hot new hipster joint that employs "mixologists" instead of bartenders—you've given up control over what's in your food and handed that control over to a bunch of folks who have less invested in your health and well-being than you do.

Sure, you can special order, you can parse the menu for the best choices, and you can quiz the waiter about what, exactly, is in the blue plate special. But you don't really know what's happening back there behind the kitchen doors, where the sizzling sound could be caused by freshly picked vegetables caressing heart-healthy canola oil or by frozen nuggets taking a bath in trans fats.

So cooking at home is not only a smart way to cut down on waste but also a smart way to stop adding to your waist.

That said, the grocery bill is always an ugly thing to look at. And over the past 3 years, prices of foods like vegetables, meat, fruit, and other high-nutrition, low-calorie treats have skyrocketed. A combination of unstable oil prices, bad weather, and a growing world population has made eating healthy more expensive.

But eating in an unhealthy way? Oh, that's still plenty cheap. In fact, junk food prices have actually decreased slightly over the past few years, which is why in many stores you can buy a couple of Twinkies for less than the cost of a single apple. Researchers at the University of Washington recently estimated the cost of a diet based on high-calorie foods versus one based on healthy, low-calorie foods. The high-calorie diet you could eat for $3.52 a day. The low-cal diet? A whopping $36.32 per diem.

Now, that sounds pretty bad. But remember, people in the United States still spend a smaller percentage of their incomes on food than almost any other people on Earth—just under 10 percent. And shopping at the grocery store—and making our own food at home—gives us a tremendous budgetary advantage. (Want to make an easy $800? Brew your own coffee each day instead of stopping for a latte on your way to work.)

The key to trimming your belly while trimming your bills is to make your kitchen the center of your home and use it to its full advantage. And we show you how to do exactly that in our Save-Money

Shopping Guide in this chapter.

Of course, you're not going to be eating at home every night. Or every morning. Or even most afternoons. And the local diner, fast-food joint, or fancy sit-down restaurant still has its magical allure even when you know you should just pack a PB&J and head out.

Restaurants know this, of course, and they also know that your dollars are tight and the competition for them is rabid. Since McDonald's introduced its dollar menu in the early 2000s, cheap restaurant food has gotten even cheaper. But remember what we said at the top of this chapter: When you eat out, you give up control of what's in your food. So being extra smart about how you approach the menu will make all the difference in keeping your wallet padded—and not the rest of you.

In this chapter, we've taken a hard look at some of the "cheap eats" out there and figured out which of them are good investments and which are just throwing your money away. Put your money in the safe deposit box, turn the lock, and read on.

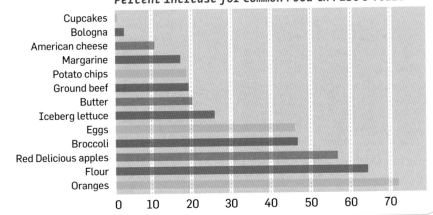

The Real Inflation Problem
Prices for junk food stay low, while health food costs continue to soar

Percent Increase for Common Food in Past 5 Years

Cupcakes
Bologna
American cheese
Margarine
Potato chips
Ground beef
Butter
Iceberg lettuce
Eggs
Broccoli
Red Delicious apples
Flour
Oranges

0   10   20   30   40   50   60   70

Your Save-Money Shopping Guide

Cut out the empty calories and maximize the quality of your supermarket score with these six rules of savvy shopping.

• **Avoid quickies.** A study published by the Marketing Science Institute found that shoppers who made "quick trips" to the store purchased an average of 54 percent more merchandise than they planned. Instead, be thoughtful in your planning—keep a magnet-based notepad on your fridge and make notes throughout the week about what you need. (And avoiding extra trips will cut down on your gasoline costs as well.)

• **Write the perfect shopping list.** Before you head out, organize your list of needs by grocery-store section: produce, dairy, meat, cleaning products, cosmetics, etc. (Rewrite the list if you need to.) Then bring a pencil and, as you add each item to your cart, tick it off from your list. No loitering, no wandering aimlessly through the store. Try to make each visit a minute or two shorter than the last—you'll find that the more time you save, the more money and calories you save too!

• **Check yourself out.** Maybe those creepy mechanical voices weird you out, or maybe you just like waiting in long lines to chat with retirees. But waiting in line for a checkout person is an invitation to caloric chaos. A study by IHL Group found that when shoppers used the self-checkout line, impulse purchases dropped by more than 16 percent for men—and more than 32 percent for women. (That's good news for your body as well. Eighty percent of candy and 61 percent of salty snacks are bought on impulse.)

• **Make Wednesday grocery night.** According to *Progressive Grocer*, only 11 percent of shoppers go to the store on Wednesdays, and only 4 per-cent of customers shop on any day after 9 P.M. If your store's open late, it might **be** the best way to avoid the crowds—and to avoid the impulse spending that accompanies being stuck in the checkout line.

• Watch your weight. Okay, so one brand of crackers costs $4 and the other $4.50. But before you assume which is cheaper, take a closer look at the net weight. You'll often find the more expensive box contains more actual food—and as such, the food is actually cheaper. Net weight is also a great way of making sure you're not paying for a lot of packaging, only to get home and discover most of what's inside the box is air.

• Eat before you shop. A 2008 study in the *Journal of Consumer Research* found that consumers are likely to spend more if their appetite is revving full throttle before making a purchase. (And it's not just food you'll spend more on. In the study, women who were given a whiff of a chocolate-scented candle were four times as likely to want to shop for a new sweater than those who weren't. Damn you, Auntie Anne's!)

Five Can't-Beat Cheap Eats

Stretch your dollar and shrink your waistline with these prudent picks

Frozen chicken breasts

Lean protein for about half the price of fresh chicken. In our taste tests, where we seasoned and grilled chicken breasts, we found it impossible to tell the difference between fresh and frozen.

Canola oil

Save the pricey olive oil for dressing salads or drizzling over grilled fish. Canola's neutral flavor is great for cooking, and it happens to have a better ratio of mono-unsaturated to saturated fat than the vaunted extra virgin. Olive oil can cost as much as a dollar per ounce, while canola oil costs about $0.25.

Dry lentils

For about the price of a bottle of water, you can boil up a massive pot of soup- and salad-ready lentils. A 1-pound bag has 11 grams of fiber and 10 grams of protein in each of its 13 servings.

Salsa

It's twice as versatile as ketchup. Look to the bottom shelf for store-brand bulk containers and you'll find a half-gallon for less than 6 bucks—a month's supply for about the price of a Chipotle burrito.

Popcorn

Paper-bag popcorns run about $3.50 for 9 ounces, versus $1.25 a pound for straight kernels. Why pay a premium for grease? Make popcorn the old fashioned way: straight from the jar. Just fill the bottom of a large saucepan with kernels and a touch of oil and cover. After it's popped, season it with herbs, citrus, or chili powder.

Cook Off The Pounds!

CUT CALORIES AND SAVE CASH WITH THESE 10 DECADENT DISHES

The best way to take control of your diet as well as your food finances is to grab a chef's knife and a sauté pan and start cooking. According to research, people consume 50 percent more calories, fat, and sodium when they eat out than when they cook at home. Add the fact that you're likely to save some serious coin with a bit of savvy shopping and you have a potent case for the power of a little down-home cooking.

In hopes of inspiring you to turn up the heat in your kitchen, we've taken a new round of 10 of America's most popular dishes and remade them, with quality nutrition, prudent spending, and maximum gustatory pleasure all considered in equal measure. As you'll see with the calorie comparisons we provide, these also happen to be 10 dishes the restaurant industry just can't seem to get right, shackled as they are with excessive amounts of fat, sugar, and sodium. To help you take back the food you love most, we built each recipe around some of the finest products in the supermarket, which will allow you to enjoy some seriously fine-dining on a shoestring.

Grilled Steak Tacos

Tacos should be a sure bet, regardless of the restaurant. But alas, not even this humble handheld street food is safe when caught in the clutches of the corporate chef. Excessive cheese and superfluous sauces ruin both the simple beauty of a taco and the nutritional integrity of a meal that should never top 500 calories. Our tacos get you back to the basics, with little more than a fiery marinade, toasted tortillas, and a scoop of salsa.

You'll Need:

- 2 chipotle peppers in adobo
- 1 cup orange juice
- 1 tsp ground cumin
- 2 cloves garlic
- 2 cups chopped fresh cilantro, plus more for garnish
- 1 lb flank steak
- ½ tsp salt
- ½ tsp pepper
- 8 corn tortillas
- ¼ cup guacamole

Salsa
- 1 red onion, minced
- 2 limes, quartered

How to Make It:

- Combine the chipotle, orange juice, cumin, garlic, and cilantro in a blender and puree. Place the steak and marinade in a resealable plastic bag and refrigerate for 30 minutes or up to 8 hours.

- Remove the steak from the marinade. Season with salt and pepper. Heat a grill, stovetop grill pan, or cast-iron skillet until hot. Cook the steak for 3 to 4 minutes per side (for medium-rare).

- Heat the tortillas until warm and pliable. It's best to do this on a hot grill or cast-iron skillet, but in a pinch, wrap the tortillas in a damp papper towel and microwave for 45 seconds.

- Slice the steak across the grain into thin pieces and divide among the tortillas. Top with guacamole, salsa, onion, extra cilantro, and a squirt of lime juice.

Makes 4 servings / Cost per serving: $3.69

Cumin has been shown to help decrease the risk of colon, stomach, and liver cancers.

250 calories
7 g fat
(1.5 g saturated)
310 mg sodium

1,110 calories
44 g fat
(13 g saturated)
2,490 mg sodium

Not That!
Chevys Grilled Steak Tacos
Price: $10.99

Save!
860 calories and $7.30!

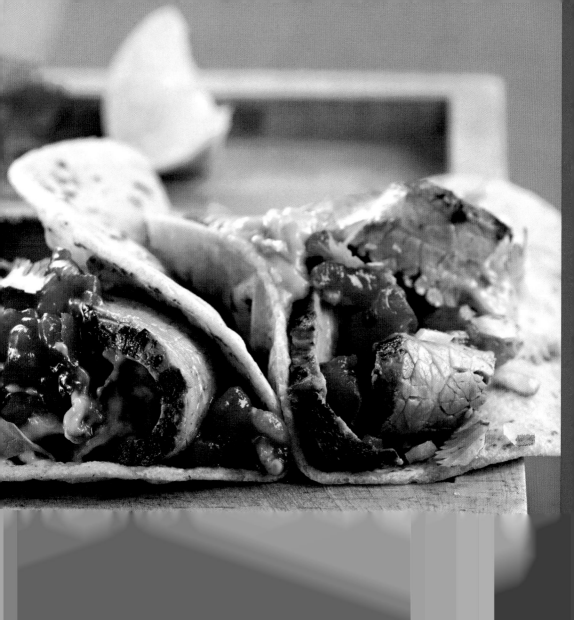

Crispy Chicken with Dijon-Caper Sauce

This dish falls somewhere between the crunchy, juicy splendors of fried chicken and the low-calorie reality of sautéed chicken. It's important that your chicken cutlets are pounded thinly and uniformly, so that the breading doesn't burn before the meat is cooked through. Ask the guy behind the meat counter to do it, or save it for home, where pounding protein can be an amazing way to work off the stress of the day.

You'll Need:

- 4 boneless, skinless chicken breasts (6 oz each)

Salt and black pepper to taste

- 2 Tbsp olive oil
- 3 egg whites, lightly beaten
- 1 ½ cup bread crumbs, preferably panko
- ¼ cup grated Parmesan
- 1 Tbsp dried Italian seasoning
- ½ cup chicken stock
- 2 Tbsp butter
- 1 Tbsp Dijon mustard
- 2 Tbsp capers

Juice of 1 lemon

- ¼ cup chopped fresh parsley

How to Make It:

- Cover the chicken breasts with parchment paper or plastic wrap and, using a meat mallet or a heavy-bottomed pan, pound the chicken until it is uniformly ¼-inch thick. Season with salt and pepper.

- Heat the oil in a large stainless steel sauté pan or cast-iron skillet over medium heat. Place the egg whites in a shallow bowl. Mix the bread crumbs, Parmesan, and Italian seasoning on a plate. Dip each breast carefully into the egg whites, then into the crumb mixture, pressing to make sure each breast is evenly coated.

- When the oil is hot, add the chicken to the pan and cook for 3 to 4 minutes on the first side before turning (the crust should be brown and crunchy). Cook for another 2 to 3 minutes, then transfer the chicken to a plate to rest.

- While the pan is still hot, add the stock and cook until reduced by half, for no more than 2 minutes. Then stir in the butter, mustard, capers, and lemon juice, using a wooden spoon to scrape up any browned bits left behind. Cut the heat and add the parsley. Serve the chicken breasts with the sauce drizzled over the top and a side of spinach sautéed with garlic and dried chiles.

Makes 4 servings /
Cost per serving: $2.97

395 calories
18 g fat

1,405 calories
76 g fat

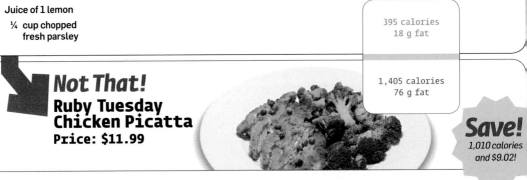

Not That!
Ruby Tuesday Chicken Picatta
Price: $11.99

Save!
1,010 calories
and $9.02!

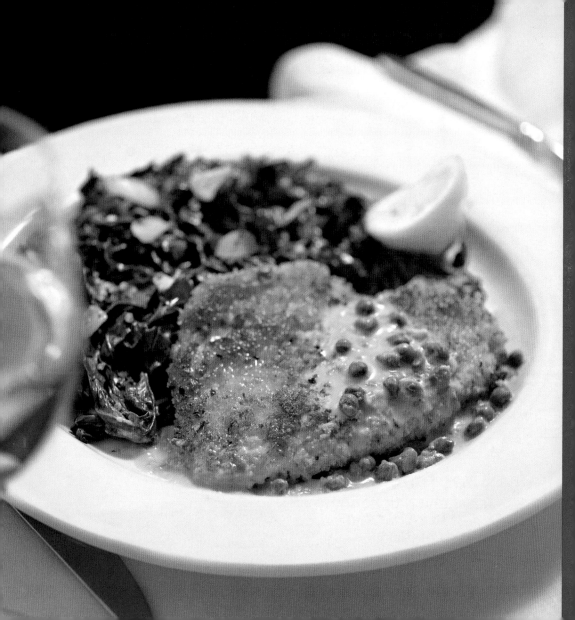

Chicken Skewers Sweet & Sour Style

When did America's chicken get so fat? After all, boneless, skinless chicken breast is among the leanest sources of protein on the planet, with little intramuscular fat. Yet restaurants across the country manage to serve up grilled chicken dinners with more calories than a 24-ounce sirloin steak. Too bad restaurants haven't embraced the skewer, a vessel that allows you to assemble a balance of meat and vegetables in a way that's incredibly easy and rewarding to cook. Plus, who doesn't like eating food off a stick?

You'll Need:

- 1 lb boneless, skinless chicken breasts, cut into bite-size chunks
- 2 cups large pineapple chunks
- 2 medium zucchini, cut into large chunks
- 2 medium red onions, cut into large chunks
- 2 red bell peppers, cut into large chunks
- Salt and black pepper to taste
- 3 Tbsp ketchup
- 1 Tbsp maple syrup
- ½ Tbsp soy sauce
- 1 Tbsp rice or apple cider vinegar
- 1 tsp sriracha or other chili sauce
- Chopped fresh cilantro (optional)

How to Make It:

- Heat a grill or stovetop grill pan until hot. Soak 8 wooden skewers in cold water for 20 minutes.
- Thread the individual ingredients onto the skewers, making sure to create a balance of chicken, pineapple, and vegetables. Season all over with salt and pepper.
- Mix the ketchup, maple syrup, soy sauce, vinegar, and sriracha. Reserve half of the mixture in a separate container to brush on after the food is cooked (you never want to brush cooked food with the same sauce you brushed on while it was raw). Use a brush to paint the other half of the glaze all over the skewers.
- Grill the skewers until lightly charred and the chicken is cooked all the way through, about 4 minutes a side. Remove from the grill and brush with the reserved sauce.

Makes 4 servings / Cost per serving: $2.85

250 calories
2 g fat
(0 g saturated)
510 mg sodium

800 calories
21 g fat
(3.5 g saturated)
943 mg sodium

Not That!
Manchu Wok Honey Garlic Chicken with Steamed Rice
Price: $5.99

Save!
Save 550 calories and $3.14!

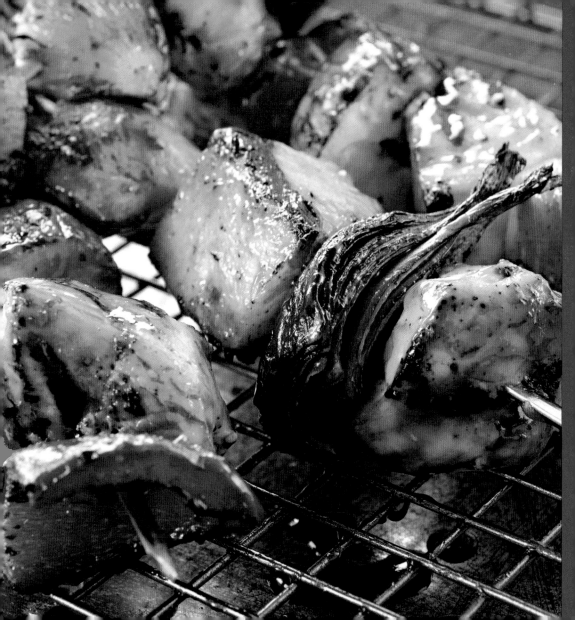

Pad Thai

It's a shame that America's largest restaurateurs haven't seen the potential for mass appeal in cuisines like Indian, Vietnamese, and Thai, since they're all among the healthiest and most delicious on the planet. Take it upon yourself to learn the basics, then—if only because it will save you from another 1,500-calorie Chinese takeout bomb.

You'll Need:

- 1 Tbsp peanut oil
- 1 cup firm tofu cubes
- 2 Tbsp minced red onion
- 2 cloves garlic, minced
- 4 scallions, whites and greens separated, sliced
- 1 tsp red pepper flakes
- 2 eggs, lightly beaten
- ½ lb medium shrimp, peeled and deveined
- 4 oz rice noodles, cooked according to package instructions
- 1 cup bean sprouts
- ¼ cup bottled pad Thai sauce
- 2 Tbsp chopped roasted peanuts
- 1 lime, cut into wedges

How to Make It:

- Heat the oil in a wok or a large nonstick pan over medium-high heat. When hot, cook the tofu until brown on all sides, about 3 to 5 minutes. Remove and reserve. Add the onion, garlic, scallion whites, and pepper flakes to the hot pan and cook until soft but not browned, about 2 minutes.

- Push the mixture to the sides of the pan, creating a well in the center; add the eggs to the well and quickly scramble until the eggs are just cooked through. Toss in the shrimp and cook until just pink, about 3 minutes. Add the noodles, bean sprouts, and sauce and toss to evenly distribute all the ingredients.

- Divide among 4 plates. Garnish with the peanuts, lime wedges, scallion greens, and more pepper flakes, if you like.

Makes 4 servings / Cost per serving: $4.09

Making sauce for pad thai from scratch is ideal (but will require fish sauce and hard-to-find tamarind paste). The bottled stuff works great in a pinch.

470 calories
15 g fat
(2 g saturated)
1,120 mg sodium

1,456 calories
68 g fat
(4 g saturated)
7,780 mg sodium

Not That!
P.F. Chang's Double Pan-Fried Noodles with Shrimp
Price: $9.75

Save!
986 calories and $5.66!

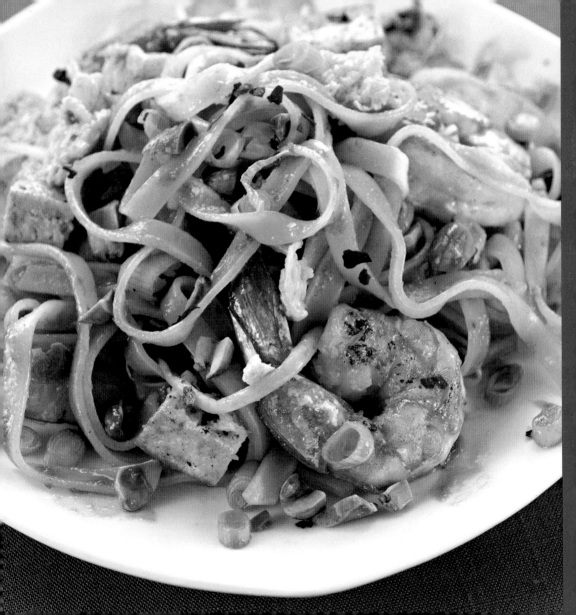

Chicken Pizzaioli

Chicken parmesan is not only one of the most popular dishes in America, but it may be the single dish that best encapsulates the Big Three behind our obesity epidemic: fried food, melted cheese, and massive portion sizes. Olive Garden's rendition represents the average plate of chicken parm—a scary proposition given the fact that it packs nearly an entire day of saturated fat and enough salt to sustain a small colony for years. To lighten things up without losing flavor, we ditch the breading (which gets soggy underneath the sauce anyway) and sear the chicken rather than fry it. A ladle of red sauce and a thin layer of bubbling mozzarella rounds the dish out—without rounding you out.

You'll Need:

- 1 Tbsp olive oil
- 4 chicken breasts (6 oz each)
- 1 tsp dried thyme or rosemary
- Salt and pepper to taste
- 1 medium yellow onion, sliced
- ½ cup chopped green olives
- 4 cloves garlic, minced
- 1 tsp red pepper flakes
- 1 28-oz can crushed tomatoes
- 1 cup grated mozzarella

How to Make It:

- Place the chicken breasts on a cutting board, cover with plastic wrap, and use a meat mallet or heavy-bottomed pan to pound the chicken into ½-inch thick cutlets. Season with thyme or rosemary and a healthy sprinkle of salt and pepper.

- Heat the oil in a large cast-iron skillet or oven-safe pan over medium high heat. When hot, add the chicken and cook for 3 to 4 minutes, until a nice crust has developed on the surface of the chicken, then flip and cook for another 3 to 4 minutes. Remove and reserve the chicken.

- Preheat the broiler. In the same pan, add the onions, olives, garlic, and chili flakes. Sauté until the onions have begun to lightly caramelize, about 5 minutes, then add the tomatoes. Cook for another 3 minutes, then slide the chicken back into the pan. Divide the mozzarella between the chicken breasts, then place the whole pan into the oven. Broil for 3 to 4 minutes, until the cheese is melted and bubbling. Serve the chicken with a generous scoop of the spicy red sauce.

Makes 4 servings /
Cost per serving: $3.56

360 calories
15 g fat
(3 g saturated)
812 mg sodium

1,090 calories
49 g fat
(18 g saturated)
3,380 mg sodium

Olive Garden Chicken Parmigiana
Price: $13.50

Save!
730 calories
and $9.94!

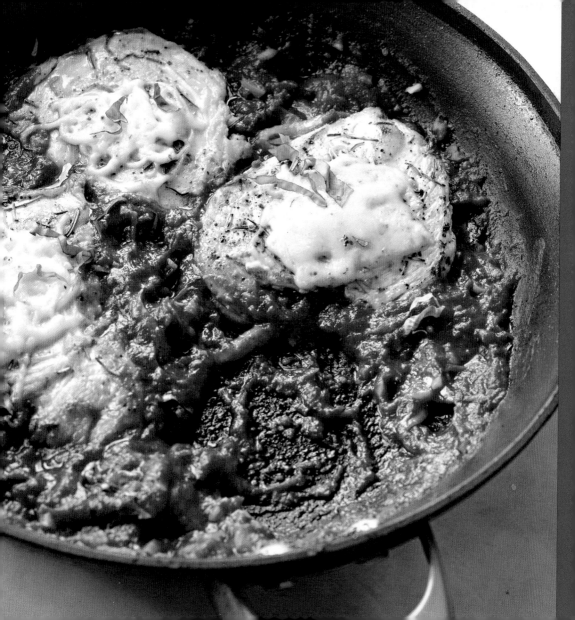

French Toast Stuffed with Strawberries

Odds are, if the word "stuffed" is in the menu description, the dish is dangerous. That's because restaurants choose to use "stuffed" as an excuse to sandwich extra quantities of the cheapest ingredients they have on hand—fat, sugar, salt—into an already-troubled creation. Case in point: IHOP's over-the-top French toast. Its stuffing technique takes a few pieces of bread and some fruit and turns them into a dish with more than half your day's caloric allotment. Done correctly, stuffing can actually be a nutritional boon: Here, it adds a dose of low-cal protein, fiber, and all the energy-boosting vitamins from fresh strawberries. Plus, it's simple enough to pull off on a weekday morning.

You'll Need:

- 1 cup low-fat ricotta or cottage cheese
- ½ cup skim milk
- 2 cups strawberries, sliced
- 2 Tbsp honey
- 2 Tbsp sliced or chopped almonds
- 1 Tbsp butter
- 2 eggs
- 1 cup milk
- ¼ tsp cinnamon
- 1 tsp vanilla extract
- 8 slices whole-wheat bread

Powdered sugar (optional)

How to Make It:

- Place the ricotta, milk, strawberries, honey, and almonds in a mixing bowl and stir gently to combine. Set aside.
- Heat the butter in a large cast-iron skillet or nonstick pan over medium heat. Beat the eggs with the milk, cinnamon, and vanilla in a shallow dish. Working one slice at a time, place the bread in the egg mixture, turning it over once to thoroughly coat, then add it directly to the hot pan. Repeat until the pan is full.
- Cook each sliced for 2 to 3 minutes per side, until a golden brown crust is formed. Remove from the pan. Divide the strawberry mixture among four slices of toast, spreading to evenly coat. Top them each with another slice to make a sandwich, then slice on the diagonal to create two equal triangles. Serve with a shake of powdered sugar or a drizzle of pure maple syrup, if you prefer.

Makes 4 servings / Cost per serving: $2.11

369 calories
12 g fat
(4 g saturated)

1,180 calories

Not That!
IHOP Stuffed French Toast
(with Strawberry Topping)
Price: $7.99

Save!
811 calories
and $5.88!

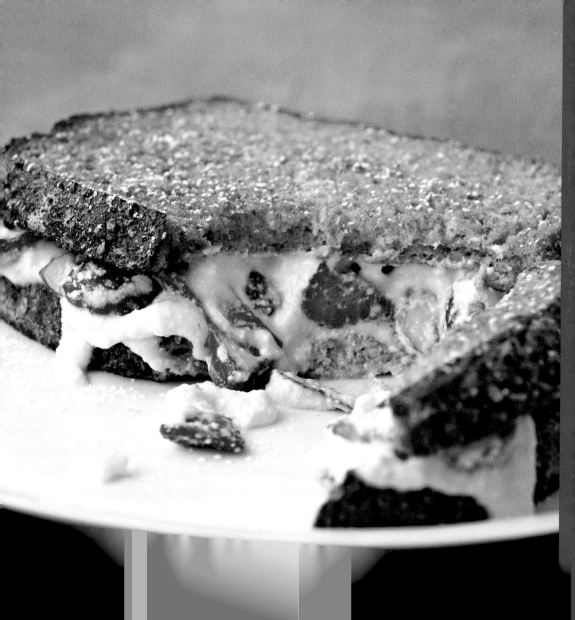

Seared Ahi with Ginger-Scallion Sauce

As much as we love ahi tuna for its profusion of lean protein and heart-strengthening, brain-boosting omega-3 fatty acids, what we love most about the fish is the fact that even a kitchen neophyte can cook it perfectly in less than 5 minutes. All it takes is pan set over high heat, a touch of oil, and a sprinkle of salt and pepper. We add bok choy to make this a more nutritious, substantial dish, but any green vegetable (spinach, broccoli, asparagus) will do. Just don't skip the ginger-scallion sauce, a ubiquitous Chinatown condiment good enough to make a pair of old socks into a memorable meal.

You'll Need:

- 1 bunch scallions, bottoms removed, finely chopped
- 2 Tbsp fresh ginger, peeled and grated
- 1 Tbsp low-sodium soy sauce
- 3 Tbsp peanut oil
- 1 Tbsp rice wine vinegar
- 16 oz ahi or other high-quality tuna steaks

Salt and pepper to taste

- ½ lb shitake mushrooms, stems removed, sliced
- 1 lb baby bok choy, stems removed

How to Make It:

- Combine the scallions, ginger, soy, 2 tablespoons of the oil, and vinegar in a mixing bowl and stir thoroughly to combine. Set aside. (Making this ahead and storing in the refrigerator is not only possible but advisable, as even 30 minutes of sitting allows the flavors to marry nicely.)

- Heat the remaining oil in a large cast-iron skillet or sauté pan. Season the tuna liberally with salt and lots of black pepper. When the oil is lightly smoking, add the tuna to the pan and sear for 2 minutes per side, until deeply browned. Remove.

- While the tuna rests, add the shitake mushrooms to the same hot pan (use another drizzle oil if the pan is dry). Cook for 2 to 3 minutes, until lightly browned, then add the bok choy. Cook for another 2 to 3 minutes, until the bok choy is lightly wilted. Season to taste with salt and pepper.

- Slice the tuna into thick strips. Divide the bok choy and mushrooms among four warm plates. Top with slices of tuna, then drizzle with the scallion-ginger sauce.

Makes 4 servings /
Cost per serving: $5.38

301 calories
12 g fat
(2 g saturated)
271 mg sodium

1,610 calories
49 g saturated fat
1,075 mg sodium

Not That!
Cheesecake Factory Wasabi Crusted Ahi Tuna
Price: $11.95

Save!
1,309 calories and $6.57!

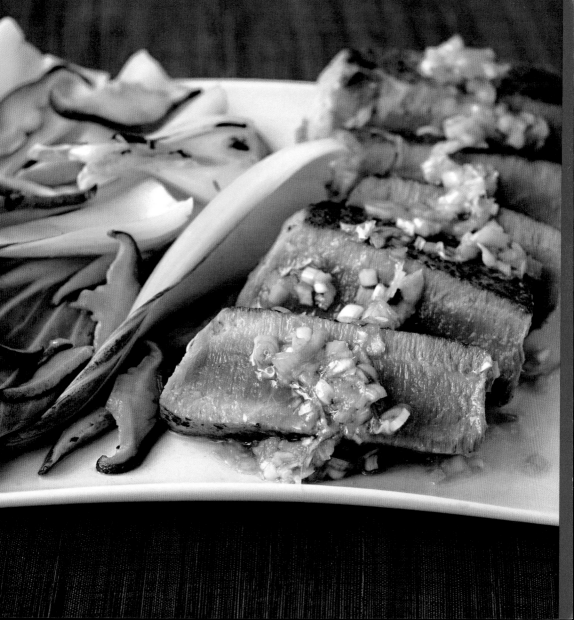

Eat This!

Turkey Burger Mediterranean Style

Thought you were doing yourself a favor by ordering the turkey burger? Think again. Whether scored from a big chain restaurant or a local dive, odds are you just ordered one of the worst items on the menu. Dark turkey packs as much fat and calories as most ground beef. Add to that the inevitable flurry of high-calorie condiments and you have a recipe for disaster. Here, we complement truly lean turkey with a barrage of big flavors—punchy olives, sweet red peppers, a layer of tangy feta cheese—that do little to compromise the overall nutritional picture. For once, you'll have a turkey burger you can eat with impunity.

You'll Need:

- 1 lb lean ground turkey
- Salt and pepper to taste
- ½ tsp dried thyme
- ½ cup feta or fresh goat cheese
- 2 cups arugula
- 4 English muffins, split and lightly toasted
- ½ cup roasted red peppers
- ¼ cup olives, chopped

How to Make It:

- Preheat a grill or grill pan. Season turkey with a few big pinches of salt and pepper, plus the dried thyme. Form the meat into four patties, being careful not to overwork the meat (which will cause the proteins to bind, making for a tough burger). Use your thumb to make a small impression in the middle of each patty (as they cook, the middle will swell up; this simple step makes for a more evenly-cooked burger).

- Cook over medium-high heat for 4 to 5 minutes on the first side, until lightly charred. Flip and immediately add the cheese to each patty. Cook for another 4 to 5 minutes, until the burgers feel firm and springy to the touch. Remove from the grill.

- Lay the arugula on the bottom of four English muffin halves. Top with the burger, then crown the burger with peppers, olives, and the other half of the English muffin.

Makes 4 servings /
Cost per serving: $2.89

```
317 calories
8 g fat
(3 g saturated)
710 mg sodium
```

```
1,126 calories
69 g fat
2,760 mg sodium
```

Not That!
Ruby Tuesday Bella Turkey Burger
Price: $8.99

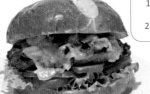

Save!
809 calories and $6.10!

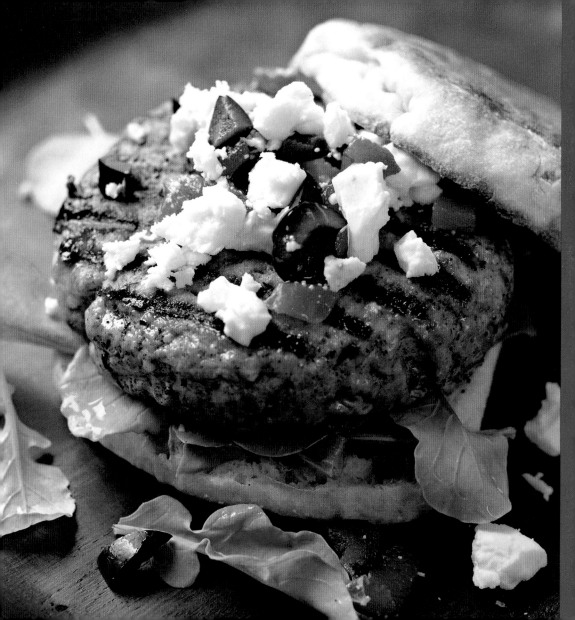

Buffalo Chicken & Blue Cheese Sandwich

Given the rate of wing consumption in this country, clearly hot sauce-slathered chicken and blue cheese is a winning combination for American palates. Problem is, most take-out wings deliver more fat than flavor, and now chains such as Chili's and Ruby Tuesday are using the high-calorie combo to fatten up their sandwiches, too. We stay true to the flavors people love—basting the chicken in hot sauce butter after grilling, topping with a yogurt-based blue cheese sauce—but manage to do what no one else out there has done yet: make Buffalo chicken into a healthy meal. Try the same technique with grilled shrimp—with or without the bread.

You'll Need:

- ¼ cup crumbled blue cheese
- ½ cup Greek-style yogurt
- Juice of half a lemon
- Salt and pepper to taste
- 4 chicken breasts (6 oz each)
- ½ Tbsp chili powder
- 1 red onion, sliced
- 2 Tbsp favorite hot sauce (Frank's Red Hot works best here)
- 2 Tbsp butter, melted in the microwave for 20 seconds
- 4 large leaves romaine lettuce
- 4 sesame buns, toasted

How to Make It:

- Preheat a grill or grill pan. While it's heating, combine the blue cheese, yogurt, and lemon juice, plus a pinch of salt and pepper. Stir to combine, and set aside.

- Season the chicken breasts with salt, pepper, and the chili powder. Add the chicken to the hot grill and cook for 4 to 5 minutes the first side, then flip. Add the onions to the perimeter of the grill (if using a grill pan, you'll need to wait until you remove the chicken to grill the onions). Cook the chicken until firm and springy to the touch, another 4 to 5 minutes. Remove, along with the grilled onions.

- Combine the hot sauce and butter and brush all over the chicken after removing from the grill. Place one large leaf of romaine on the base of each bun. Top with a chicken breast, then spoon over the blue cheese sauce. Top with grilled onions and the top half of the bun.

*Makes 4 servings /
Cost per serving: $3.81*

387 calories
15 g fat
(5 g saturated)
872 mg sodium

1,560 calories
86 g fat
(14 g saturated)
4,010 mg sodium

Not That!
Chili's Buffalo Chicken Ranch Sandwich
Price: $8.79

Save!
1,173 calories and $4.98!

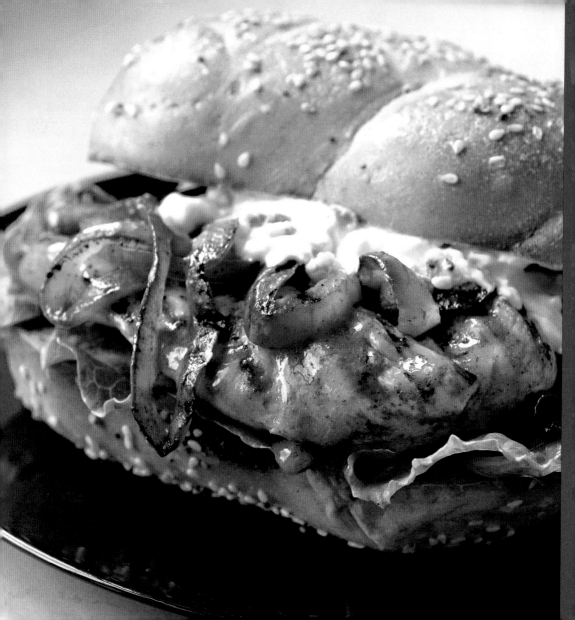

Eat This!
Seared Sirloin with Red Wine Mushrooms

Do you really want to go out and spend $20 or $30 on a steak dinner only to find out the beef was of dubious origin and the nutritionals look more like Dow Jones updates than calorie counts? That's what's in store for you when you seek out your beef fix at one of our country's largest national chains. We not only guarantee that this recipe will slash your bill by 75 percent, but that your taste buds will thank you many times over. Skip the grill and cook on cast iron instead—it not only gives your steak a marvelous crust in a matter of minutes, but it helps form the basis for this knockout mushroom sauce. Cook this when you need to impress someone—even if it's just yourself.

You'll Need:

- 1 Tbsp olive oil
- 4 sirloin steaks or petite filets (6 oz each)
- Salt and black pepper to taste
- 2 shallots, minced
- 2 cloves garlic, minced
- ½ lb white or cremini mushrooms, cleaned, stems removed, and sliced
- 1 cup red wine
- 1 cup low-sodium beef stock
- 2 tsp fresh rosemary, chopped

How to Make It:

- Preheat the oven to 400°F. Heat the oil in a large cast-iron or oven-safe skillet over high heat. Season the steaks with salt and plenty of black pepper and add to the hot pan. Sear the first side for 3 to 4 minutes, until a deep brown crust has developed, then flip. Place the pan in the oven to finish cooking (about 6 to 8 minutes for medium rare; an instant-read thermometer inserted into the thickest part will read 140°F). Remove from the oven and transfer the steaks to a cutting board to rest.

- Using a potholder, place the pan back on the stove over medium heat. Add the shallots, garlic, and mushrooms and cook for 3 to 4 minutes, until the mushrooms have begun to caramelize. Add the red wine and the stock, using a wooden spoon to scrape the bottom of the pan. Cook for another 2 to 3 minutes, until the alcohol has burned off and the liquid has reduced by about half. Stir in the rosemary.

- Divide the steaks among four plates, top with mushrooms, and spoon over the sauce.

Makes 4 servings /
Cost per serving: $4.47

405 calories
12 g fat
(5 g saturated)
677 mg sodium

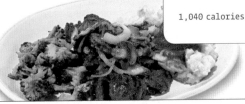

1,040 calories

Not That!
IHOP Sirloin Steak Tips Dinner
Price: $12.99

Save!
635 calories
and $8.52!

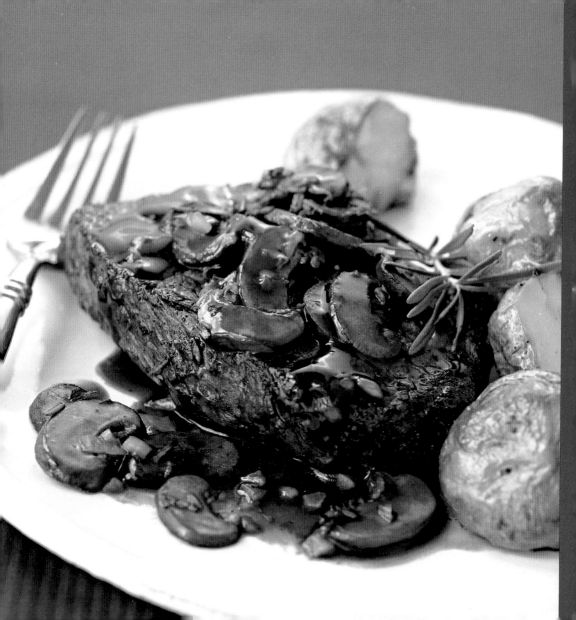

Index

Boldface page references indicate photographs.
Underscored references indicate boxed text.

A

A&W food, 76–77, **76–77**
Additives, food, 36
Alcohol, 44, **44**, 47. *See also specific type*
Almonds, **50**, 53
Appetizers, 72, **72**, 244–45, **244–45**
Applebee's food, xxi, **xxi**, xxvii, **xxvii**, 9, 11–12, 78–79, **78–79**, 295
Arby's food, 80–81, **80–81**
Asparagus, 292, **293**
Atlanta Bread Company food, 82–83, **82–83**
Au Bon Pain food, 84–85, **84–85**
Auntie Anne's food, 86–87, **86–87**, 272, **272**
Avocado, **50**, 52, 292, **292**

B

Bac-Os, 20, **21**
Bagels, 42, 85, **85**, 127, **127**, 301, **301**
Baja Fresh food, 71, **71**, 88–89, **88–89**
Baked goods, 5. *See also specific type*
Ballpark (arena) food, 270–71, **270–71**
Bananas, 46, **46**, 291, **291**
Barley, 42, **42**
Bars, cereal and energy, 218–19, **218–19**
Baskin-Robbins ice cream, 90–91, **90–91**, 223–24, 296
Beef. *See also* Burgers
  at Arby's, 80–81, **80–81**
  at ballpark, 270, **270**
  at Boston Market, 98, **98**
  at Chipotle, 114–15, **114–15**
  for Christmas, 266–67, **266–67**
  at cocktail party, 268, **268**
  frozen entrées, 242–43, **242–43**
  Grilled Steak Tacos, 314, **315**
  healthy choices, 31
  for mental acuity, 47
  at Outback Steakhouse, xxiii, **xxiii**, 67, **67**, 152–53, **152–53**, 297
  at P.F. Chang's, 160–61, **160–61**
  at Romano's Macaroni Grill, 168–69, **168–69**
  at Ruby Tuesday, xxiii, **xxiii**
  Seared Sirloin, 332, **333**
  at T.G.I. Friday's, 180, **180**
  worst, 67, **67**
Beer, 258–59, **258–59**, 267, **267**, 269–70, **269–70**
Beets, 294, **294**

Bell peppers, **50**, 53, 289, **289**, 291, **291**
Ben & Jerry's ice cream, xxix, **xxix,** 92–93, **92–93**
Betty Crocker's Bac-Os, 20, **21**
Beverages. *See also specific type*
  calories in, 285–86
  Coldstone Creamery, 69, **69**
  for illness management and prevention, 43
  Jamba Juice, 138–39, **138–39**
  Orange Julius, 272, **272**
  Smoothie King, 174–75, **174–75**, 273, **273**
  Starbucks, 176–77, **176–77**, 299
  Wendy's, 14, 16
  worst, 69, **69**
Blackberries, 294, **295**
Blimpie food, 61, **61**, 94–95, **94–95**
Blueberries, 295, **295**
Blue-colored foods, 294–95, **294–95**
Bob Evans food, 96–97, **96–97**
Boston Market food, 98–99, **98–99**
Breads
  breakfast, 198–99, **198–99**
  French Toast, 324, **325**
  multigrain, 6
  sandwich, 210–11, **210–11**
Breakfast food
  at Au Bon Pain, 84–85, **84–85**
  at Bob Evans, 96–97, **96–97**
  breads, 198–99, **198–99**
  at Denny's, 122, **122**
  at Dunkin Donuts, 126–27, **126–27**
  French Toast, 324, **325**
  frozen entrées, 232–33, **232–33**
  at Hardee's, 64, **64**
  healthy sandwiches choices, 28
  at IHOP, 70, **70**, 132–33, **132–33**
  importance of, 41
  at Jack in the Box, 136–37, **136–37**
  at Krispy Kreme, 142–43, **142–43**
  at McDonald's, 10
  at Panera Bread, 156–57, **156–57**
  skipping, avoiding, 284
  at Subway, 178–79, **178–79**
  at Tim Horton's, 184–85, **184–85**
  worst, 64, **64**, 70, **70**
Breyer's ice cream, xxix, **xxix**
Broccoli, 293, **293**
Brussels sprouts, 292, **293**
Burger King food, xx, **xx,** 9, 100–101, **100–101**, 296, 300–301, **300–301**

Burgers
  Burger King, xx, **xx,** 100–101, **100–101**, 296, 301, **301**
  Cheesecake Factory, 106–7, **106–7**
  Denny's, 68, **68**
  fast-food, 18, **19**, 29, 62, **62**
  Five Guys, 128–29, **128–29**
  Hardee's, 130, **130**
  In-N-Out Burger, 134–35, **134–35**
  McDonald's, 146–47, **146–47**, 303, **303**
  restaurant, 30, 68, **68**
  at T.G.I. Friday's, 181, **181**
  Wendy's, xx, **xx,** 188, **188**
  worst, 62, **62**, 68, **68**

C

California Pizza Kitchen food, xxv, **xxv,** 59, **59**, 102–3, **102–3**
Calories, 4–5, 10–11, 285–86
Candy, 22, 46, 230–31, **230–31**, 270, **270**, 274–77, **274–77**
Canola oil, 312
Cantaloupe, 290, **290**
Carl's Jr. food, 9, 104–5, **104–5**
Carrots, **46**, 47, 290, **290**
Cereal bars, 218–19, **218–19**
Cereals, 196–97, **196–97**
Champagne, 268, **268**
Cheese, 202–3
Cheesecake Factory food, 66–67, **66–67**, 73, **73**, 75, **75**, 106–7, **106–7**
Chevys Fresh Mex food, 108–9, **108–9**
Chicken. *See* Poultry
Chick-fil-A food, 110–11, **110–11**
Children's food
  at Burger King, 300–301, **300–301**
  color of, 288–95, **289–95**
  daily requirements and, 281
  at Dunkin' Donuts, 300–301, **300–301**
  food pyramid and, 282–83
  healthy choices, 33
  at KFC, 302–3, **302–3**
  at McDonald's, 302–3, **302–3**
  nutritional guidelines, 284–87
  present-day, 280–82
  restaurant report card, 295–99
  at Subway, 304–5, **304–5**
  at Taco Bell, 304–5, **304–5**
  worst restaurant food, 59, **59**

Chile peppers, 41, **41**
Chili's food, xxiv, **xxiv**, 112–13, **112–13**, 296
Chinese food
    Panda Express, 154–55, **154–55**, 272, **272**
    P.F. Chang's, 66, **66**, 160–61, **160–61**
    worst entrée, 66, **66**
Chipotle food, 114–15, **114–15**
Chips, 222–23, **222–23**
Chocolate, 40, **40**, 44, **44**
Chocolate milk, 45
Christmas food, 266–67, **266–67**
Clams. *See* Fish and seafood
Cocktail party food, 268–69, **268–69**
Coffee, 39, 41
Coffee drinks, 252–53, **252–53**
Coldstone Creamery ice cream and beverages, 69, **69**, 116–17, **116–17**
Condiments, 208–9, **208–9**
Cookies, 228–29, **228–29**
Cooking, 287. *See also* Homemade food
Corn, 291, **291**
Cosi food, 118–19, **118–19**
Crackers, 220–21, **220–21**

D

Dairy Queen food, 120–21, **120–21**
Dark chocolate, 40, **40**, 44, **44**
Deli meats, 16, 18, 204–5, **204–5**
Denny's food, 68, **68**, 122–23, **122–23**
Depression-management food, 40
Dessert, worst, 74, **74**
Dietary fat, 6
Dips, 224–25, **224–25**
Domino's Pizza food, xxviii, **xxviii**, 63, **63**, 124–25, **124–25**, 296
Doritos, 24, 25
Doughnuts, 26, **27**, 142–43, **142–43**, 184–85, **184–85**, 300, **300**
Dunkin' Donuts food, 126–27, **126–27**, 296, 300–301, **300–301**

E

Eggplant, 294, **295**
Eggs, 39, **39**, 48, **49**
Energy bars, 218–19, **218–19**
Energy-boosting food, 42
Energy drinks, 47, 252–53, **252–53**
Exercise-boosting and recovery food, 45

F

Fast food, worst, 62, **62**
Fats, 6
Fish and seafood
    at Cheesecake Factory, 75, **75**
    clams, 42, **42**
    at Cosi, 118–19, **118–19**
    frozen entrées, 238–39, **238–39**
    healthy choices, 30
    at Long John Silver's, 144–45, **144–45**
    at McDonald's, 16, **17**
    Pad Thai, 320, **321**
    at Red Lobster, 166–67, **166–67**, 298
    at Ruby Tuesday, 170–71, **170–71**
    salmon, 40
    sardines, 46
    Seared Ahi, 326, **327**
Five Guys food, 62–63, **62–63**, 128–29, **128–29**
Flaxseed, 47
Food. *See also* Homemade food; *specific type*
    additives, 36
    calories in, 4–5, 10–11
    changes to, 4–5
    color of, 288–95, **289–95**
    costs, 309, 310
    for depression management, 40
    for energy boost, 42
    for exercise boost and recovery, 45
    healthy choices, 28–33, 36, 38
    for illness management and prevention, 43
    labels, 2–3, 6–7, 12
    for mental acuity, 46–47
    for metabolism boost, 41
    multigrain, 6
    nutritious, 36, 38, 48, **49–50**, 51–53
    preservatives, 36
    pyramid, 282–83
    for sexual desire boost, 44
    for stress management, 38–39
    swaps, xx–xxix, **xx–xxix**
    terminology in industry, 6–7
    whole, 286–87
    worst, 58–75, **59–75**
Food hybrid, worst, 63, **63**
Food industry, 6–13. *See also* Restaurant food
Food, labels, 2–3
French fries, xxvi, **xxvi,** 32, 62–63, **62–63**, 271, **271**
Fruits. *See specific type*

G

Garlic, 40, **40**, 46, **46**, **50**, 51
Gin, 269, **269**
Grains, 212–13, **212–13**. *See also specific type*
Grapefruit, **49**, **51**, 289, **289**
Grapes, 294, **294**
Greek yogurt, **50**, 52
Green-colored food, 292–93, **292–93**
Green tea, **49**, 51
Guava, 289, **289**
Gum, chewing, 39, **39**

H

Ham, 82, **82**
Hardee's food, 64, **64**, 130–31, **130–31**
High-fructose corn syrup (HFCS), 13, 26
Holiday food, 262–63. *See also specific holiday*
Homemade food
    Buffalo Chicken, 330, **331**
    Chicken Pizzaioli, 322, **323**
    Chicken Skewers, 318, **319**
    Crispy Chicken, 316, **317**
    food costs and, 309, 310
    French Toast, 324, **325**
    Grilled Steak Tacos, 314, **315**
    health and, 308–9
    Pad Thai, 320, **321**
    recipe overview, 314
    Seared Ahi, 326, **327**
    Seared Sirloin, 332, **333**
    Turkey Burger, 328, **329**
    weight loss and, 308–9
Honey, 43, **43**
Hot dogs, 76, **76**, 86, **86**, 206–7, **206–7**, 269, **269**, 270, **270**

I

Ice cream
    at ballpark, 271, **271**
    Baskin-Robbins, 23–24, 90–91, **90–91**, 296
    Ben & Jerry's, xxix, **xxix,** 92–93, **92–93**
    Breyer's, xxix, **xxix**
    Cold Stone Creamery, 116–17, **116–17**
    healthy sundae choices, 33
    McDonald's, 272, **272**
    supermarket brands, xxix, **xxix,** 246–47, **246–47**

IHOP food, 70, **70**, 132–33, **132–33**, 297
Illness management and prevention, food for, 43
In-N-Out Burger food, 134–35, **134–35**

J

Jack in the Box food, 136–37, **136–37**
Jamba Juice beverages, 138–39, **138–39**
Juices, 47, 250–51, **250–51**
Junk food costs, 310

K

Kale, 293, **293**
KFC food, xxvi, **xxvi**, 9, 140–41, **140–41**, 297, 302–3, **302–3**
Kidney beans, 42, **42**
Kiwi, 43, **43**, 293
Krispy Kreme food, 142–43, **142–43**

L

Labels, food, 2–3, 6–7, 12
Lattes, venti, 47
Lentils, dry, 312
Lettuce, 292, **292**
Long John Silver's food, 144–45, **144–45**

M

Mall food, 272–73, **272–73**
Margarita, 269, **269**
McDonald's food, 10, 14, **15**, 16, **17**, 146–47, **146–47**, 272, **272**, 297, 302–3, **302–3**
Meals, 41, 287. *See also specific food*
Meats. *See specific type*
Mental acuity, food promoting, 46–47
Metabolism-boosting food, 41
Mexican food
    Baja Fresh, 71, **71**, 88–89, **88–89**
    Chevys Fresh Mex, 108–9, **108–9**
    Chili's, xxiv, **xxiv**, 112–13, **112–13**, 296
    Chipotle, 114–15, **114–15**
    fajitas, xxiv, **xxiv**
    Grilled Steak Tacos, 314, **315**
    On the Border, xxiv, **xxiv**, 150–51, **150–51**
    Taco Bell, 23, 182–83, **182–83**, 299, 304–5, **304–5**
    worst entrée, 71, **71**
Milk, chocolate, 45
Mixers, drink, 256–57, **256–57**

Movie theater food, 274–75, **274–75**
Mrs. Fields food, 273, **273**
Multigrain food, 6

N

Nachos, 271, **271**
Noodles, 212–13, **212–13**
    Pad Thai, 320, **321**
Nutritional guidelines, 284–87
Nutrition information, 3, 11–12

O

Obesity, 12–13, 36, 281–82
Olive Garden food, xxii, **xxii**, 11, 148–49, **148–49**, 297
Olives, 43
On the Border food, xxiv, **xxiv**, 150–51, **150–51**
Orange-colored food, 290, **290**
Orange Julius beverages, 272, **272**
Oranges, 290, **290**
Outback Steakhouse food, xxiii, **xxiii**, 11–12, 67, **67**, 72, **72**, 152–53, **152–53**, 297
Oysters, 44

P

Panda Express food, 154–55, **154–55**, 272, **272**
Panera Bread food, xxvii, **xxvii**, 156–57, **156–57**
Papa John's food, 158–59, **158–59**, 298
Pasta
    at Cheesecake Factory, 75, **75**
    frozen entrées, 236–37, **236–37**
    healthy choices, 29
    at Olive Garden, xxii, **xxii**, 148–49, **148–49**, 297
    at Romano's Macaroni Grill, xxii, **xxii**, xxv, **xxv**
    at Sbarro, 172, **172**
Peas, 293, **293**
P.F. Chang's food, 66, **66**, 160–61, **160–61**
Pies, 264–65, **264–65**
Pineapple, 291, **291**
Pizza
    at ballpark, 271, **271**
    Domino's Pizza, xxviii, **xviii**, 124, **124**, 296
    frozen, 234–35, **234–35**
    Papa John's, 158–59, **158–59**, 298
    Pizza Hut, xxviii, **xxviii**, 162–63, **162–63**, 298
    Sbarro, 173, **173**, 273, **273**
    Subway, 305, **305**

Taco Bell, 23
Uno Chicago Grill, 72–73, **72–73**
    worst, 72–73, **72–73**
Pizza Hut food, xxviii, **xxviii**, 162–63, **162–63**, 298
Plums, 295, **295**
Popcorn, 275, **275**, 312
Portions, 5, 285
Potatoes, 264–65, **264–65**, 266–67, **266–67**, 290, **290**. *See also* French fries
Poultry
    at A&W, 77, **77**
    at Applebee's, xxi, **xxi**, 78–79, **78–79**
    at Atlanta Bread Company, 83, **83**
    at Baja Fresh, 88–89, **88–89**
    at Blimpie, 94–95, **94–95**
    at Boston Market, 99, **99**
    Buffalo Chicken, 330, **331**
    at Burger King, 300, **300**
    at California Pizza Kitchen, xxv, **xxv**, 102–3, **102–3**
    at Carl's Jr., 104–5, **104–5**
    at Cheesecake Factory, 73, **73**, 107, **107**
    at Chevys Fresh Mex, 108–9, **108–9**
    Chicken Pizzaioli, 322, **323**
    Chicken Skewers, 318, **319**
    at Chick-fil-A, 110–11, **110–11**
    at Chili's, xxiv, **xxiv**, 112–13, **112–13**
    Crispy Chicken, 316, **317**
    at Dairy Queen, 120–21, **120–21**
    at Domino's Pizza, 125, **125**
    for energy boost, 42
    frozen chicken breast, 312
    frozen chicken entrées, 240–41, **240–41**
    grilled chicken breast, 42
    at Hardee's, 131, **131**
    healthy choices, 31, 42
    at KFC, 140–41, **140–41**, 297, 302–3, **302–3**
    at McDonald's, 14, **15**, 297, 302, **302**
    at On the Border, xxiv, **xxiv**, 150–51, **150–51**
    at Panda Express, 154–55, **154–55**, 272, **272**
    at Quiznos, 164–65, **164–65**, 273, **273**
    at Subway, 272, **272**
    at Taco Bell, 304, **304**
    at T.G.I. Friday's, 181, **181**
    turkey, 264–65, **264–65**
    Turkey Burger, 328, **329**
    at Uno Chicago Grill, xxi, **xxi**, 186–87, **186–87**
    at Wendy's, 189, **189**
    wings, xxi, **xxi**, 330, **331**
    worst chicken entrée, 73, **73**

Preservatives, food, 36
Pretzels, 86–87, **86–87**, 272, **272**, 274, **274**
Purple-colored food, 294–95, **294–95**

Q

Quinoa, **49**, 52
Quiznos food, 164–65, **164–65**, 273, **273**, 298

R

Radish, 294, **294**
Red Bull drink, 45
Red-colored food, 289, **289**
Red Lobster food, 11, 166–67, **166–67**, 298
Restaurant food. *See also specific restaurant*
  for children, report card on, 295–99
  nutrition and, 11–12, 56–57
  truth about, 14, 16, 18, 20, 22–24
  worst, 58–75, **59–75**
Ribs, worst, 67, **67**
Romano's Macaroni Grill food, xxii, **xxii**, xxv,
  xxv, 168–69, **168–69**
Ruby Tuesday food, xxiii, **xxiii,** 170–71,
  170–71, 298

S

Salad dressing, 226–27, **226–27**
Salads
  Applebee's, xxvii, **xxvii**
  Chevys Fresh Mex, 109, **109**
  Chipotle, 115, **115**
  healthy choices, <u>32</u>
  On the Border, 151, **151**
  Panera Bread, xxvii, **xxvii**
  T.G.I. Friday's, 65, **65**
  worst, 65, **65**
Salmon. *See* Fish and seafood
Salsa, <u>312</u>
Salt, 7, 9–10
Sandwiches
  A&W, 77, **77**
  Arby's, 80–81, **80–81**
  Atlanta Bread Company, 82–83, **82–83**
  Au Bon Pain, 84–85, **84–85**
  Baja Fresh, 88, **88**
  Blimpie, 61, **61**, 94–95, **94–95**
  Boston Market, 99, **99**
  breads, 210–11, **210–11**
  Carl's Jr., 104–5, **104–5**

Cheesecake Factory, 66–67, **66–67**
Chick-fil-A, 110–11, **110–11**
Così, 118–19, **118–19**
Dairy Queen, 120, **120**
Denny's, 123, **123**
Domino's Pizza, 125, **125**
Hardee's, 130–31, **130–31**
healthy breakfast choices, <u>28</u>
KFC, 9, 140, **140**
Panera Bread, 156–57, **156–57**
Quiznos, 164–65, **164–65**, 273, **273**, 298
salami, 16, 18
Starbucks, 176–77, **176–77**
Subway, 10, 178–79, **178–79**, 272, **272**,
  299, 302, **302**
Wendy's, 189, **189**
worst, 66–67, **66–67**
worst "healthy," 61, **61**
Sardines. *See* Fish and seafood
Sauces, 214–15, **214–15**
Sausages, 206–7, **206–7**
Sbarro food, 172–73, **172–73**, 273, **273**
Seafood. *See* Fish and seafood
Serving sizes, 5, 285
Sexual desire, food boosting, 44
Shopping strategies, 194–95, 311–12
Sides, 62–63, **62–63**, 244–45, **244–45**
Skittles candy, 22
Smoothie King beverages, 174–75, **174–75**,
  273, **273**
Snack food, 244–45, **244–45**, 274–77, **274–77**
Snacking strategies, 284–85
Soda, 47, 271, **271**
Soda tax, 8
Sodium, 7, 9–10
Soups, 216–17, **216–17**
Spinach, 45, **45**, 292, **292**
Spreads, 224–25, **224–25**
Squash, 290, **290**, 291, **291**
Starbucks food and beverages, 176–77,
  176–77, 299
Stouffer's food, 60, **60**
Stress-management food, 38–39
Subway food, 10, 20, 22, 178–79, **178–79**,
  272, **272**, 299, 304–5, **304–5**
Supermarket food, 60, **60**, 192–93.
  See also specific food
Supersized food, 4
Sweeteners, 6
Swiss chard, **49**, 53

T

T.G.I. Friday's food, 65, **65**, 180–81, **180–81**,
  299
Taco Bell food, 23, 182–83, **182–83**, 299,
  304–5, **304–5**
Tea, 43, 45, 254–55, **254–55**.
  See also Green tea
Thanksgiving food, 264–65, **264–65**
Tim Horton's food, 184–85, **184–85**
Tofu
  Pad Thai, 320, **321**
Tomatoes, 289, **289**
Trans fat, 5, 7
Treats, frozen, 248–49, **248–49**.
  See also Ice cream
Turkey. *See* Poultry
Type 2 diabetes, 282

U

Uno Chicago Grill food, xxi, **xxi**, 72–73, **72–73**,
  74, **74**, 186–87, **186–87**

V

Vegetables. *See specific type*
Vending machine food, 276–77, **276–77**
Vodka, 268, **268**

W

Watermelon, 46, **46**, 289, **289**
Weight loss, 38
Wendy's food and beverages, xx, **xx**, xxvi, **xxvi,**
  14, 16, 62, **62**, 188–89, **188–89**, 299
White chocolate, 40, **40**
Whole foods, 286–87
Wine, 39, **39**, 266, **266**
Wings, chicken, xxi, **xxi,** 330, **331**

Y

Yellow-colored food, 291, **291**
Yogurt, 41, **41**, 200–201, **200–201**.
  See also Greek yogurt

Z

Zucchini, **292**, 293